MW00396328

COGNITIVE THERAPY OF PERSONALITY DISORDERS

ALSO AVAILABLE

For Professionals

Cognitive and Behavioral Theories in Clinical Practice
*Edited by Nikolaos Kazantzis, Mark A. Reinecke,
and Arthur Freeman*

Cognitive-Behavioral Strategies in Crisis Intervention, Third Edition
Edited by Frank M. Dattilio and Arthur Freeman

Cognitive Therapy for Adolescents in School Settings
Torrey A. Creed, Jarrod Reisweber, and Aaron T. Beck

Cognitive Therapy of Anxiety Disorders: Science and Practice
David A. Clark and Aaron T. Beck

Cognitive Therapy of Depression
Aaron T. Beck, A. John Rush, Brian F. Shaw, and Gary Emery

Cognitive Therapy of Substance Abuse
*Aaron T. Beck, Fred D. Wright, Cory F. Newman,
and Bruce S. Liese*

Cognitive Therapy with Children and Adolescents, Second Edition:
A Casebook for Clinical Practice
Edited by Mark A. Reinecke, Frank M. Dattilio, and Arthur Freeman

Cognitive Therapy with Inpatients: Developing a Cognitive Milieu
*Edited by Jesse H. Wright, Michael E. Thase,
Aaron T. Beck, and John W. Ludgate*

Group Cognitive Therapy for Addictions
*Amy Wenzel, Bruce S. Liese, Aaron T. Beck,
and Dara G. Friedman-Wheeler*

Schizophrenia: Cognitive Theory, Research, and Therapy
Aaron T. Beck, Neil A. Rector, and Paul Grant

The Integrative Power of Cognitive Therapy
Brad A. Alford and Aaron T. Beck

For General Readers

The Anxiety and Worry Workbook: The Cognitive Behavioral Solution
David A. Clark and Aaron T. Beck

Cognitive Therapy of Personality Disorders

THIRD EDITION

Edited by

Aaron T. Beck
Denise D. Davis
Arthur Freeman

THE GUILFORD PRESS
New York   London

© 2015 The Guilford Press
A Division of Guilford Publications, Inc.
370 Seventh Avenue, Suite 1200, New York, NY 10001
www.guilford.com

Paperback edition 2016

All rights reserved

No part of this book may be reproduced, translated, stored in a retrieval
system, or transmitted, in any form or by any means, electronic, mechanical,
photocopying, microfilming, recording, or otherwise, without written permission
from the publisher.

Printed in the United States of America

This book is printed on acid-free paper.

Last digit is print number: 9 8 7 6 5 4 3

The authors have checked with sources believed to be reliable in their efforts to
provide information that is complete and generally in accord with the standards
of practice that are accepted at the time of publication. However, in view of the
possibility of human error or changes in behavioral, mental health, or medical
sciences, neither the authors, nor the editors and publisher, nor any other party
who has been involved in the preparation or publication of this work warrants
that the information contained herein is in every respect accurate or complete,
and they are not responsible for any errors or omissions or the results obtained
from the use of such information. Readers are encouraged to confirm the
information contained in this book with other sources.

Library of Congress Cataloging-in-Publication Data

Cognitive therapy of personality disorders / edited by Aaron T. Beck, Denise D.
Davis, Arthur Freeman.—Third edition.
     pages cm
   Includes bibliographical references and index.
   ISBN 978-1-4625-1792-3 (hardback)
   ISBN 978-1-4625-2581-2 (paperback)
   I. Beck, Aaron T., editor of compilation.   II. Davis, Denise D., editor of
compilation.   III. Freeman, Arthur, 1942– editor of compilation.
   RC554.B43 2015
   616.85′8—dc23

                                                              2014014448

About the Editors

Aaron T. Beck, MD, is the founder of cognitive therapy, University Professor Emeritus of Psychiatry at the University of Pennsylvania, and President Emeritus of the Beck Institute for Cognitive Behavior Therapy. He is the recipient of numerous awards, including the Albert Lasker Clinical Medical Research Award, the American Psychological Association (APA) Lifetime Achievement Award, the American Psychiatric Association Distinguished Service Award, the Robert J. and Claire Pasarow Foundation Award for Research in Neuropsychiatry, and the Institute of Medicine's Sarnat International Prize in Mental Health and Gustav O. Lienhard Award. Dr. Beck has worked extensively with personality disorders and has been an investigator on two studies using cognitive therapy with borderline personality disorder.

Denise D. Davis, PhD, is Associate Professor of the Practice of Psychology at Vanderbilt University, where she is Associate Director of Graduate Training in Clinical Science. She is a Founding Fellow, Diplomate, and certified Trainer and Consultant of the Academy of Cognitive Therapy (ACT). Dr. Davis was the founding Associate Editor of the journal *Cognitive and Behavioral Practice* prior to serving the first full term as that journal's Editor. Her research and clinical interests include ethics, psychotherapy termination, and cognitive therapy of personality disorders.

Arthur Freeman, EdD, ABPP, is Professor of Behavioral Medicine at Midwestern University, where he is Executive Director of the Clinical Psychology Programs at both the Downers Grove, Illinois, and Glendale, Arizona, campuses. He is a past president of the Association for Behavioral and Cognitive Therapies and the International Association for Cognitive Psychotherapy and a Distinguished Founding Fellow of the ACT. With over 100 chapters and articles, his work has been translated into 20 languages and he has lectured in 45 countries. Dr. Freeman's research and clinical interests include marital and family therapy, and cognitive-behavioral treatment of depression, anxiety, and personality disorders.

Contributors

Arnoud Arntz, PhD, Department of Clinical Psychology, University of Amsterdam, Amsterdam, The Netherlands

Aaron T. Beck, MD, Department of Psychiatry, University of Pennsylvania, Philadelphia, Pennsylvania; Beck Institute for Cognitive Behavior Therapy, Bala Cynwyd, Pennsylvania

Judith S. Beck, PhD, Department of Psychology in Psychiatry, University of Pennsylvania, Philadelphia, Pennsylvania; Beck Institute for Cognitive Behavior Therapy, Bala Cynwyd, Pennsylvania

Wendy T. Behary, LCSW, The Cognitive Therapy Center of New Jersey, Springfield, New Jersey

Lindsay Brauer, PhD, Department of Psychiatry and Behavioral Neuroscience, University of Chicago, Chicago, Illinois

David A. Clark, PhD, Department of Psychology, University of New Brunswick, Fredericton, New Brunswick, Canada

Daniel O. David, PhD, Department of Clinical Cognitive Sciences, Babes-Bolyai University, Cluj-Napoca, Romania

Denise D. Davis, PhD, Department of Psychology, Vanderbilt University, Nashville, Tennessee

Robert A. DiTomasso, PhD, ABPP, Department of Psychology, Philadelphia College of Osteopathic Medicine, Philadelphia, Pennsylvania

Jay C. Fournier, PhD, Department of Psychiatry, University of Pittsburgh School of Medicine, Pittsburgh, Pennsylvania

Arthur Freeman, EdD, ScD, ABPP, ACT, Department of Behavioral Medicine and Clinical Psychology Programs, Midwestern University, Downers Grove, Illinois

Gina M. Fusco, PsyD, Foundations Behavioral Health and First Home Care, Doylestown, Pennsylvania

Anil Gündüz, MD, Department of Psychiatry, Marmara University,
Istanbul, Turkey

Catherine A. Hilchey, BSc, Department of Psychology,
University of New Brunswick, Fredericton, New Brunswick, Canada

Pawel D. Mankiewicz, DClinPsy, National Health Service, South Essex
Partnership University NHS Foundation Trust, Clinical Psychology Services,
Disability Resource Centre, Dunstable, United Kingdom

Damon Mitchell, PhD, Department of Criminology and Criminal Justice,
Central Connecticut State University, New Britain, Connecticut

Christine A. Padesky, PhD, Center for Cognitive Therapy,
Huntington Beach, California

James L. Rebeta, MTh, PhD, Department of Psychiatry, Weill Cornell
Medical College, New York–Presbyterian Hospital, White Plains, New York

Mark A. Reinecke, PhD, Division of Psychology, Northwestern University,
Chicago, Illinois

Julia C. Renton, DClinPsy, National Health Service, South Essex
Partnership University NHS Foundation Trust, Clinical Psychology Services,
Disability Resource Centre, Dunstable, United Kingdom

Bradley Rosenfield, PsyD, Department of Psychology, Philadelphia College
of Osteopathic Medicine, Philadelphia, Pennsylvania

Karen M. Simon, PhD, Cognitive Behavioral Therapy of Newport Beach,
Newport Beach, California

Mehmet Z. Sungur, MD, Department of Psychiatry, Marmara University,
Istanbul, Turkey

Raymond Chip Tafrate, PhD, Department of Criminology and Criminal Justice,
Central Connecticut State University, New Britain, Connecticut

Michael T. Treadway, PhD, Center for Depression, Anxiety and Stress Research,
McLean Hospital/Harvard Medical School, Belmont, Massachusetts

Preface

By definition, personality disorders are deeply embedded in an individual's sense of self, often exacting a significant toll in the life of that person and impacting his or her social networks, including caregivers. Terms such as "tough," "problematic," "challenging," "unremitting," and even "intractable" have all been used to describe the course of treating individuals with personality difficulties. As we complete this third edition of *Cognitive Therapy of Personality Disorders*, we appreciate these fundamental realities. At the same time, we believe that "inspired," "collaborative," and "hopeful" are apt ways to describe the evolution and promise of cognitive therapy as a treatment for disorders of personality.

In 1988, when Aaron Beck first asked Arthur Freeman to collaborate on a volume on treating clients with personality disorders, there were few treatment manuals designed to help this high-profile, low-success group of patients. Most of the literature at the time was based on a psychodynamic perspective that conceptualized disorders of personality as "neurosis," or "neurotic styles" (Shapiro, 1965). Inspired by the incredible impact of *Cognitive Therapy of Depression* (Beck, Rush, Shaw, & Emery, 1979) and *Anxiety Disorders and Phobia: A Cognitive Perspective* (Beck & Emery with Greenburg, 1985), the natural next frontier for testing Beck's cognitive therapy model was the treatment of personality disorders. Accumulating evidence from clinical trials of treatments for symptomatic disorders such as depression or anxiety provided further impetus for the work, as there were always patients who dropped out or didn't respond in typical ways to the treatment protocols. Often these patients also had known or suspected personality disorders. Given the clear clinical need and relative lack of tested treatments, it seemed reasonable to explore ways to extend and adapt the cognitive model for treating this population. There was no shortage of challenging patients, and the early adopters of cognitive therapy grappled with ways to achieve progress and overcome roadblocks. Much creative thinking occurred in case conference discussions, where ideas were proffered and then taken back to the consulting rooms to test for clinical value.

Beck and Freeman decided to summarize this clinical perspective and make it available for wider clinical testing. They began by enlisting the help of a few of the superb therapists who were trained or strongly influenced by Beck's work at the Center for Cognitive Therapy at the University of Pennsylvania. This small cadre of nine early associates of the Beck Center (now Founding Fellows of the Academy of Cognitive Therapy) collaboratively shaped their insights about how the cognitive model could be adapted for patients with personality disorders. Together they produced the first edition of *Cognitive Therapy of Personality Disorders* in 1990, the pioneer effort that outlined a comprehensive cognitive approach for each of the personality disorders described in DSM-III-R. Our colleagues reviewed the work and called it "useful," "scholarly," "clinically valuable," and "an advancement of the therapy of this difficult group." The active, problem-oriented treatment methods comprised by cognitive therapy enlivened the options for patients with complex or intractable problems, and this approach was widely embraced by the growing corps of therapists.

After the successful reception of that first edition, Beck and Freeman were asked to develop a second edition. They thought about what to revise, correct, modify, or change based on the reviews of the book, and on findings from ongoing work in the field. Continuing with the collaborative approach, they decided to invite one of the contributors from the first volume, Denise Davis, to serve as contributor and general editor. In her role as coeditor and contributing author, she helped shape the direction of revisions, bridged the work from the first to second editions, and ensured integration and continuity of "voice" throughout the new volume. We reassembled a small group of 10 contributors, carrying forward the basic foundation with several of the same authors, but also adding new contributors for new dimension and perspective in the work. Rather than simply a light rehash of what we had said 14 years earlier, the text was advanced both theoretically and clinically. Once again, we had the enveloping experience of inspiration and hope in what our contributors and we produced. And, once again, the professional reviews were most positive.

In 2012, The Guilford Press asked us to consider a third edition of *Cognitive Therapy of Personality Disorders*. Was there more to say? Were there new data that could inform our treatment formulations? What had we not covered in the previous editions that would be relevant to further improving care for patients with personality disorders? After much consideration, we decided to proceed, with Davis taking on the role of lead editor.

We had a huge challenge. DSM-5 was on the way, with much fanfare, disagreement, and uncertainty about its content, particularly its treatment of personality disorders. What was the DSM task force going to leave in, and what were they going to leave out? We prodded our friends for information, but even those who knew didn't really know. We decided to maintain our clinical focus and produce another text designed and focused on the daily work of the frontline therapist. We moved ahead with anticipation of updates in DSM-5, and integrated this new information as soon as it was released. Based on our experience as clinicians, researchers, editors, and consumers of the scholarly literature, we chose to include several disorders that had been moved over the years to the back of DSM, and others that had been totally dismissed. For example, in our combined century of clinical practice, we had all seen many patients that fit the criteria (delineated in earlier editions of DSM) of passive–aggressive personality. So we included this clinical entity in our discussion to help practicing clinicians understand, conceptualize, and treat it in their patients. Similarly, we decided that inclusion of the depressive personality could address an important gap in the literature.

From the outset, we endeavored to retain the richness and detail that had been well received in the second edition, while also providing a comprehensive and substantial update that is well integrated across the chapters. The result is a third edition that is approximately 65% new material. The new edition retains the two-section format from the second edition (beginning with theory, research, and general clinical methods, then moving to clinical applications to specific personality disorders), but also includes a new third section on comorbidity and clinical management. In total, five chapters offer totally new content that did not appear in previous editions—on the topics of neural mechanisms of maladaptive schemas and modes, diversity and culture, depressive personality disorder, symptomatic comorbidity, and clinical management. The chapters on the research overview, clinical assessment, dependent personality disorder, narcissistic personality disorder, histrionic personality disorder, and antisocial personality disorder have each been completely rewritten under new or combined authorship. Coverage of paranoid personality disorder has been combined with schizotypal and schizoid personality disorders in a single chapter. In addition, the existing chapters on theory, general principles and specialized techniques, and therapeutic alliance are all substantially updated.

So what did we add and how did we keep the text to a practical length? To keep from ending up with a two-volume set, we chose to delete tables of diagnostic criteria, as these can easily be located elsewhere; trimmed historical discussions; and focused on providing new case illustrations and details relevant to successful clinical interventions. To the chapters on clinical applications for specific disorders, each author has added comments on key treatment goals, lifespan or developmental considerations, termination issues specific to that disorder, common challenges with that disorder, and tips for clinician self-care. The fundamental chapters on theory and basic clinical methods as well as clinical applications chapters have been refreshed and expanded to integrate newer technical developments that are compatible with cognitive therapy and relevant to personality disorders:

motivational interviewing, mindfulness, schema role plays and other experiential exercises, schema-focused feedback, building of functional core beliefs and personal models for resilience, values clarification, and specific strategies for managing the therapeutic alliance. Of special note, Aaron Beck's well-articulated continuity hypothesis is further detailed in his updated chapter on theory, incorporating his latest insights on how primal needs give rise to behavioral strategies that form basic traits of personality, and how personality disorders arise from hypertrophied and inflexibly activated schemas and modes. As in previous editions, Beck's steadfastly compassionate stance and masterful integration of theory and clinical illustration provide an inspiring, hopeful, and essential grounding in his vision of the conceptual model of cognitive therapy. We believe a solid understanding of this fundamental theory is key to effective conceptualization and flexible use of the clinical methods presented throughout the text.

In the 25 years since publication of the first edition, cognitive therapy has been widely adopted as a therapeutic model, on a worldwide scale. So it seems fitting that the list of contributing authors has more than doubled for this edition. Given this larger group of contributors, we decided that it made most sense to link authorship with specific chapters. Some of the previous authors were unable to contribute to this third edition, and we thank them for their efforts, which helped to raise the standard of our work and the field. We would like to acknowledge three specific persons who have contributed to all three volumes: Judith Beck, Christine Padesky, and Karen Simon. In regrouping for this edition, we added new topics already mentioned and invited new authors to join us. We are delighted that this highly esteemed group of clinicians and scientists includes international representation from five different countries in addition to the United States, weaving in cultural nuances that help to deepen our understanding of personality. At the same time, we see that application of the cognitive model is extremely consistent across the globe, providing evidence of its transcultural viability.

We are extremely grateful for the efforts of so many who have worked hard to bring this work this far, advancing psychotherapy generally and cognitive therapy specifically. We are inspired by the visionary wisdom of The Guilford Press, and humbled to see our students and our students' students quoted in the text. We continue to learn from our patients and are encouraged by their response to our efforts. Speaking on behalf of our contributors, we are all inspired by the resilience, brilliance, and unwavering kindness of senior editor Aaron Beck, without question one of the giants and geniuses of our era. We hope you find the ideas presented in this third edition of *Cognitive Therapy of Personality Disorders* to be engaging, informative, useful, and, most of all, a source of hope for your work in helping those who strive to overcome disorders of personality.

Acknowledgments

Cognitive therapy has grown from its humble beginnings to become the fastest-growing psychotherapy in the world. I am particularly proud of this revised edition of *Cognitive Therapy of Personality Disorders* because it represents the collaborative effort of many of the most productive members of my professional family (including, of course, my daughter Judith). I want to express my appreciation to the various contributors to the book and particularly to Denise Davis, Art Freeman, Susan Blassingame, Lucas Zullo, and Kelly Devinney, who brought the revised edition to fruition.

—AARON T. BECK

Tim Beck and Art Freeman have provided many years of encouragement and inspired leadership in the development of cognitive therapy. I want to express my deepest personal thanks to Tim and Art for their friendship and encouragement across editions of this project. Their confidence is indeed a treasured gift. The contributors to this volume have all been wonderful, enlightening, and responsive to the tight timeline and detailed requests. I am most grateful for having had the opportunity to learn from their work. Wendy Behary and Judith Beck were fabulous coauthors on the chapters that we rewrote together. I also wish to thank my beloved collaborator in life, Charlie Sharbel, for the joy, space, and continuing support that made immersion in this project possible.

—DENISE D. DAVIS

In 1977, I began working at the Center for Cognitive Therapy at the University of Pennsylvania, thereby beginning almost four decades of collaboration with Tim Beck. This was a turning point in my life, both personally

and professionally. Tim has been a colleague, counselor, collaborator, supporter, critic, and friend, and it has been my privilege and honor to be working with him. Denise Davis has likewise been a valued colleague, friend,
and collaborator for 35 years. My colleagues, students, and friends at Philadelphia College of Osteopathic Medicine and now Midwestern University
have been a resource for my thinking and conceptualizing and responsible
for making my work satisfying, enjoyable, and even fun. I thank them all.

—ARTHUR FREEMAN

Contents

PART II. CLINICAL APPLICATIONS

PART III. COMORBIDITY AND CLINICAL MANAGEMENT

COGNITIVE THERAPY OF PERSONALITY DISORDERS

PART I

THEORY, RESEARCH, AND CLINICAL METHODS

CHAPTER 1

Overview of Cognitive-Behavioral Therapy of Personality Disorders

Daniel O. David
Arthur Freeman

"Normal" human personality is composed of several personality traits. Indeed, each individual has a personal profile consisting of few central traits, several principal traits, and many secondary traits (see Hogan, Johnson, & Briggs, 1997; John, Robinson, & Pervin, 2010; Matthews, Deary, & Whiteman, 2003).

If we evaluate the personality traits in terms of performance (e.g., How well does the individual's response measure up to particular standards?), then we talk about aptitudes (e.g., intelligence, creativity). If we evaluate the personality traits in terms of social values, then we talk about characterological traits (e.g., generosity, aggressiveness). Finally, if we evaluate the personality traits in terms of dynamism and energy, then we talk about temperamental traits (e.g., explosiveness/impulsivity, inhibition; see Hogan et al., 1997; John et al., 2010).

There are many models of human personality. We do not review them here, as this is not the aim of the chapter (for a comprehensive review, see Hogan et al., 1997; John et al., 2010). We only mention here that one of the most comprehensive and empirically supported models of human personality is the "Big Five" model (see Costa & McCrae, 1992). According to this model, human personality is composed of five factors: (1) openness, (2) conscientiousness, (3) extraversion, (4) agreeableness, and (5) neuroticism. Each factor includes a variety of more specific personality traits.

For example, the extraversion factor includes such personality traits like positive feelings, assertiveness, dynamism, and so on (see Matthews et al., 2003).

There are many psychological models of personality disorders (for a review, see Millon, Millon, Meagher, Grossman, & Ramnath, 2004). Probably the first organized models were based on a psychoanalytical approach, later and further developed as a dynamic–psychoanalytical paradigm. The humanistic–existential–experiential paradigm also proposed various models of disorders of personality. Obviously, the cognitive-behavioral paradigm has its own models of personality disorders. However, while the first two paradigms—the dynamic–psychoanalytic and the humanistic–existential-experiential models—are not explicitly related to the mainstream psychopathology as concerning personality disorders (e.g., the DSM system), the cognitive-behavioral paradigm is consistent with (although not necessary dependent on) the mainstream models of psychopathology regarding personality disorders. For example, the cognitive therapy model of personality disorder (A. Beck, Chapter 2, this volume) views personality disorder based on the DSM system and as a hypertrophy of traits that originate in an adaptive context but become exaggerated and prepotent over the course of development.

THE COGNITIVE-BEHAVIORAL APPROACH TO PERSONALITY DISORDERS

The cognitive-behavioral therapy (CBT) framework/paradigm has a set of interrelated theoretical principles (i.e., CBT architecture) and a set of techniques that can be organized into clinical strategies included in more or less manualized clinical protocols. Indeed, from this general CBT framework, various CBT psychological treatments can be derived based on (1) general and/or specific models related to various clinical conditions, thus promoting theoretically driven techniques (i.e., *systemic CBT psychological treatments*); and/or (2) a multicomponential combination of CBT techniques for a specific clinical condition, with less theoretical integration, derived pragmatically from the general CBT theoretical principles rather than from a CBT general and/or specific model of that clinical condition (i.e., *multicomponential CBT psychological treatments*).

Among the empirically investigated systemic CBT psychological treatments—each organized like a "CBT school of thought"—we can mention alphabetically acceptance and commitment therapy (ACT; Hayes, Strosahl, & Wilson, 2011), dialectic behavior therapy (DBT; Dimeff & Linehan, 2001), and schema therapy (ST; Young, Klosko, & Weishaar, 2003). Obviously, we should include here cognitive therapy (CT; Beck, 1976; J. Beck, 1995) and rational-emotive behavior therapy (REBT; DiGiuseppe, Doyle, Dryden, & Backx, 2013; Ellis, 1994), which, although are the foundational approaches of the general CBT paradigm (see below), were also investigated as systemic CBT psychological treatments. Finally, there is a plethora of multicomponential CBT psychological treatments, organized more like a pragmatic therapeutic package that are less theoretically driven and/or integrated (check the Research-Supported Psychological Treatments list of the American Psychological Association, Division 12; *www.div12. org/PsychologicalTreatments/index.html*).

CBT Theoretical Foundations

Beck's CT (Beck 1963, 1976) and Ellis's REBT (Ellis, 1957, 1962, 1994) have established the foundational structure of the modern CBT paradigm. Congruent with earlier models of behavior therapy, they did not treat personality disorder symptoms as an expression of an underlying illness/disorder/conflict, but rather as learned human responses to specific or general stimuli. However, innovatively and differently from both the older behavior therapy and the extant medical approaches, the individual's responses (e.g., subjective, cognitive, behavioral, psychophysiological)—be they learned or an expression of a broader underlying disorder—were not treated in the same way. The cognitive component has been much emphasized and often promoted as a preliminary "cause" of the others. However, it does not mean that the causality is unidirectional. Both Beck (by his concept of "mode"— Beck, 1996; see also Chapter 2, this volume) and Ellis (by his concept of "interdependency"—Ellis, 1957, 1994) were careful to argue that all types of responses are strongly interrelated, forming a multidimensional interactive psychological structure. Thus, the ABC model (Ellis, 1994; but see also J. Beck, 1995) has arguably emerged explicitly as a general foundation of the CBT architecture (see Figure 1.1).

The "A" refers to various <u>a</u>ctivating events, whether external and/or internal. "B" refers to the individual's <u>b</u>eliefs more generally to our information processing (i.e., cognitions) in the forms of beliefs and thoughts. Initially, both Ellis (1957, 1962, 1994) and Beck (1963, 1976) emphasized conscious information processing (i.e., explicit cognitions in the form of beliefs and thoughts); it might function unconsciously (i.e., functional cognitive unconscious), but by specific techniques (e.g., thought monitoring or

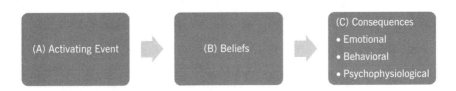

FIGURE 1.1. The general ABC model of CBT.

imagery), these cognitions can be made consciously accessible. The "C" refers to various consequences in the form of the individual's subjective, behavioral, and/or psychophysiological responses. Typically, distorted cognitions are associated with dysfunctional consequences (e.g., dysfunctional/ unhealthy feelings, maladaptive behaviors), while nondistorted cognitions are associated with functional consequences (e.g., functional/healthy feelings, adaptive behaviors). Once generated, a C could become a new A, thus further priming metabeliefs/secondary beliefs (B') that generate metaconsequences/secondary consequences (C').

Starting from this general cognitive architecture of CBT, particular cognitive models have been developed depending on (1) the type of cognitions emphasized at B; (2) the sequence of clinical strategies (e.g., first changing A and/or changing B and/or targeting directly the C); and (3) how the therapist, guided by the patient, deals with various clinical conditions and events.

For example, concerning the type of cognitions, we can make a distinction between "cold" cognitions and "hot" cognitions (for details, see Wessler, 1982, and the derivative work of David & Szentagotai, 2006). Cold cognitions refer to descriptions of reality (e.g., "My wife is not at home") and the individual's interpretations/inferences (e.g., "She is out cheating on me"). Hot cognitions refer to how we evaluate/appraise these descriptions and inferences about the reality (e.g., "My wife should not cheat on me and if it happens, it is awful and the worst thing possible"). Both cold and hot cognitions could be more surface beliefs (i.e., automatic thoughts/ self-statements) or more core beliefs. Beck's CT was initially more focused on descriptions and inferences (e.g., see the "cognitive errors" described by Beck, Rush, Shaw, & Emery, 1979), thus connecting itself more to general attribution theory (see Weiner, 1985). Later, CT, and other CBT psychological treatments like ST and DBT, focused on both cold and hot cognitions that are often integrated phenomenologically (i.e., how they arise in the mind of the client). Indeed, various scales of distorted cognitions (e.g., Automatic Thoughts Questionnaire [Hollon & Kendall, 1980]; Dysfunctional Attitudes Scale [Weissman, 1979]; Young Schema Questionnaire [Young & Brown, 1994]) contain both hot and cold cognitive items. REBT makes a clear distinction between descriptions/inferences and appraisals (i.e., evaluations). Irrational beliefs (e.g., "My wife should not cheat on me and if it happens it is awful.) and rational beliefs (e.g., "I would like my wife not to cheat on me and I am doing my best to avoid it, but I can accept that sometimes things are not under my control; if it happens, it is very bad, but not the worst thing ever") are seen as appraisals, thus relating them to the more general appraisal theory (see Lazarus, 1991). Indeed, REBT considers, based on the appraisal theory (Lazarus, 1991), that unless appraised, the cold cognitions (e.g., descriptions/inferences) do not generate feelings, although they could directly generate behaviors.

The sequence of clinical strategies in CT typically focuses first on the automatic thoughts (most of them expressed as descriptions and inferences—including mental imagery—and/or as a mixture of cold and hot cognitions) and later on core beliefs (i.e., coded in our mind as schemas). At some point, CT focuses on activating events by problem-solving strategies and/or on the consequences of the beliefs by behavioral and/or coping techniques (see J. Beck, 1995). However, the interactive nature of the core elements is different for each individual. For one individual the sequence may be cognition–affect–behavior, for another the sequence may be behavior–affect–cognition, and for a third the sequence may be affect–cognition–behavior. For a comparison, REBT focuses on altering dysfunctional consequences by changing irrational beliefs first and then, if not successfully altered during the process of restructuring irrational beliefs, on changing the cold cognitions. The process is first focused on the surface beliefs in the forms of specific irrational self-statements and later on general irrational core beliefs. After the cognitive restructuring process, REBT would focus on the other components like the activating events/A (e.g., by problem-solving strategies) and/or consequences C (e.g., by behavioral techniques and/or coping strategies; see DiGiuseppe et al., 2013). ACT (Hayes et al., 2011), mindfulness-based CT (Segal, Williams, & Teasdale, 2002), and other so-called third-wave CBT have challenged the need of changing the content of distorted cognitions to achieve a more adaptive change at the emotional and behavioral level by arguing that we need to modify (i.e., cognitively restructure) the function of distorted cognitions—to neutralize and to cognitively defuse them—by acceptance and mindfulness techniques.

There are also variations among CBTs regarding how psychotherapists deal with the clinical conditions (for a debate, cf. Ellis, 2003; Padesky & Beck, 2003). CT argues for very specific and detailed models for each clinical disorder (J. Beck, 1995; Beck, Freeman, & Davis, 2004). REBT (see DiGiuseppe et al., 2013) and more recently ST (see Bamelis, Evers, Spinhoven, & Arntz, 2014) have supported more general models dealing with various clinical conditions, arguing that while these specific models can be valid, underneath the specificity there are core common psychological processes expressed in distorted core beliefs. These distorted core beliefs can interact differently for various clinical conditions (see David, Lynn, & Ellis, 2010). The process is similar to what is seen in neuroscience, where a large variety of symptoms and disorders can be reduced and/or explained by a few classes of neurotransmitters and their interrelations.

David (in press) has recently tried to unify these specific models, by extending the classical ABC architecture of the CBT paradigm, based on a cognitive science and cognitive neuroscience framework, thus trying to move the field from various "CBT schools of thought" to an integrative and multimodal CBT (IM-CBT; see also David, Matu, & David, 2013). It is "integrative" because the interrelated theoretical principles are better organized in a coherent CBT theory (i.e., a CBT general model) that can accommodate various CBT schools and their general and/or specific models. It is multimodal because various techniques and clinical strategies (from CBT and/or other psychotherapy tradition) are derived and/or conceptualized based on the integrative CBT theory, rather than being components, more or less related to one another, derived from various CBT general principles, organized pragmatically to deal with a clinical condition in a multicomponential CBT package. Thus, IM-CBT emphasizes a theoretically driven (i.e., integrative) multimodal approach toward helping patients deal with various psychological conditions.

According to the IM-CBT framework (see Figure 1.2) there are two types of core beliefs. The first type is related to cold cognitions. Here we can include the Beckian general core beliefs like "unlovability" and "helplessness," coded in the human mind as schemas (see A. Beck, Chapter 2, this volume; J. Beck, 1995). The second type is related to hot cognitions. Here we can include the Ellisian general irrational core beliefs expressed as "demandingness" ("Things *must* be done my way"), "catastrophizing" ("It is the worst thing possible"), "frustration intolerance," ("I cannot bear these demands on me"), and "global evaluation of human worth" (for acting or believing in that way shows that the person is a totally worthless

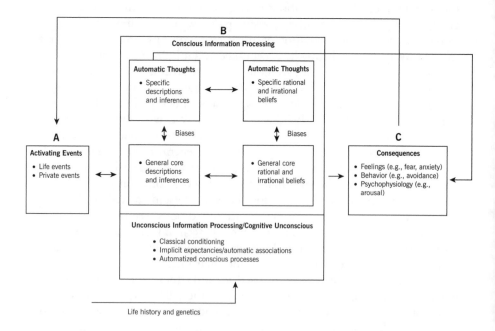

FIGURE 1.2. The modern architecture of CBT. From David (in press). Copyright by Wiley-Blackwell. Reprinted by permission.

individual), coded in the human mind as schemas (DiGiuseppe, 1996, called them "evaluative schemas"; but see also Szentagotai et al., 2005). Phenomenologically, these cold and hot core beliefs could come into our conscious mind in a mixed way. Various core beliefs interact to bias the information processing of events, thus generating specific automatic thoughts that lead to dysfunctional consequences (see Szentagotai & Freeman, 2007). Automatic thoughts, both hot and cold, may come to our conscious mind unintentionally (automatically) and are typically related to the activating event. Indeed, as mentioned above, many scales measuring automatic thoughts and core beliefs contain items referring to both cold and hot cognitions (e.g., Automatic Thoughts Questionnaire, Dysfunctional Attitudes Scale, Young Schema Questionnaire). However, from a psychological mechanistic view, they are different processes and thus, future studies should investigate them as such. The source of core beliefs is related to both environment/ education and biological (e.g., genetic/evolutionary) predisposition (A. Beck, Chapter 2, this volume; J. Beck, 1995; David & DiGiuseppe, 2010). The genetic/evolutionary predispositions have been specially emphasized in relationship to general irrational core beliefs.

Based on IM-CBT, the coping mechanisms are not different cognitive and/or behavioral processes. They are the regular cognitive and behavioral processes that have a different function, namely to help us cope with various feelings and experiences (see Lazarus, 1991).

Finally, the IM-CBT also adds the concept of unconscious information processing at the level of the individual's beliefs. It is a kind of structural cognitive unconscious, containing information coded in formats that are not usually consciously accessible. It can generate dysfunctional consequences directly (e.g., classical conditioning) and/or indirectly (i.e., the output of classical conditioning becomes an A in the A-B-C process; for details, see David, 2003). This information is embedded in the nonconscious, automatic core brain structures like the amygdala (see Treadway, Chapter 4, this volume) and cannot be directly changed on the sole basis of classical cognitive restructuring techniques. However, behavioral techniques (e.g., exposure) and reappraisals based on new experiential information are promising methods to alter the strength of cognitive neural networks that modify input to the core system (Treadway, Chapter 4, this volume).

CBT Applications to Personality Disorders

In the case of personality disorders, the main etiopathogenetic mechanisms should be related to our core beliefs, which are shaped through key developmental experiences and some of which might be based on biological predispositions (A. Beck, Chapter 2, this volume; Young et al., 2003). However, each school of therapy is focused on its main hypothesized core beliefs.

The CT model is mainly focused on the cold general core beliefs and the mechanisms to cope with them (e.g., intermediate beliefs in the form of evaluations, positive and negative assumptions, and rules; A. Beck, Chapter 2, this volume). One can, therefore, see the issue as one of the individual's interpretations or parenthetic views. For example, if an individual were self-focused as a result of the life experience in his or her family of origin, he or she may believe that "I am special." The key issue is not the idea of the individual's specialness, but how he or she completes the sentence. It may be completed in a variety of ways, each determining a different emotional, behavioral, and social outcome.

"I am special (therefore others should give me all that I demand)."
"I am special (and I have to always do things for others to maintain my special status)."
"I am special (and anyone who does not recognize and agree must be punished)."
"I am special (and I will never get the special treatment that I deserve and was given to me by my early caretakers and that would be awful and unlivable)."
"I am special (and regarded as odd by others, and so will never fit in or be understood)."
"I am special (and more clever than most, so I can get away with things others cannot)."

The focus on altering the initial idea of specialness can be a fruitless goal. Does the therapist challenge and dispute the individual's specialness (What about high self-esteem? Shall we build unconditional self-acceptance rather than self-esteem?)? Does the therapist look at the patient's reality? Many readers of this text would endorse the idea that "I am special by virtue of being able to seek, attain, show interest in, and read this book." Thus, the therapeutic focus is on considering the meaning embedded in the belief, and how it impacts an individual's adaptive functions.

ST originated in CT, but expanded the original theory. Thus, ST identified more core beliefs (i.e., early maladaptive schemas) and added several mechanisms of coping with them. DBT also started from behavioral skills training, and expanded it by adding new theoretical mechanisms (e.g., biological diathesis related to the reactivity of the arousal system) and new clinical strategies and techniques to cope with cognitive and emotional distress (e.g., acceptance and mindfulness). REBT is mainly focused on general irrational core beliefs and their interaction to one another (e.g., demandingness + catastrophizing) and on their role (e.g., primary generative mechanisms vs. coping processes) in the primary and secondary/meta-consequences.

Key Features of the CBT Clinical Intervention

The CBT intervention for personality disorders typically includes (1) clinical assessment; (2) cognitive conceptualization; (3) technical interventions; and (4) building and using the therapeutic relationship, much the same as treatment for symptomatic disorders.

However, various adaptations for patients with personality disorders deserve note. Based on the current DSM-5, the clinical assessment can be focused on both categorical and dimensional aspects. For some personality disorders (e.g., antisocial personality disorder) clinical interviews and psychological tests based on self-report should be complemented by psychological tests based on clinicians' (or other relevant persons') report and external and corroborative data.

As concerning the cognitive conceptualization, it is often more dynamic in the case of personality disorders, including (for details, see David, in press) a connection among (1) the cognitive conceptualization of the current problems, (2) the cognitive conceptualization of the past problems, and (3) the cognitive conceptualization of the problems expressed in the therapeutic relationship/setting (see also Figure 8.2 in Brauer & Reinecke, Chapter 8, this volume). This process is similar to the one found in short-term dynamic therapies, although based on clear-cut cognitive conceptualizations as opposed to interpretations or interpolations of dynamic unconscious data. Doing this, the patients can understand how they historically developed their current problems and can even face them directly and experientially ("here and now") as they move through the therapy sessions.

The CBT intervention for personality disorders is typically longer than the CBT intervention for other clinical conditions and often includes more experiential techniques, creating a multimodal approach. As in the case of other clinical conditions, the interventions could be delivered individually or in group.

The therapeutic relationship is characterized by collaboration, congruence, empathy, and genuineness (Davis & J. Beck, Chapter 6, this volume). For personality disorders the relationship must be often used as a vehicle for change, and as a modeling procedure, rather than only as a context of implementing a CBT intervention. Indeed, the therapeutic relationship is often used to generate strong experiences during and subsequent to the session related to the patient's past experiences or current life experiences.

EMPIRICAL SUPPORT FOR CBT IN THE TREATMENT OF PERSONALITY DISORDERS

Barlow (2004) has proposed a clear distinction between "psychotherapy" (i.e., a general psychological intervention in mental health) and "psychological treatment" (i.e., an intervention designed for specific clinical conditions). We further develop this framework, arguing that while "CBT framework" (e.g., IM-CBT) refers to a comprehensive theory and a set of multimodal techniques derived and/or underlined by this integrative theory, CBT psychological treatments refer to (more or less manualized) clinical protocols—often theoretically driven—designed for specific clinical conditions. Furthermore, David and Montgomery (2011) argued that a real evidence-based psychotherapy (i.e., evidence-based psychological treatment) should be validated both in terms of the efficacy/effectiveness of the clinical protocol and the support for the theory underlying the proposed clinical protocol.

Psychotherapy and Personality Disorders

In general, there is strong support for the use of psychotherapy for personality disorders in terms of efficacy and effectiveness (for details, see Hadjipavlou & Ogrodniczuk, 2010). Arnevik and colleagues (2010) found that eclectic psychotherapy implemented in private practice is comparable to a more comprehensive day hospital and outpatient follow-up treatment. Moreover, Mulder, Joyce, and Frampton (2010) found that patients treated for major depression also improved in regard to an identified personality disorder. Thus, personality disorders are neither stable nor treatment resistant. Recent analyses also support the cost-effectiveness of psychotherapy for personality disorders. Indeed, Soeteman and colleagues (2011) found that short-term day hospital psychotherapy and short-term inpatient psychotherapy are more cost-effective than long-term day hospital psychotherapy, long-term inpatient psychotherapy, and long-term outpatient psychotherapy for patients with avoidant, dependent, and obsessive–compulsive personality disorders. Pasieczny and Connor (2011) found DBT to be cost-effective in a routine public mental health setting (e.g., including the treatment of patients with borderline personality disorder). Finally, van Asselt and colleagues (2008) found ST cost-effective in the treatment of borderline personality disorder.

CBT Psychological Treatments for Personality Disorders

Most of the investigated psychological treatments for personality disorders are CBT. Among them, the best investigated are DBT, ST, CT, and multicomponential CBT. As concerning the clinical conditions (for a review, see Dixon-Gordon, Turner, & Chapman, 2011), the most investigated personality disorder is borderline personality disorder. In recent years, some trials have focused on the other personality disorders (e.g., avoidant personality disorder). We still miss rigorous trials for schizoid and schizotypal personality disorders. A recent meta-analysis of psychological interventions for antisocial personality disorder (Gibbon et al., 2010) concluded that there is not enough evidence to argue for the use of psychological treatments in adults with antisocial personality disorder, although CBT psychological treatments (or containing CBT modules) seem promising (see Mitchell, Tafrate, & Freeman, Chapter 16, this volume).

The empirical support of CBT for personality disorders will be examined here based on the CBT psychological treatments derived from it and mainly from an intervention point of view (see also Matusiewicz, Hopwood, Banducci, & Lejuez, 2010). Some CBT psychological treatments have an underlying theoretical model that is consistent with the general CBT framework and the techniques and clinical strategies are derived from the specific model; we call them systemic CBT psychological treatments. Other CBT psychological treatments are based on the general CBT theory, containing a mixture of CBT techniques and clinical strategies, more pragmatically and less theoretically related/integrated; we will call them multicomponential CBT psychological treatments.

Systemic CBT Psychological Treatments

DBT is one of the CBT psychological treatments that have a clear theoretical model and techniques consistent with this model. DBT has been well validated mainly for borderline personality disorder. Indeed, its efficacy and effectiveness have been investigated in various randomized clinical trials and it is recognized as an evidence-based treatment by both National Institute for Health and Clinical Excellence Guidelines (NICE Guidelines) and the Research-Supported Psychological Treatments of the American Psychological Association, Division 12. Lynch and colleagues (2007) found that DBT added to medication is better than medication alone in a sample of older adults suffering from depression with comorbid personality disorders. However, although the impact of DBT on borderline personality disorder is seen as very good, recent analyses added some cautionary ideas. In a recent Cochrane Review, Stoffers and colleagues (2012) argued that none of the investigated psychological treatments (i.e., DBT, mentalization-based treatment in a partial hospitalization setting, mentalization-based treatment outpatient, transference-focused therapy, multicomponential CBT, dynamic deconstructive therapy, interpersonal psychotherapy, and interpersonal psychotherapy for borderline personality disorder) displayed a robust evidence base, although there are some important beneficial clinical effects. Similarly, Springer, Lohr, Buchtel, and Silk (1996) found that a brief inpatient DBT psychological treatment for a sample of patients with mixed personality disorder is, in general, not better than a discussion group (although DBT group considered the intervention more beneficial in lives outside the hospital).

ST is another CBT psychological treatment that has a clear theoretical model and techniques consistent with this model. ST has been investigated in randomized clinical trials for various personality disorders. The study of Gisen-Bloo and colleagues (2006) found that ST was superior to transference-focused therapy for borderline personality disorder (and even more cost-effective) and Farrell, Shaw, and Webber (2009) found ST superior to treatment as usual for borderline personality disorder. In the Bamelis and colleagues (2014) study it was found that ST provided better results than either psychological treatment as usual or a humanistic–existential–experiential approach (i.e., a Rogerian approach in the form of clarification-oriented therapy) for a mixed group of personality disorders (e.g., avoidant, dependent, obsessive–compulsive, histrionic, narcissistic, and paranoid personality disorders). For borderline personality disorder, individual ST seemed to have the same efficacy as combined group–individual ST, but with a lower dropout rate (Dickhaut & Arntz, 2014). However, Dickhaut and Arntz (2014) noted that when the psychotherapists delivering the group sessions are trained in group psychotherapy, the speed of recovery in combined specialized group–individual ST was higher in comparison to individual ST. Ball, Maccarelli, LaPaglia, and Ostrowski (2011) compared individual drug counseling with dual-focus ST for 105 patients who were substance dependent with versus without specific personality disorders. They found that individual drug counseling impacted the symptoms of personality disorders more than dual-focus ST, thus questioning the need of dual-focus ST for patients who were substance dependent with comorbid personality disorders. Some ST research (see Renner et al., 2013) also investigated the mechanisms of change underlying ST psychological treatment. For example, the reduction in global distress in adults with personality disorders and/or personality disorder symptoms was accompanied by a decrease in maladaptive schemas and coping and a slight increase in adaptive schema; however, the reduction in maladaptive schemas did not remain significant after controlling for distress.

CT, together with REBT, is the foundational approach of the CBT framework. However, several CT-oriented psychological treatments were specifically developed for personality disorders. For example, Davidson and colleagues (2006; see also Davidson, Tyrer, Norrie, Palmer, & Tyrer, 2010) compared treatment as usual with treatment as usual as routinely delivered in the UK National Health service plus CT (BOSCOT study) in the case of patients with borderline personality disorder. Adding CT improved the outcome in several domains (e.g., less anxiety, less distress, less dysfunctional cognitions), while other domains were not affected (e.g., frequency of nonsuicidal self-injury, interpersonal functioning, global functioning, psychopathology symptoms, inpatient hospitalization, emergency room visits, cost-effectiveness). Cottraux and colleagues (2009) found that CT for patients with borderline personality disorder was superior to Rogerian counseling in several outcomes (e.g., more rapid improvement in hopelessness, impulsivity, global symptoms severity); however, Matusiewicz and colleagues (2010) noted that the results of this study should be interpreted cautiously because of the high rate of dropouts. Manual-assisted CT seems effective for borderline personality disorder (see Evans et al., 1999; Morey, Lowmaster, & Hopwood, 2010; Weinberg, Gunderson, Hennen, & Cutter, 2006) when used in combination to treatment as usual; in samples with mixed diagnoses its effect is less stable (for a detailed analysis, see Matusiewicz et al., 2010). Finally, Rees and Pritchard (in press) found preliminary support for a brief CT intervention for avoidant personality disorder and Emmelkamp and colleagues (2006) found CT superior to short dynamic therapy for avoidant personality disorder.

Besides these standard CBT psychological treatments, which showed very good, preliminary good, and/or promising effects, two new emerging systemic CBT psychological treatments should be mentioned. A recent public-sector pilot study analyzing treatment as usual argued that borderline personality symptoms could be treated more efficiently with the addition of 12 two-hour ACT group sessions to the treatment as usual consisting of support, medication management, and crisis contact as needed (Morton, Snowdon, Gopold, & Guymer, 2012). The study also found that psychological flexibility, emotional regulation skills, and mindfulness mediated the changes in symptoms of borderline personality disorder. Those researching ACT should build on these encouraging preliminary results to investigate more of the theoretically driven psychological treatments for personality disorders in rigorous large-scale randomized trials.

A study by Fuller, DiGiuseppe, O'Leary, Fountain, and Lang (2010) used REBT as the main therapeutic component in a multicomponential psychological treatment (16 two-hour group sessions) for adult outpatients ($N = 12$) diagnosed with 29 symptomatic and 43 personality disorders. Positive results (pre–post) were found for reducing trait anger, anger symptoms, and depression symptoms. Other theoretically driven empirical studies have shown a systematic association between irrational beliefs and various personality disorders (Lohr, Hamberger, & Bonge, 1988). Spörrle, Strobel, and Tumasjan (2010) found that irrational beliefs have an effect on life satisfaction even beyond the Big Five personality factors. Finally, Sava (2009) found strong associations between general irrational core beliefs measured by the Attitude and Belief Scale–II (DiGiuseppe, Leaf, Exner, & Robin, 1988) and early maladaptive schemas measured by the Young Schema Questionnaire. Taking all these together, REBT should be investigated in large-scale randomized trials for its efficacy and/or effectiveness in the treatment of personality disorders. Given that the NICE Guidelines for antisocial personality disorder argue for a preventive action focused on children with disruptive disorders, and that REBT is considered a probably efficacious treatment for disruptive behavior in children (see the Division 52 list of evidence-based treatments), such a study would be useful.

Multicomponent CBT Psychological Treatments

Various multicomponent cognitive-behavioral treatments have been investigated for borderline personality disorder and antisocial personality disorder (see Matusiewicz et al., 2010). Muran, Safran, Samstag, Wallner, and Winston (2005) found that CBT seems useful for reducing the symptoms and dysfunctionality (e.g., interpersonal problems) in a sample of patients with complex personality disorders. System training for emotional predictability and problem solving (STEPPS)—based on a behavioral skills training approach (Blum et al., 2008)—seems effective for reducing symptoms in patients with borderline personality disorder either alone and/ or in combination with treatment as usual. Emotional regulation group treatment (REGT)—based on an acceptance skills training approach— can also generate clinically important reductions in symptoms of nonsuicidal patients with borderline personality disorder (Gratz & Gunderson, 2006). Cognitive-behavioral group therapy (CBGT) has been investigated for avoidant personality disorder (see Alden, 1989; Renneberg, Goldstein, Phillips, & Chambliss, 1990). This type of psychological treatment typically includes exposure, cognitive restructuring, and social skills training. In general, CBGT has been found efficacious in reducing symptoms of avoidant personality disorder and many comorbid problems (e.g., anxiety).
     Summarizing, although overall studies support the role of CBT psychological treatment for personality disorders, there is need for more rigorous replication studies and place for new CBT psychological treatments.

Other Psychological and Pharmacotherapy Treatments

By contrast to CBT, the efficacy and effectiveness of psychological treatments derived from the dynamic–psychoanalytical paradigm for personality disorders is mixed. For example, Town, Abbass, and Hardy (2011) argued that short-term psychodynamic psychotherapy may be considered an efficacious evidence-based treatment for a large range of personality disorders, based on results of eight randomized trials of moderate quality. On the other hand, Leichsenring and Rabung (2011) found, after analyzing 10 controlled studies, that long-term psychodynamic psychotherapy is better than short-term psychotherapies in complex mental disorders, including personality disorders. However, more recently, Smit and colleagues (2012), after analyzing 11 trials, argued that the effectiveness of long-term psychoanalytical psychotherapy is limited and conflicting. For example, they found that for personality pathology the combined Hedges'g, at the longest follow-up for each study, was nonsignificant ($g = 0.17$, with a 95% confidence interval: -0.25 to 0.59). Clarke, Thomas, and James (2013) recently found that cognitive analytic therapy ($N = 38$) is more effective than treatment as usual ($N = 40$) in improving symptoms and interpersonal difficulties in patients with a personality disorder. Thus psychological treatments for personality disorders, derived from a dynamic–psychoanalytical tradition, seem to work in the form of short-term dynamic therapy and/or in combination with CBT (i.e., cognitive analytic therapy). The impact of long-term dynamic–psychoanalytical treatments for personality disorders is, at this time, debatable.

The results of studies investigating the use of pharmacotherapy for the treatment of personally disorders are mixed. Pharmacotherapy with mood stabilizers, second-generation antipsychotics, and omega-3 fatty acids can target some symptoms of borderline personality disorder and associated psychopathology (see Bellino, Rinaldi, Bozzatello, & Bogetto, et al., 2011; Lieb, Völlm, Rücker, Timmer, & Stoffers, 2010; Stoffers et al., 2010); however, they do not impact on the core symptoms and overall severity of borderline personality disorder. Regarding antisocial personality disorder, after analyzing eight existing trials, there are no firm conclusions about the efficacy of pharmacotherapy (Khalifa et al., 2010).

CONCLUSION

Personality disorders are important clinical conditions that impact other psychological and/or medical clinical conditions. Summarizing the current state of the art, at this moment CBT seems to be the best validated form of psychological intervention for a variety of personality disorders. Although CBT appears promising in the treatment of personality disorders, a number of patients do not fully respond to the intervention and/or the results are not yet completely convincing. Most studies are focused on borderline personality disorder and only a few of them on the other personality disorders, so our conclusions are framed with this caution in mind. Most of the studies are focused on a category of personality disorders (i.e., efficacy paradigm), although studies focused on patients with mixed (Bamelis et al., 2014; Springer et al., 1996) or comorbid personality disorders (Muran et al., 2005) exist (i.e., effectiveness paradigm). Various CBT psychological treatments derived from the general CBT framework (e.g., IM-CBT) are not equally well validated. Some have more empirical support than others. Future studies should further test the existing clinical protocols, such as those outlined in this volume, and even develop new more powerful ones. The new studies should investigate both the efficacy (i.e., how psychotherapy works in controlled conditions), to obtain internal validity, and the effectiveness (e.g., how psychotherapy works in real clinical practice), to obtain external validity. As concerning effectiveness, to fit the real-life contexts, it is expected that more studies will focus on comorbid personality disorders, personality disorders with other comorbid disorders, and even mixed samples (e.g., patients with various personality disorders). The transdiagnostic approach (i.e., the dimensional component of personality disorders) should be an important line of study, consistent with the programmatic research of the National Institutes of Health. Cost-effectiveness analyses will also be very important, in a health system influenced by limited resources and by health insurance companies. Future studies should also explore the role of preventive CBT interventions for personality disorders by focusing on child and adolescent pathology and/or traits (see also the NICE Guidelines for antisocial personality disorder).

In general, the specific theories underlying the clinical protocols are less rigorously investigated than the efficacy and/or effectiveness of the clinical protocols. Therefore, future studies should also focus on theory testing, preferably guided by an etiopathogenetic point of view, rather than by a symptomatic point of view. Only by integrating well-validated theories expressed in efficacious CBT psychological treatments can we promote a rigorous evidence-based approach in the field of personality disorders (see David & Montgomery, 2011).

As there are preliminary evidences for the efficacy and effectiveness of psychological treatments derived from other psychotherapy paradigms (e.g., dynamic–psychoanalytical), CBT should act as a platform for psychotherapy integration, also preparing for integration with other nonpsychological treatments (i.e., pharmacotherapy) when they are evidence based. A multilevel analysis of the CBT outcomes (e.g., including the neurobiological level) is important for an integration between psychological and pharmacological treatments, although, taking the state of pharmacotherapy reviewed here into account, at this time the psychological treatments are the first-line interventions for personality disorders.

CHAPTER 2

Theory of Personality Disorders

Aaron T. Beck

Cognitive therapy for any disorder depends on the conceptualization of the disorder and its adaptation to the unique features of a specific case. This chapter presents an overall theory of personality disorders within the broad context of their origin, development, and function of personality. This exposition focuses initially on how personality processes are formed and operate in the service of adaptation. Before presenting a synopsis of our theory of personality disorders, we review our concepts of personality and link them to the disorders.

We start the discourse with a speculative, evolutionary-based explanation of how the prototypes of our personality patterns could be derived from our phylogenetic heritage. Those genetically determined "strategies" that facilitated survival, resource conservation and expansion, and reproduction would presumably be favored by natural selection. Derivatives of these primitive strategies can be observed in an exaggerated form in the symptom syndromes, such as anxiety disorders and depression, and in personality disorders, such as the dependent personality disorder. Personality disorders, as well as symptom disorders, thus represent an exaggeration of adaptive personality strategies.

Our discussion then progresses along the continuum from evolutionary-based strategies to a consideration of how information processing, including affective processes, is antecedent to the operation of these strategies. In other words, evaluation of the particular demands of a situation precedes and triggers an adaptive (or maladaptive) strategy. How a situation is evaluated depends in part, at least, on the relevant underlying beliefs.

Those beliefs are embedded in more or less stable structures, labeled "schemas," that select and synthesize incoming data. The psychological sequence progresses then from evaluation to affective and motivational arousal, and finally to selection and implementation of a relevant strategy. We regard the basic structures (schemas) on which these cognitive, affective, and motivational processes depend as the fundamental units of personality. Although the schemas are not observable by introspection, the content of beliefs is accessible, and the functional processes can be detected.

Personality "traits" identified by adjectives such as "dependent," "withdrawn," "arrogant," or "extraverted" may be conceptualized as the overt expression of these underlying structures. By assigning meanings to events, the cognitive structures start a chain reaction culminating in the kinds of overt behavior (strategies) that are attributed to personality traits. Behavioral patterns that we commonly ascribe to personality traits or dispositions ("honest," "shy," "outgoing") consequently represent interpersonal strategies developed from the interaction between innate dispositions and environmental influences. Each strategy has a specific, adaptive goal-oriented function.

Attributes such as dependency and autonomy, which are conceptualized in motivational theories of personality as basic drives, may be viewed as a function of a conglomerate of basic schemas. In behavioral or functional terms, the attributes may be labeled "basic strategies." These specific functions may be observed in an exaggerated way in some of the overt behavioral patterns attributed, for example, to the dependent or schizoid personality disorders. The nature of these behavioral patterns may be further understood in terms of regulatory functions that are internalized (self-monitoring and inhibiting) or externalized (reacting, competing, demanding).

We then move on to the topic of activation of the schemas (and modes) and their expression in behavior. Having laid the groundwork for our theory of personality, we go on to review the relation of these structures to psychopathology. The pronounced activation of dysfunctional schemas lies at the core of the former Axis I disorders, such as depression. The more idiosyncratic, dysfunctional schemas displace the more reality-oriented, adaptive schemas in functions such as information processing, recall, and prediction. In depression, for example, the mode that is organized around the theme of self-negation becomes dominant; in anxiety disorders, the personal danger mode is hyperactive; in panic disorders, the mode relevant to imminent catastrophe is mobilized.

The typical dysfunctional beliefs and maladaptive strategies expressed in personality disorders make individuals susceptible to life experiences that impinge upon their cognitive vulnerability, particularly with regard to expanding or sustaining resources. Thus, the dependent personality disorder is characterized by a sensitivity to external loss of love and security; the narcissistic by trauma to self-esteem from external sources; the histrionic by failure to externally engage others for attention and emotional security. The cognitive vulnerability is based on beliefs that have an adaptive element, but have become extreme, rigid, and imperative. We speculate that these dysfunctional beliefs have originated as the result of the interaction between the individual's genetic predisposition and exposure to undesirable influences from other people or cultural experiences and specific traumatic events. Thus, in the course of development, certain key strategies become hypertrophied and emerge as specific, or blended personality disorders.

THE EVOLUTION OF INTERPERSONAL STRATEGIES

Our theory of personality disorders takes into account the role of our evolutionary history in shaping our patterns of thinking, feeling, and acting. We can better understand personality structures, functions, and processes if we examine attitudes, feelings, and behavior in the light of their possible relation to ethological strategies.

Much of the behavior we observe in nonhuman animals is generally regarded as "programmed." The underlying processes are programmed and are expressed in overt behavior. The development of these programs frequently depends on the interaction between genetically determined structures and experience. Similar developmental processes may be assumed to occur in humans (Gilbert, 1989). It is reasonable to consider the notion that long-standing cognitive–affective–motivational programs influence our automatic processes: the way we construe events, what we feel, and how we are disposed to act. The programs involved in cognitive processing, affect, arousal, and motivation may have evolved as a result of their ability to sustain life and promote reproduction.

As people move through successive stages in life, they confront a variety of challenges and problems as well as incentives and opportunities. Individuals are born with a cluster of needs: for sustenance, protection, and help that persist throughout life. These hardwired needs are expressed in the form of cravings, urges, and drives that press for satisfaction. Individuals are also predisposed not only to crave the necessities of life but also to maintain attachments to the human resources essential for success and survival in a competitive and sometimes hostile environment. In addition to automatic defensive responses such as the fight–flight reaction, people have innate structures to perceive and respond to less immediate threats and needs. Automatic strategies in infancy such as crying and smiling, for example, evoke caring responses from the caregivers.

In accordance with the evolutionary mandate for survival and perpetuation of their genetic heritage, individuals are hardwired not only to experience a variety of cravings, urges, and drives but also to selectively attend to caretakers and, at a higher level of maturation, to potential mates. The activation of the various needs is contingent in part on the proximity of human resources. In infancy, the presence of a caregiver is the catalyst for the expression of all need for nurturance. This need persists in a modified form throughout life.

Natural selection presumably brought about some kind of fit between programmed behavior and the demands of the environment or culture. However, our environment has changed more rapidly than have our automatic adaptive strategies—largely as a result of our own modifications of our social milieu. Thus, strategies of predation, competition, and sociability that were useful in the more primitive surroundings do not always fit into the present niche of a highly individualized and technological society, with its own specialized cultural and social organization. A bad social fit may be a factor in the development of behavior that we diagnose as a "personality disorder."

Regardless of their survival value in more primitive settings, certain of these evolutionary-derived patterns become problematic in our present culture because they interfere with the individual's personal goals or conflict with group norms. Thus, highly developed predatory or competitive strategies that might promote survival in primitive conditions may be ill suited to a social milieu and may eventuate in an "antisocial personality disorder." Similarly, a kind of exhibitionistic display that would have attracted helpers and mates in the wild may be excessive or inappropriate in contemporary society. In actuality, however, these patterns are most likely to cause problems if they are inflexible and relatively uncontrolled.

The symptom syndromes can also be conceptualized in terms of evolutionary principles. For example, the fight–flight pattern, although presumably adaptive in archaic emergency situations of physical danger, may form the substrate of either an anxiety disorder or a chronic hostile state. The same response pattern that was activated by the sight of a predator, for example, is also mobilized by threats of psychological traumas such as rejection or devaluation (Beck & Emery, 1985). When this psychophysiological response—perception of danger and arousal of the autonomic nervous system—is triggered by exposure to a broad spectrum of potentially aversive interpersonal situations, the vulnerable individual may manifest a diagnosable anxiety disorder.

Similarly, variability of the gene pool could account for individual differences in personality. Thus, one individual may be predisposed to freeze in the face of danger, another to attack, a third to avoid any potential sources of danger. These differences in overt behavior, or strategies—any of which may have survival value in certain situations—reflect relatively enduring characteristics that are typical of certain "personality types" (Beck et al., 1985). An exaggeration of these patterns may lead to a personality disorder; for example, the avoidant personality disorder may reflect a strategy of withdrawing from or avoiding any situation involving the possibility of social disapproval.

Resources

The major route to the necessities of life is via bonding with other people. Alternatively, individuals depend on their own capabilities to confront challenges of everyday life themselves. However, people crave acceptance by their intimates and by their peer group. The devastating impact of rejection is a token of the importance of interpersonal resources. The dependence on intimate and group relationships appears to be a powerful evolved component of the innate drives. In primordial eras, acceptance, drive, and integration into the tribe were crucial for privileges, nourishment, and reproduction.

People also capitalize on their own inherited resources to maximize their utilization of external resources as well as to function autonomously. Entitlement plays a large role in individuals striving to gain access to resources. Individuals who are of high status and privilege are entitled, and this represents secure access to resources and protection from harm. Being high on the totem pole means not only being a "superior person" but also implies entitlement to another side of life and society, where pleasure is more assured, pain is minimized, and reproduction is more likely.

There are other forms of entitlement besides status. For example, a child may feel entitled to care from his or her parents. A spouse may feel entitled to closeness, intimacy, support, and so on from his or her partner. Diminishing of a relationship (resources) means an attenuation of entitlement. Somebody who is banished from a group or rejected by a lover no longer is entitled to the various benefits that these relationships can bring.

Entitlement and privilege are related to the strength of a bond with other people and groups. When an individual is ultimately bonded to a group, he or she is entitled to the group's support. When an individual is strongly bonded to another individual, then again he or she is entitled. In general, the pressure for entitlement is a strong force for an individual's attempt to increase the bonding with other individuals, or to increase the status with other individuals, in service of the drive toward emotional and physical security.

Strategies

Why do we apply the term "strategy" to characteristics that have been traditionally labeled "personality traits" or "patterns of behavior"? Strategies in this sense may be regarded as forms of programmed behavior that are designed to serve biological goals. Although the term implies a conscious, rational plan, it is not used in that sense here. Rather, we use it as ethologists employ it—to denote highly patterned, stereotyped behaviors that promote individual survival and reproduction (Gilbert, 1989). These patterns of behavior may be viewed as having an ultimate goal of survival and reproduction: "reproductive efficacy" or "inclusive fitness." More than 200 years ago, Erasmus Darwin, grandfather of Charles Darwin (1791, cited in Eisely, 1961), described these evolutionary strategies as expressions of hunger, lust, and security.

Although animals are not aware of the ultimate goal of these biological strategies, they are conscious of subjective states that reflect their mode of operation: hunger, fear, or sexual arousal, and the rewards and punishments for their fulfillment or nonfulfillment (namely, pleasure or pain). Humans are also prompted to eat to relieve the pangs of hunger and obtain satisfaction. We seek sexual relations to reduce sexual tension as well as to gain gratification. We "bond" with other people to relieve loneliness and to achieve the pleasure of camaraderie and intimacy. In sum, when we experience internal pressure to satisfy certain short-range wishes, such as obtaining pleasure and relieving tension, we may, to some degree at least, be fulfilling long-range evolutionary goals.

In humans, the term "strategy" can be analogously applied to forms of behavior that may be either adaptive or maladaptive, depending on the circumstances. Egocentricity, competitiveness, exhibitionism, and avoidance of unpleasantness may all be adaptive in certain situations but grossly maladaptive in others.

Individuals are equipped with a repertoire of innate strategies to exploit and expand interpersonal resources. Each of these interpersonal strategies represents a special sector of the personality, commonly referred to as traits. Each of the strategies (or traits) is tailored to draw on the relevant resources. The strategies are activated in response to the various cravings, urges, and drives and are reinforced by pleasure when the urges are satisfied. On the other hand, failure of a strategy is followed by pain. For example, acceptance by a romantic partner is rewarded by gratification, whereas rejection brings dejection.

Although there are numerous potentially maladaptive strategies such as submissiveness, aggressiveness, and shyness, these do not rise to the level to justify their being included as personality disorders in the official classification systems. Other strategies of a positive nature such as kindness, generosity, and self-sacrifice do not eventually develop into personality disorders, even when exaggerated. The strategies that do transition into personality disorders are inflexible, overgeneralized, and overly intrusive. These excessive strategies interfere with adjustment to others and reduce well-being. In addition, the disorder may manifest when certain inflexible strategies occur in the absence of other moderating strategies. For example, narcissism may develop when competitive strategies are reinforced, without moderating elements of empathy or social reciprocity.

Figure 2.1 provides a graphic illustration of the evolutionary model for development of personality disorders and symptom syndromes. Adaptive efforts to satisfy basic goals may become overdeveloped in a number of ways that result in a maladaptive progression toward different disorders. Specific overdeveloped strategies lay the foundation of the personality disorder and impact evaluations of risk and loss, increasing vulnerability to anxiety and affective disorders. With the development of symptomatic disorders, the basic cognitive content of schemas becomes more embedded and salient, solidifying the cognitive foundation of the personality disorder.

To further detail this model, the personality disorders may be grouped according to their main resources: interpersonal (sociotrophic—outer focused) or individualistic (autonomous—inner focused), as depicted in Table 2.1. The predominant drives include compete, attach, attract, protect, control, defend, and critique. All of these drives serve one of two primary functions—to expand or protect personal resources or domains—and are linked to innate strategies. The strategies are unique and are used as diagnostics for observing and understanding the evolutionary function of each disorder.

Of the disorders driven by a goal of expanding personal domains, the narcissistic personality disorder is typified by a strategy to outcompete others for status and to self-advertise and demand special treatment. The goal of attachment or bonding is achieved through assertion of neediness and pleasing (dependent personality disorder), attraction and engagement (histrionic). Individuals with antisocial personality disorder pursue the goal of expanding their domain through strategies of competition, somewhat similar to the narcissistic personality. They regard others as fair game for

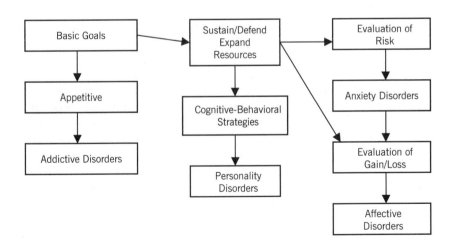

FIGURE 2.1. Goals, strategies, evaluation, and disorders.

TABLE 2.1. Evolutionary Model for Personality Disorders

Disorder	Resources	Drive	Functional strategy
Narcissistic	Groups	Compete; expand	Assert specialness
Dependent	Others	Attach; expand	Assert needs; please others
Histrionic	Others; Groups	Attract; expand	Engage; entertain
Avoidant	Others	Protect	Avoid devaluation
Antisocial	Own skills	Compete; expand	Deceive, cheat, rob
Obsessive–compulsive	Own skills	Control; expand	Set up standards, systems
Paranoid	Self	Defend; protect	Hypervigilance; counterattack
Schizoid	Self	Protect	Isolate; detach
Passive–aggressive	Self	Control; protect	Resist external control; argue
Depressive	Self	Critique; protect	Complain, surrender, retreat, brood

exploitation, objects for physical attack, and deprivation of their possessions, but appear more individualistic in their detachment from social opinion, in sharp contrast with narcissistic individuals. Individuals with obsessive–compulsive personality disorder rely on internally derived systems of control and evaluations to expand their personal domain. The capacity for organizing problem solving and efficacy are adaptive when used appropriately, but become a problem when overused.

Of the disorders characterized by a drive to achieve safety, the avoidant personality disorder may be viewed in terms of a strategy of protection against especially challenging social situations and potential devaluation. On the other hand, individuals with this personality disorder crave a relationship with other people, making them especially sensitive to the potential for rejection, criticism, or ridicule. They shun situations in which they don't feel completely safe. In fact, a factor analysis of the Personality Belief Questionnaire showed a common factor for both avoidant and dependent disorders (Fournier, DeRubeis, & Beck, 2011).

The paranoid personality disorder is characterized by defensiveness. This represents an exaggeration of the normal process of vigilance and protection from potentially harmful individuals. Patients with this disorder focus on their own resources to satisfy their needs, and are prone to personalize threats and counterattack when they perceive some encroachment on their territory. Isolation is the main feature of the schizoid personality disorder. These individuals are characterized by a lack of interest in other people and a strategy of emotional and physical detachment and aloofness. Individuals with schizotypal disorder are similar in many ways to both paranoid and schizoid persons, although their strategies are highly idiosyncratic and socially unusual. The borderline disorder appears to manifest drives and patterns of behavior that are characteristic of the broad range of personality disorders, often producing conflicting motives and significant distress. Thus, these two disorders are not included in Table 2.1. We do include conceptualization of the clinically meaningful disorders of passive–aggressive personality and depressive personality. Both rely on the autonomous resources (self), and are driven by the goal of protecting their domains, through control by indirect resistance or argumentation (passive–aggressive), or criticism, retreat, and brooding (depressive).

It may also be useful to consider the concepts of internalizing and externalizing when observing clinical signs of the various strategies. Internalizing strategies generally involve inhibition and overcontrol, whereas externalizing strategies reflect opportunistic or expressive behaviors that are undercontrolled (e.g., impulsive, reactive, hyperactive, aggressive). As noted by Fournier (Chapter 3, this volume), these dimensions are independent, and it is possible that some personality disorder strategies are externalizing/undercontrolled (e.g., antisocial, histrionic), and some are primarily internalizing/overcontrolled (e.g., avoidant, depressive). Some disorders may arguably reflect low levels of both internalizing and externalizing features (e.g., schizoid), or high levels of both (e.g., borderline, passive–aggressive). The overlap with grouping by main resources (autonomous or sociotropic) is only partial, and may offer further explanation of differences within those groups. Although this conceptualization remains to be confirmed by research, it may provide a clinically helpful method to recognize patterns, gather further data, communicate with patients, and develop treatment interventions.

We suggest that such goals and strategies may be analyzed in terms of their possible antecedents in our evolutionary past. The dramatic behavior of the histrionic personality, for example, may have its roots in the display rituals of nonhuman animals, the antisocial in predatory behavior, and the dependent in the attachment behavior observed throughout the animal kingdom (cf. Bowlby, 1969). By viewing people's maladaptive behavior in such terms, we can review it more objectively and reduce the tendency to stamp it with pejorative labels such as "neurotic" or "immature."

The concept that human behavior can be viewed productively from an evolutionary perspective was developed fully by McDougall (1921). He elaborated at length on the transformation of "biological instincts" into "sentiments." His writing paved the way for some of the current biosocial theorists such as Buss (1987), Scarr (1987), and Hogan (1987). Buss has discussed the different types of behaviors displayed by humans, such as competitiveness, dominance, and aggression, and traced their similarity to the behaviors of other primates. Particularly, Buss focuses on the role of sociability in humans and other primates.

Hogan (1987) postulates a phylogenetic heritage, according to which biologically programmed mechanisms emerge in developmental sequence. He views culture as providing the opportunity through which genetic patterns may be expressed. He regards the driving force of adult human activity, such as the investment in acceptance, status, power, and influence, as analogous to that observed in primates and other social mammals, as well as in humans. He emphasizes the importance of "fitness" in his evolutionary theory of human development.

Scarr specifically emphasizes the role of genetic endowment in determining personality. She states:

> Over development, different genes are turned on and off, creating maturational change in the organization of behavior as well as maturation changes in patterns of physical growth. Genetic differences among individuals are similarly responsible for determining what experiences people do and do not have in their environments. (1987, p. 62)

INTERACTION BETWEEN THE GENETIC AND THE INTERPERSONAL

The processes highlighted in the personality disorders can also be clarified by studies in the field of developmental psychology. Thus, the kind of clinging behavior, shyness, or rebelliousness observed in the growing child may persist through the developmental period (Kagan, 1989). We predict that these patterns persist into late adolescence and adulthood and may find continued expression in certain of the personality disorders, such as the dependent, avoidant, or passive–aggressive types.

Regardless of the ultimate origin of the genetically determined prototypes of human behavior, there is strong evidence that certain types of relatively stable temperaments and behavioral patterns are present at birth (Kagan, 1989). These innate characteristics are best viewed as "tendencies" that can become accentuated or diminished by experience. Furthermore, a continuous, mutually reinforcing cycle can be set up between an individual's innate patterns and the patterns of other significant people. Deoxyribonucleic acid (DNA) does not determine personality type and view of the world, but rather these innate tendencies are shaped and changed by interactions that are embedded in an evolving culture, and occur across the lifespan.

For example, an individual with a large potential for care-eliciting behavior may evoke the care-producing behavior of other people, so that his or her innate patterns are maintained long beyond the period that such behavior is adaptive (Gilbert, 1989). Sue, a patient whom we discuss in detail later, was described by her mother as having been more clinging and demanding of attention than her siblings practically from the time of birth. Her mother responded by being especially nurturing and protective. Throughout her childhood developmental period and into adulthood, Sue succeeded in attaching herself to stronger people who would respond to her expressed desires for continuous affection and support. However, her older brothers jealously picked on her, laying the foundation for a later belief: "I cannot maintain the affection of a man," and struggles with the fear that she was unlovable. Because of these beliefs, she tended to avoid situations in which she could be rejected.

Until now we have been speaking of "innate tendencies" and "behavior" as though those characteristics can account for individual differences. Actually, our theory stipulates that integrated cognitive–affective–motivational programs decide an individual's behavior and differentiate that individual from other people. In older children and in adults, shyness, for example, is a derivative of an infrastructure of attitudes such as "It's risky to stick your neck out," a low threshold for anxiety in interpersonal situations, and a motivation to hang back with new acquaintances or strangers. These beliefs may become fixed as a result of the repetition of traumatic experiences that seem to confirm them.

Because we can observe only the overt behavior of other people, the question arises as to how our conscious internal states (thoughts, feelings, and wishes) are related to the strategies. If we examine the cognitive and affective patterns, we see a specific relationship between certain beliefs and attitudes on the one hand and behavior on the other. It follows logically that a dependent personality disorder characterized by clinging behavior would stem from a cognitive substrate based in part on the fear of abandonment, avoidant behavior from a fear of being hurt, and passive–aggressive patterns from a concern about being dominated. The clinical observations from which these formulations are derived are discussed in subsequent chapters.

Despite the powerful combination of innate predispositions and environmental influences, some individuals manage to change their behavior and modify the underlying attitudes. Not all shy children grow into shy adults. The influences of key people and purposeful experiences in cultivating more assertive behaviors, for example, may shift a shy person toward greater assertiveness and gregariousness, particularly if there is a cultural "pull" that broadly rewards this change. As we see in subsequent chapters in this book, even strongly maladaptive patterns may be modified by focusing therapy on testing these attitudes and forming or strengthening more adaptive attitudes.

Our formulation until now has addressed, briefly, how innate endowment can interact with environmental influences to produce quantitative distinctions in characteristic cognitive, affective, and behavioral patterns to account for individual differences in personality. Each individual has a unique personality profile, consisting of varying degrees of probability of responding in a particular way to a particular degree to a particular situation.

A person entering a group including unfamiliar people may think "I'll look stupid," and will hang back. Another person may respond with the thought "I can entertain them." A third may think "They're unfriendly and may try to manipulate me," and will be on guard. When differing responses are characteristic of individuals, they reflect important structural differences represented in their basic beliefs (or schemas). The basic beliefs, respectively, would be "I am vulnerable because I am inept in new situations," "I am entertaining to all people," and "I am vulnerable because people are unfriendly." Such variations are found in normal, well-adjusted people, and provide a distinctive coloring to their personalities.

However, these kinds of beliefs are far more pronounced in the personality disorders; in the example just mentioned, they characterize the avoidant, histrionic, and paranoid disorders, respectively. Individuals with personality disorders show the same repetitive behaviors in many more situations than do other people, beyond what could be culturally normative. The typical maladaptive schemas in personality disorders are evoked across many or even most situations, have a compulsive quality, and are less easy to control or modify than their counterparts in other people. Any situation that has a bearing on the content of their maladaptive schemas will activate those schemas in preference to more adaptive ones. For the most part, these patterns are self-defeating in terms of many of these individuals' important goals. In sum, relative to other people, their dysfunctional attitudes and behaviors are overgeneralized, inflexible, imperative, and resistant to change.

ORIGIN OF DYSFUNCTIONAL BELIEFS

Given that the personality patterns (cognition, affect, and motivation) of people with personality disorders deviate from those of other people, the question arises: How do these patterns develop? To address this question— albeit briefly—we need to return to the nature–nurture interaction. Individuals with a particularly strong sensitivity to rejection, abandonment, or thwarting may develop intense fears and beliefs about the catastrophic meaning of such events. A patient, predisposed by nature to overreact to the more commonplace kinds of rejection in childhood, may develop a negative self-image ("I am unlovable"). This image may be reinforced if the rejection is particularly powerful, occurs at a particularly vulnerable time, or is repeated. With repetition, the belief becomes structuralized.

The patient mentioned earlier, Sue, developed an image of herself as inept and inadequate because her siblings always criticized her whenever she made a mistake. To protect herself as much as possible from pain and suffering, she tended to avoid situations in which this could occur. Her overgeneralized attitude was "If I allow myself to be vulnerable in any situation, I will get hurt."

INFORMATION PROCESSING AND PERSONALITY

The way people process data about themselves and others is influenced by their beliefs and the other components of their cognitive organization. When there is a disorder of some type—a symptom syndrome or a personality disorder —the orderly utilization of these data becomes systematically biased in a dysfunctional way. This bias in interpretation and the consequent behavior is shaped by dysfunctional beliefs.

The various strategies may be utilized in an adaptive or maladaptive way. The functional application of strategies, or the typical traits we see in action, is based on an adaptive system of beliefs. Beliefs in their various forms represent the content of cognitive schemas. When the schema is activated, the content (belief) becomes salient in the stream of consciousness and influences information processing. As hypothetical constructs, the schemas are not observable by introspection but their content (beliefs) is readily accessible. For the sake of simplicity, we will use the term "belief" for both schema and belief.

Let us return to the example of Sue, who had both dependent and avoidant personality disorders and felt great concern about being rejected. In a typical scenario, she heard noises coming from the next room, where her boyfriend, Tom, was attending to some chores. Her perception of the noise provided the raw data for her interpretation. This perception was embedded in a specific context—her knowledge that Tom was in the next room putting up some pictures. The fusion of the stimulus and the context constituted the basis for information.

Because raw sensory data, such as noises, have limited informational value, they need to be transformed into some kind of meaningful configuration. This integration into a coherent pattern is the product of structures (schemas) operating on raw sensory data within a specific context. Sue's instant thought was "Tom is making a lot of noise." In most instances, people might conclude their information processing at this point, with the storing of this inference in short-term memory. But because Sue was rejection prone, she was disposed to infer important meanings from such situations, and to apply internalizing protective strategies. Consequently, her information processing continued and she attached a personalized meaning: "Tom is making a lot of noise *because he's angry at me.*"

Such an attribution of causality is produced by a higher order of structuring that attaches significance to events. A component (schema) of this higher-level system would be her belief: "If an intimate of mine is noisy, it means he's angry at me." This type of belief represents a conditional schema ("If . . , then") in contrast to a basic schema ("I am unlovable"). In this case, it was possible that Tom was angry with Sue. However, because Sue's basic belief was very strong, she was apt to make this interpretation whenever an intimate such as Tom was noisy, whether or not he actually was angry. Furthermore, prominent in the hierarchy of her beliefs was the formula "If an intimate is angry, he will reject me," and at a more generalized level, "If people reject me, I will be all alone," and "Being alone will be devastating." Beliefs are organized according to a hierarchy that assigns progressively broader and more complex meanings at successive levels.

This example illustrates a concept from cognitive psychology—namely, that information processing is influenced by a "feedforward" mechanism (Mahoney, 1984). At the most basic level, Sue had a belief that she was unlovable. This belief was manifested by a disposition to assign a consistent meaning when a relevant event occurred (Beck, 1964, 1967). The belief took a conditional form: "If men reject me, it means I'm unlovable." For the most part, this belief was held in abeyance if she was not exposed to a situation in which personal rejection by a man could occur. This belief (or schema) would supersede other more reasonable beliefs (or schemas) that might be more appropriate, however, when a situation relevant to this belief occurred (Beck, 1967). If there were data that could conceivably indicate that Tom was rejecting her, then her attention became fixed on the notion of her unlovability. She molded information about Tom's behavior in a way to fit this schema, even though other formulas might fit the data better— for example, "Loud hammering is a sound of exuberance." Because Sue's rejection schema was hypervalent, it was triggered in preference to other schemas, which seemed to be inhibited by the hypervalent schema.

Of course, Sue's psychological processes continued beyond her conclusion about being rejected. Whenever a schema of personal loss or threat is activated, there is a consequent activation of an affective component; in Sue's case intense sadness. A negative interpretation of an event is linked to an affect that is congruent with it, activating the associated strategy. In Sue's case, she might tiptoe around Tom out of fear that he was thinking of breaking up with her, or attempt to please him in some safe way. Although it might appear adaptive for her to rush out to pick up a man-lover's pizza for their lunch, this behavior was actually motivated by her fearful thoughts about his anger, and the maladaptive pressure to assert her need for his approval and avoid any devaluation. The maladaptive nature was further evident in that Sue was trying to lose weight and personally wanted to avoid things like heavy meat-and-cheese pizza for lunch.

Although phenomena such as thoughts, feelings, and wishes may flash only briefly into our consciousness, the underlying structures responsible for these subjective experiences are relatively stable and durable. Furthermore, these structures are not in themselves conscious, although we can, through introspection, identify their content. Nonetheless, through conscious processes such as recognition, evaluation, and testing of their interpretations (basic techniques of cognitive therapy), people can modify the activity of the underlying structures and, in some instances, substantially change them.

CHARACTERISTICS OF SCHEMAS

It seems desirable at this point to review the place of schemas in personality and to describe their characteristics. The concept of "schema" has a relatively long history in 20th-century psychology. The term, which can be traced to Bartlett (1932, 1958) and Piaget (1926, 1952), has been used to describe those structures that integrate and attach meaning to events. The concept of schemas is similar to the formulation by George Kelly (1955) of "personal constructs." In relationship to a theory of psychopathology, the concept of schemas was first applied to depression (Beck, 1964, 1967) and eventually to other disorders such as anxiety disorders but has been used less frequently in discussing personality disorders. As noted, the schemas are not observable by introspection, although the belief contents can be discerned. For simplicity, we use the term "belief" to refer to schemas and their cognitive contents. Schemas also have a variety of properties in addition to their content: activation, degree of charge, permeability, and accommodation.

In the field of psychopathology, the term "schema" has been applied to structures with a highly personalized idiosyncratic content that are activated during disorders such as depression, anxiety, panic attacks, and obsessions, and become prepotent. When hypervalent, these idiosyncratic schemas displace and probably inhibit other schemas that may be more adaptive or more appropriate for a given situation. They consequently introduce a systematic bias into information processing (Beck, 1964, 1967; Beck et al., 1985).

The typical schemas of the personality disorders resemble those that are activated in the symptom syndromes, but they are operative on a more continuous basis in information processing. In dependent personality disorder, the belief "I need help" will be activated whenever a problematic situation arises, whereas in depressed persons it will be prominent only during the depression. In personality disorders, the schemas are part of normal, everyday processing of information.

The term "belief" includes attitudes, assumptions, and expectations. Beliefs may take either a conditional or unconditional form. Unconditional beliefs—for example, "I am needy" or "Other people are dangerous"—are emotionally laden constructs. Beliefs in conditional form—for example, "If my boyfriend rejects me, it means I am unlovable"—impose meaning on an event. The conditional belief is often biased since it is derived from exaggerated unconditional beliefs. For example, "If my wife is distant, it means she does not love me" is conditional. Beliefs may also be formed as injunctions: "I must get my house in order" and "People should pay attention to me." There is often a sequence from the meaning—assumption—belief to the imperative belief. For example, an individual with histrionic behavior had the belief "If I don't entertain people, they will ignore me." She consequently would follow an imperative to tell jokes and make up stories. When people were not amused, she had the thought "I am boring." The sequence was conditional belief → instructional belief. When a person's interpretation or review of information has a high significance for the individual, there is a shift in information processing from the conditional belief to unconditional belief.

When the conditional beliefs provide the meaning of events, the dynamic force of strategies is self-instruction. These may take the form of "should" or "must." An example would be "I must compel them to show me respect." Different imperatives are directed at other people: "I must show respect to my elders." The more complete sequence would be situation → conditional belief → self-instruction → strategy. For example, a situation of seeing an elderly person standing in a subway might trigger the conditional belief that "If I am a good citizen, I should show courtesy to elders," followed by the self-instruction that "I should get up and give him my seat," followed by the appropriate behavior. This sequence would be different for someone with antisocial personality, however. The situation of seeing an elderly person standing in a subway might trigger the conditional belief that "If I can move to the right position, I can pick his pocket," followed by the self-instruction that "I should take advantage of this easy opportunity," followed by behavior consistent with the self-instruction.

At the most primal level the formation of beliefs starts at the earliest stage of perception. The individual receives a host of stimuli, many of which are labeled "good" or "bad." As the perceptions accumulate over time they develop into generalizations (beliefs). Since these generalizations are based on perceptions they may take on the full force and veridicality of reality. They are not only credible but they also influence information processing leading to credible interpretations of events. The content is a fusion of a number of cognitive constructs, labeled beliefs for convenience. It consists of consolidated memories, goals, expectancies, and rules. The underlying concept is represented by the belief. The beliefs (or more precisely the schemas) are generally adaptive and lead to the requisite interpretation of a situation and the activation of the appropriate strategy. When the schemas become activated, the belief becomes operative in providing the content of an interpretation.

Rapid cognitive processing is facilitated by the use of opposing categories to sort information, and then apply relevant formulas or algorithms. This creates consistent belief systems—for example, that friends are safe and strangers are dangerous—that support a coherent way of filtering experiences. Each of the personality disorders shows a characteristically extreme set of bipolar or dichotomous belief systems that operate as a sort of triage for sorting and preparing to respond to events, with predominant beliefs related to the patient's most salient goals. For example, dependent patients may believe that being helped/loved is essential, while being abandoned/rejected is disastrous. In life, this formula is selected as a filter so that events are viewed through the lens of acceptance or rejection. Obsessive–compulsive patients hold the categorical conditional beliefs that "If I follow systems, rules, and evaluations, I will function optimally," and "If I don't follow the systems, things will fall apart." Antisocial patients may believe "If I take advantage of other people, it proves I am strong and powerful," and "If I cannot prey on other people, it means I'm weak and will be exploited." The avoidant patient tends to believe "If I expose myself to unpleasant feelings, they will get out of control and cause pain," and "If I can control and avoid my feelings, I will be fine." The polarity of a paranoid patient holds "If I am suspicious of other people's motives, they cannot hurt me," and "If I am not suspicious, I am vulnerable." Patients with narcissistic personality disorder may believe "If I am famous, my life will be a superior success," contrasted with "If I'm not famous, my life will be an inferior failure."

When a person enters a new situation, a relevant schema is activated according to a sensitivity threshold. The degree of charge to the schema determines the power of the interpretation and whether it is prepotent and likely to supersede or inhibit more appropriate schemas in processing information. If it is hypersalient, the schema determines the interpretation to be correct (confirmational). Since the belief is tied to the strategy, an exaggerated belief can lead to an exaggerated strategy. Thus, the key to understanding the formation of personality disorders lies in the understanding of the beliefs. For example, the highly charged belief "I cannot manage anything on my own" would be reflected in the formation of dependent personality disorder. The belief "I must avoid unpleasant feelings at all costs" would be central to avoidant personality disorder.

PERSONALITY AND MODES

The blueprint for cognitive therapy of personality disorders is forged from an understanding of schemas and modes and how they operate. Personality may be conceptualized as a relatively stable organization composed of schema systems and modes. Systems of interlocking structures (schemas) are responsible for the sequence extending from the reception of a stimulus to the end point of a behavioral response. The integration of environmental stimuli and the formation of an adaptive response depend on these interlocking systems of specialized structures. Separate but related systems are involved in memory, cognition, affect, motivation, action, and control. The basic processing units, the schemas, are organized according to their functions (and also according to content). Different types of schemas have varying functions. For example, the cognitive schemas are concerned with abstraction, interpretation, and recall; the affective schemas are responsible for the generation of feelings; the motivational schemas deal with wishes and desires; the instrumental schemas prepare for action; and the control schemas are involved with self-monitoring and inhibiting or directing actions. Some subsystems composed of cognitive schemas are concerned with self-evaluation; others are concerned with evaluation of other people. Other such subsystems are designed to store memories, either episodic or semantic, and provide access to them. Still other subsystems function to prepare for forthcoming situations and provide the basis for expectancies, predictions, and long-range forecasts.

Modes refer to the network of cognitive, affective, motivational, and behavioral components that organize response patterns when activated by specific challenges or in pursuit of life goals (J. Beck, 1995; Beck & Haigh, 2014). Cognitive components of a mode include embedded beliefs, rules, and expectancies, as well as complex concepts such as identity. Affective responses, strategies, and motivation are also components of the mode. This network of components functions as an integrated organization, characterized by features of individual schemas. Modes have varying levels of activation from minimal to maximal, depending on relevance to specific beliefs in the schema, and can become overly activated and hypertrophied, causing problems in adaptation. However, there are many more adaptive modes than there are maladaptive ones. Modes implement the evolved needs, which are experienced as cravings, urges, and drives, and satisfaction of these drives is accomplished through the use of personal or interpersonal resources. For example, the narcissistic person might be excited by a competitive situation. The belief "I need to be better than others" is activated followed by an urge to demonstrate superiority.

There is a continuum between adaptation and dysfunctionality of specific modes. Modes relevant to psychopathology can be labeled according to their diagnostic classification of personality disorders. The narcissistic mode is concerned with beliefs and urges for increased status, the dependent mode is directed to relief seeking and bonding, the obsessive–compulsive mode on control of self and others, the antisocial mode on preying on others for gratification, the avoidant mode on evading relatively unpleasant situations, the schizoid mode on isolation from the stress of others, the paranoid mode on protection from assumed sinister individuals, the passive–aggressive mode on preserving autonomy and freedom, and the depressive mode on loss or fault recognition.

Modes operate within a situational context. In general, the modes are proactive as well as reactive. They seek opportunities for need satisfaction, and are reinforced by the reward systems, such as when the narcissistic person seeks out positions of power as well as reacts to competitive opportunities to demonstrate power to an audience. The histrionic person may be on the lookout for opportunities to connect with other people. When an opportunity occurs, the activation level of this mode rises to higher levels. The activation may shift from one mode to another depending on the circumstances, and depending on the availability of other schema modes. There would be, for example, a shift from the histrionic mode to a dependent mode during a visit to a physician. The modes in personality disorders tend to be more highly charged than the adaptive modes, and thus more easily triggered. Their exaggerated beliefs lead to inappropriate, inflexible, and dysfunctional strategies. This accounts for the pervasive and inflexible features associated with personality disorders of all types. For example, the histrionic patient might not make an appropriate contextual shift during a physician's visit, and instead behave seductively, misperceiving the situation as an opportunity to garner sexual attention. Building up the strength and availability of alternative, more adaptive schema modes is an essential aspect of cognitive intervention.

THE ROLE OF AFFECT IN PERSONALITIES

Discussion of cognitive and behavioral patterns may seem to slight the subjective aspects of our emotional life—our feelings of sadness, joy, terror, and anger. We are aware that we are likely to feel sad when we are separated from a loved one or experience a loss of status, pleased when we receive expressions of affection or reach a goal, and angry when we are unfairly treated. How do these emotional—or affective—experiences fit into the scheme of personality organization? What is their relationship to basic cognitive structures and strategies? According to our formulation, the affects related to pleasure and pain play a key role in the mobilization and maintenance of the crucial strategies. The survival and reproductive strategies appear to operate in part through their attachment to the pleasure–pain centers. As pointed out previously, activities that are directed toward survival and reproduction lead to pleasure when successfully consummated and to "pain" when thwarted. The appetitive urges related to eating and sex create tension when stimulated and gratification when fulfilled. Other emotional structures producing anxiety and sadness, respectively, reinforce the cognitive signals that alert us to danger or accentuate the perception that we have lost something of value (Beck et al., 1985). Thus, the emotional mechanisms serve to reinforce behaviors directed toward survival and bonding through the expectation and experience of various types of pleasure. At the same time, complementary mechanisms serve to dampen potentially self-defeating or dangerous actions through the arousal of anxiety and dysphoria (Beck et al., 1985). Other automatic mechanisms, those associated with the control system and involved in modulating behavior, are discussed below.

THE INTERNAL CONTROL SYSTEM

We know that people do not give in to every impulse, whether it is to laugh, cry, or hit somebody. Another system—the "control system"—is operative in conjunction with the action system to modulate, modify, or inhibit impulses. This system also is based on beliefs, many or most of which are realistic or adaptive. Although the impulses constitute the "wants," these beliefs constitute the "dos" or the "don'ts" (Beck, 1976). Examples of such beliefs are "It is wrong to hit somebody weaker or bigger than you," "You should defer to authorities," and "You should not cry in public." These beliefs are automatically translated into commands: "Don't hit," "Do what you're told," and "Don't cry." The prohibitions thus exercise a counterforce to the expression of the wishes. Sue had specific personal beliefs—here, in particular, "If I ask Tom too much for reassurance, he will get mad at me" (a prediction). Hence, she inhibited her wish to run into the next room and ask him whether he still loved her.

In therapy, it is important to identify those beliefs (e.g., "I'm unlikable") that shape the personal interpretations, those in the instrumental system that initiate action (e.g., "Ask him if he loves me"), and those in the control system that govern anticipations and consequently facilitate or inhibit action (Beck, 1976). The control or regulatory system plays a crucial— and often unrecognized—role in personality disorders and consequently deserves further elaboration. The control functions can be divided into those concerned with self-regulation—that is, inner-directed—and those involved with relating to the external, primarily social, environment. The self-directed regulatory processes of particular relevance to the personality disorders are concerned with the way people communicate with themselves. The internal communications consist of self-monitoring, self-appraisal and self-evaluation, self-warnings, and self-instructions (Beck, 1976). When exaggerated or deficient, these processes become more conspicuous, and may be observed in the form of internalizing or externalizing strategies. People who monitor themselves too much tend to be inhibited—we see this in the avoidant personality, as well as in anxiety states—whereas too little inhibition facilitates impulsivity.

Self-appraisals and self-evaluations are important methods by which people can determine whether they are "on course." Whereas self-appraisal may simply represent observations of the self, self-evaluation implies making value judgments about the self: good–bad, worthwhile–worthless, lovable–unlovable. Negative self-evaluations are found overtly in depression but may operate in a more subtle fashion in most of the personality disorders.

In normal functioning, this system of self-evaluations and self-directions operates more or less automatically. People may not be aware of these self-signals unless they specifically focus their attention on them. These cognitions may then be represented in a particular form labeled "automatic thoughts" (Beck, 1967). As noted earlier, these automatic thoughts become hypervalent in depression, and they are expressed in notions such as "I am worthless" or "I am undesirable."

The self-evaluations and self-instructions appear to be derived from deeper structures: namely, the self-concepts or self-schemas. In fact, exaggerated negative (or positive) self-concepts may be the factors that move a person from being a "personality type" into having a "personality disorder." For example, the development of a rigid view of the self as helpless may move a person from experiencing normal dependency wishes in childhood to "pathological" dependency in adulthood. Similarly, an emphasis on systems, control, and order may predispose a person to a personality disorder in which the systems become the master instead of the tool—namely, obsessive–compulsive personality disorder.

In the course of maturation, we develop a medley of rules that provide the substrate for our self-evaluations and self-directions. These rules also form the basis for setting standards, expectations, and plans of action for ourselves. Thus, a woman who has a rule with content such as "I must always do a perfect job" may be continuously evaluating her performance, praising herself for attaining a specific goal, and criticizing herself for falling short of the mark. Because the rule is rigid, she cannot operate according to a practical, more flexible rule, such as "The important thing is to get the job done, even if it isn't perfect." Similarly, people develop rules for interpersonal conduct: The dos and don'ts may lead to marked social inhibition, such as we find in avoidant personalities. These people also will feel anxious at even entertaining thoughts of violating a rule such as "Don't stick your neck out."

TRANSITION TO PERSONALITY DISORDER

When people develop a symptomatic disorder, they tend to process information selectively and in a dysfunctional way. Basic beliefs that the patient held prior to developing depression or anxiety become much more plausible and pervasive, solidifying the cognitive foundation of the personality disorder. Beliefs such as "If you aren't successful, you are worthless," or "A good parent should always satisfy her children's needs," become more absolute and extreme. Moreover, certain aspects of the negative self-image become accentuated and broadened, so that the patient begins to perseverate in the thought "I am worthless," or "I am a failure." Negative thoughts that were transient and less powerful prior to the depression become prepotent and dominate the patient's feelings and behavior (Beck, 1963).

Some of the more specific conditional beliefs become broadened to include a wider spectrum of situations. The belief or attitude "If I don't have somebody to guide me in new situations, I won't be able to cope" becomes extended to "If somebody strong isn't accessible at all times, I will flounder." As the depression increases, these beliefs may be broadened to "Since I'm helpless, I need somebody to take charge and take care of me." The beliefs thus become more absolute and more extreme.

The ease with which these patients accept their dysfunctional beliefs during depression or anxiety disorders suggests that they have temporarily lost the ability to reality-test their dysfunctional interpretations. For example, a depressed patient who gets the idea "I am a despicable human being" seems to lack the capacity to look at this belief, to weigh contradictory evidence, and to reject the belief even though it is unsupported by evidence. The cognitive disability seems to rest on the temporary loss of access to and application of the rational modes of cognition by which we test our conclusions. Cognitive therapy aims explicitly to "reenergize" the reality-testing system. In the interim, the therapist serves as an "auxiliary reality tester" for the patient. Depressed patients differ also in the way that they automatically process data. Experimental work (Gilson, 1983) indicates that they rapidly and efficiently incorporate negative information about themselves but are blocked in processing positive information. Dysfunctional thinking becomes increasingly prominent, and it becomes more difficult to apply the corrective, rational cognitive processes.

As pointed out earlier, the way people use data about themselves and others is influenced by their personality organization. When there is a disorder of some type—a clinical (symptom) syndrome (formerly Axis I) or personality disorder (formerly Axis II)—the orderly processing of these data becomes systematically biased in a dysfunctional way. The bias in interpretation and the consequent behavior is shaped by the patients' dysfunctional beliefs and attitudes.

THE COGNITIVE SHIFT

The shift in the cognitive functions in the transition from a personality disorder into an anxiety state and then to depression is illustrated by Sue's experience. As far back as Sue could remember, she had questions about her acceptability. When her relationship with Tom was threatened, these sporadic self-doubts became transformed into continuous worry. As she moved into depression, her belief that she might be undesirable shifted to the belief that she *was* undesirable.

Similarly, Sue's attitude about the future shifted from a chronic uncertainty to a continuous apprehension, and ultimately—as she became more depressed—to hopelessness about her future. Furthermore, she tended to catastrophize about the future when anxious but accepted the catastrophe as though it had already occurred when she became depressed.

When she was not clinically depressed or anxious, Sue was capable of accessing some positive information about herself: She was a "good person," a considerate and loyal friend, and a conscientious worker. As she became anxious, she could credit herself with these positive qualities, but they seemed less relevant—perhaps because they apparently did not assure her of a stable relationship with a man. With the onset of her depression, however, she had difficulty in acknowledging or even thinking of her positive assets; even when she was able to acknowledge them, she tended to disqualify them, as they were discordant with her self-image.

We have already noted that patients' dysfunctional beliefs become more extreme and rigid as the affective disorders develop. Prior to this, Sue would only occasionally endorse the belief "I can never be happy without a man." As her anxiety and depression developed, this belief moved to "I will always be unhappy if I don't have a man."

The progression of cognitive dysfunction from the personality disorder to anxiety and then to depression is illustrated by the gradual impairment of reality testing. When in an anxious state, Sue was able to view a few of her catastrophic concerns with some objectivity. She could see that the thought "I will always be alone and unhappy if this relationship breaks up" was only a thought. When she became depressed, the idea that she would indeed always be unhappy was no longer simply a possibility; it was, for her, reality—a fact.

In therapy, the long-standing beliefs that form the matrix of the personality disorder are the most difficult to change. The beliefs that are associated only with the affective and anxiety disorders are subject to more rapid amelioration because they are less stable. Thus, it is possible for a person to shift from a depressive mode to a more normal mode with psychotherapy, chemotherapy, or simply with the passage of time. There is a shift in energy—or cathexis—from one mode to the other. When this shift takes place, the features of the "thinking disorder" in depression (systematic negative bias, overgeneralization, personalization) greatly diminish. The "normal" mode of the personality disorder is more stable than the depressive or anxious mode. Because the schemas in the normal mode are denser and more heavily represented in the cognitive organization, they are less amenable to change. These schemas give the normal personality and the personality disorder their distinctive characteristics. Within each personality disorder, certain beliefs and strategies are predominant and form a characteristic profile.

COGNITIVE PROFILES

One simple way to approach the personality disorders is to think of them in terms of certain vectors. Following the formulation of Horney (1950), we can view these interpersonal strategies in terms of how personality types relate to and act toward other people, and how they use interpersonal space. Individuals may move or place themselves against, toward, away from, above, or under others. The dependent moves *toward* and often *below* (submissive, subservient). Another "type" *stays still* and may obstruct others: the passive–aggressive. The narcissists position themselves *above* others. The compulsive may move *above* in the interest of control. The schizoid moves *away,* and the avoidant moves *closer* and then *backs off.* The histrionic personalities use the space to *draw others* toward them. As we shall see, these vectors may be regarded as the visible manifestations of specific interpersonal strategies associated with specific personality disorders. This simplified sketch presents one way of looking at personality types and personality disorders—in terms of the way individuals position themselves in relation to other people. Insofar as this patterning is regarded as dysfunctional, the diagnosis of personality disorder is deemed to be justified when it leads to (1) problems that produce suffering in the patient (e.g., avoidant personality) or (2) difficulties with other people or with society (e.g., antisocial personality). However, many people with a diagnosed personality disorder do not regard themselves as having such a disorder. Individuals generally regard their personality patterns as undesirable only when they lead to symptoms (e.g., depression or anxiety) or when they seem to interfere with important social or occupational aspirations (as in the case of the dependent, avoidant, or passive–aggressive personalities).

When confronted with situations that interfere with the operation of their idiosyncratic strategy—for example, when a dependent person is separated from or threatened with separation from a significant other, or the obsessive–compulsive is thrown into an unmanageable situation—then the person may develop symptoms of depression or anxiety. Other people with personality disorders may regard their own patterns as perfectly normal and satisfactory for them but acquire a diagnostic label because their behavior is viewed negatively by other people, as in the case of narcissistic, schizoid, or antisocial personalities.

The observable behaviors (or strategies), however, are only one aspect of the personality disorders. Each disorder is characterized by dysfunctional or asocial behavior and by a composite of beliefs and attitudes, affect, and strategies. It is possible to provide a distinctive profile of each of the disorders based on their typical cognitive, affective, and behavioral features, indicating the clinical signs that might be observed by the clinician. Although this typology is presented in pure form, it should be kept in mind that specific individuals might show features of more than one personality type.

OVERDEVELOPED AND UNDERDEVELOPED PATTERNS

Individuals with a personality disorder tend to show certain patterns of behavior that are hypertrophied, or overdeveloped, and other patterns that are underdeveloped. The obsessive–compulsive disorder, for example, may be characterized by an excessive emphasis on control, responsibility, and systematization, and a relative deficiency in spontaneity and playfulness. As illustrated in Table 2.2, the other personality disorders similarly show a heavy weighting of some patterns and a light representation of others. The deficient features are frequently the counterparts of the strong features. It is as though when one interpersonal strategy is overdeveloped, the balancing strategy fails to develop properly. One can speculate that as a child becomes overinvested in a predominant type of behavior, it overshadows and perhaps weakens the development of other adaptive behaviors.

As will be shown in the subsequent chapters on each of the personality disorders, certain overdeveloped strategies may be a derivative from or compensation for a particular type of self-concept and a response to particular developmental experiences, including evolving cultural demands. Also, as indicated previously, genetic predisposition may favor the development of a particular type of pattern in preference to other possible patterns. Some children, for example, appear to be oriented toward entertaining, whereas others appear shy and inhibited from the early stages of development. Thus, the narcissistic personality may develop as an individual who genetically tends toward extroversion and hyperactivity, fights fiercely to overcome a chronic sense of unworthiness, and is able to capitalize on inherited resources such as athletic skill to achieve culturally defined superiority. The obsessive–compulsive personality may develop in a temperamentally sensitive individual's response to chaotic conditions in childhood—as a way of bringing order to a disordered environment. A paranoid personality may be formed in response to early experiences of betrayal or deception; a passive–aggressive personality may develop in response to manipulation by others. The dependent personality often represents a fixation on a close attachment that, for a variety of reasons, may have been reinforced by family members rather than normally attenuated over the developmental period. Similarly, a histrionic personality may be evoked from experiences of being

TABLE 2.2. Cognitive Profiles of Personality Disorders

Personality disorder	View of self (core beliefs)	View of others (core beliefs)	Conditional/predictive and imperative beliefs	Overdeveloped strategies (behaviors)	Underdeveloped strategies (behaviors)
Avoidant	Socially inferior Vulnerable to devaluation and emotional stress "I'm awkward." "I'm unwanted." "I'm unlovable." "I can't take it."	Critical Demeaning Superior "They look down on me." "They are powerful and will be critical of me."	"I don't have friends, so I must be unlikable." "If people notice me, they will reject or humiliate me." "If I was confident, they might like me." "Be careful." "Don't look weird."	Anticipate and avoid attention or discomfort Inhibit emotional expression, passive Escape Ruminate and wish for relationships	Social risk taking Self-assertion Casual social interactions Expressive communications
Dependent	Vast needs Weak, fragile, incompetent without support Vulnerable to abandonment "I'm needy." "I'm helpless." "I'm unlovable."	Idealized Nurturing Supportive Capable "They are strong and can help me." "They have it figured out."	"If I don't have someone to lean on, I'm lost." "If I have people around me, I'm safe and happy." "Do whatever it takes to make the relationship last." "Don't risk it on your own."	Strong attachment Help seeking Clinging Inhibit self Defer decisions Rely on others People pleasing	Healthy separateness Self-expression Skill and interest development Self-reliance
Passive–aggressive	Self-sufficient Vulnerable to manipulation "I need control." "I deserve more." "I'm trapped." "I'm a loser."	Intrusive Demanding Dominating "They are controlling and will push me around."	"If I give up my options, I'll be the loser." "Give them an inch, and they'll take a mile." "Agree and then do what you want." "Hold your ground, don't give in."	Indirect control Passive resistance Surface submissiveness Circumvent rules or expectations	Assertiveness Cooperation Negotiation Acceptance of limits
Obsessive–compulsive	Accountable Fastidious	Casual Incompetent	"If I'm not in control, then things will fall apart."	Being thorough Doing it "right"	Spontaneity Playfulness

	View of self	View of others	Beliefs	Strategy	Adaptive
	Vulnerable to mistakes "I'm responsible." "I'm an example."	Self-indulgent "They are irresponsible."	"People *should* do better, try harder." "It's all on me." "I must take control."	Locate and punish imperfections Rule adherence Dictate "shoulds" Restrain impulses	Creative exploration Discern reasonable standards and exceptions
Paranoid	A loner Vulnerable to pillaging Righteous, noble Clever "I'm a target." "I'm no fool."	Deceitful Malicious Discriminatory Abusive motives "They want to harm me or steal from me."	"If I let them, others will take advantage of me." "If I stay alert, I can defend myself." "Don't trust anyone." "Defend your turf."	Suspiciousness Vigilance Hide; secretive Counterattack	Trust Relaxation Acceptance Openness
Schizotypal	A loner Vulnerable to alien forces Different Supernaturally attuned "I'm unique." "I have special gifts."	Unfriendly Hostile "They don't care about me and might hurt me." "They don't understand the powerful forces."	"If I'm different, others will admire me and leave me alone." "If I use my powers, the forces will protect me." "Be unusual." "Get away from people." "Protect your gifts." "Don't let anyone too close."	Put on a mask Keep distance "Sense" the supernatural Cultivate unusual appearance Use magical tools and talismans	Develop personal connections Congregate with others Follow social convention
Schizoid	A loner Oddball, misfit Self-sufficient Vulnerable to social pressure "I'm not normal." "I need space." "I'm happier alone."	Demanding Unkind, hostile "People ask too much." "They will pick on me if they have the chance." "I don't really like them."	"If I open up, people will see how odd I am and tease or reject me." "I don't enjoy people, so there is no point in being social." "Avoid contact." "Get loose of them." "Let them do their thing without me."	Physical isolation Unresponsiveness Solitary activity Inhibit affect Detachment	Tolerance of social proximity Informal social exchange Expressive affect Mild emotional risks

(continued)

TABLE 2.2. *(continued)*

Personality disorder	View of self (core beliefs)	View of others (core beliefs)	Conditional/predictive and imperative beliefs	Overdeveloped strategies (behaviors)	Underdeveloped strategies (behaviors)
Antisocial	Strong, clever Autonomous Invulnerable "I make my own rules." "I'm smart." "I'm entitled." "I need excitement."	Weak, stupid, vulnerable Rule bound "Only fools follow the rules." "Another person's weakness is my opportunity."	"It's stupid to work if you can use the system." "If I don't (sell drugs), someone else will." "If I happen to hurt someone, there's no point in worrying about it." "Take advantage of the chance." "Get what you want." "Have some fun."	Manipulation Deception Opportunism Predation Thrill seeking	Responsibility Empathy Rule adherence Behavioral inhibition
Narcissistic	Special, superior Entitled Majestic Vulnerable to loss of status "I'm better than others." "I'm extraordinary, powerful, perfect."	Inferior Admirers "They look up to me." "They wish they could be me." "Most people are insignificant and not worth my time."	"Since I'm special, I *deserve* special rules." "If someone challenges me, I must come out on top." "If I have the right things, it shows my superiority." "Demand the best." "Don't let anyone ahead of you." "Protect your image."	Compete, boast Use others Manipulate for power and status Aggrandize self Attack challengers Bully inferiors Transcend rules and ordinary limits	Share the stage Show empathy and consideration Inhibit impulses to brag, compete, or dominate others Social reciprocity
Histrionic	Glamorous Entertaining	Seducible Receptive	"If I'm not admired, I might go insane."	Magnify emotions Display sexuality	Reflective observation

	Self-View	Other-View	Strategies	Behaviors	Adaptive Capacities
	Inadequate Vulnerable to neglect and approval. "I need attention and approval." "I'm unworthy."	Admirers "They are easy to manipulate." "They can make me feel better about myself."	"If I'm seductive, they will notice me." "Use your charms." "Express your feelings." "Make them meet your needs."	Somatic complaints Impulsive reactions Tantrums Perform for attention	Impulse control Distress tolerance Social reciprocity Sexual discretion
Depressive	Immutably worthless Vulnerable to loss and meaninglessness "I'm pathetic." "I can't change." "I'm incompetent."	Foolish and delusional "People are basically selfish and stupid." "They are worse than me."	"If I am hopeful, I will only be let down." "If others are incompetent, then I'm not as bad by comparison." "Don't expect much, and you won't be disappointed." "There's no point."	Critical appraisal Complaints Avoidance goals Worry, brood Procrastination Passive surrender	Attention to strengths and positive emotion Repair negative moods Hopeful anticipation
Borderline	Defective Vulnerable to abuse, betrayal, neglect "I'm bad." "I don't know me." "I'm weak and overwhelmed." "I can't help myself."	Warm, nurturing yet untrustworthy "They are strong and caring but might turn and use, hurt, or abandon me."	"If I'm alone, I won't be able to cope." "If I trust someone, I'll be abused or abandoned." "If my feelings are ignored or dismissed, I will lose control." "Demand what you need." "Fight back." "Get relief now."	Subjugate self Alternate inhibition with dramatic protest Punish others Expel tension with reckless, self-damaging actions	Trusting attachment Self-assertion and limit setting Modulated anger Distress tolerance Impulse control

rewarded for successful exhibitionism—for example, entertaining others to get approval and affection. It should be noted that different pathways might lead to personality disorders. Narcissistic, obsessive–compulsive, paranoid, and even antisocial personality disorder, for example, may develop either as a compensation or as a fear (i.e., as a result of a sense of chaos, manipulation, or victimization) as a result of reinforcement of the relevant strategies by significant others or through both methods.

One cannot overlook the importance of identification with other family members. Some individuals *seem* to adopt certain dysfunctional patterns of their parents or siblings and build on them as they grow older. In other individuals, personality disorders seem to evolve from the inheritance of a strong predisposition. Thus, research by Kagan (1989) indicates that a shyness exhibited early in life tends to persist. It is possible that an innate disposition to shyness could be so reinforced by subsequent experience that instead of simply being nonassertive, the individual develops into an avoidant personality. It is useful to analyze the psychological characteristics of individuals with personality disorders in terms of their views of themselves and others, their basic beliefs, their basic strategies, and their main affects. In this way, therapists can obtain specific cognitive–behavioral–emotive profiles that help them to understand each disorder and that facilitate treatment.

SPECIFIC COGNITIVE PROFILES

Avoidant Personality Disorder

People diagnosed as having avoidant personality disorder, using DSM-5 criteria, have the following key conflict: They would like to be close to others and to live up to their intellectual and vocational potential, but they are afraid of being hurt, rejected, and unsuccessful. Their strategy (in contrast to the dependent) is to back off—or avoid getting involved in the first place. A key word to describe this personality disorder is "hypersensitive."

- *Self-view:* They see themselves as socially inept and incompetent in academic or work situations.

- *View of others:* They see others as potentially critical, uninterested, and demeaning.

- *Beliefs:* Not infrequently, persons with this disorder have these *core* beliefs: "I am no good . . . , worthless . . . , unlovable. I cannot tolerate unpleasant feelings." These beliefs feed into the next (higher) level of *conditional* beliefs: "If people got close to me, they would discover the 'real me' and would reject me—that would be intolerable" and "If I undertake something new and don't succeed, it would be devastating." The next level, which dictates their behavior, consists of *instrumental* or self-instructional beliefs such as "It is best to stay clear of risky involvement," "I should avoid unpleasant situations at all costs," and "If I feel or think of something unpleasant, I should try to wipe it out by distracting myself or taking a fix (drink, drug, etc.)."

• *Threats:* The main threats are of being discovered to be a "fraud," being put down, demeaned, or rejected.

• *Strategy:* Their main strategy is to avoid situations in which they could be evaluated. Thus, they tend to hang back on the fringes of social groups and avoid attracting attention to themselves. In work situations, they tend to avoid taking on new responsibilities or seeking advancement because of their fear of failure and of subsequent reprisals from others.

• *Affect:* The main affect is dysphoria, a combination of anxiety and sadness, related to their deficits in obtaining the pleasures they would like to receive from close relationships and the sense of mastery from accomplishment. They experience anxiety, related to their fear of sticking their necks out in social or work situations.

Their low tolerance for dysphoria prevents them from developing methods for overcoming their shyness and asserting themselves more effectively. Because they are introspective and monitor feelings continually, they are acutely sensitive to their feelings of sadness and anxiety. Ironically, despite their hyperawareness of painful feelings, they shy away from identifying unpleasant thoughts—a tendency that fits in with their major strategy and is labeled "cognitive avoidance." Their low tolerance for unpleasant feelings and their sensitivity to failure and rejection pervade all of their actions. Unlike the dependent person, who handles fear of failure by leaning on others, the avoidant person simply lowers expectations and stays clear of any involvement that incurs a risk of failure or rejection.

Dependent Personality Disorder

Individuals with dependent personality disorder have a picture of themselves as helpless and therefore try to attach themselves to some stronger figure who will provide the resources for their survival and happiness. Key words to describe this personality disorder are "clingy" and "compliant."

• *Self-view:* They perceive themselves as needy, weak, helpless, and incompetent.

• *View of others:* They see the strong "caretaker" in an idealized way: as nurturing, supportive, and competent. In contrast to the avoidant personality, who stays clear of "entangling relationships" and consequently does not gain social support, the dependent personality can function quite well as long as a strong figure is accessible.

- *Beliefs:* These patients believe that "I need other people—specifically, a strong person—in order to survive." Furthermore, they believe that their happiness depends on having such a figure available. They believe that they need a steady, uninterrupted flow of support and encouragement. As one dependent patient put it, "I cannot live without a man" and "I can never be happy unless I am loved." In terms of the hierarchy of beliefs, their *core* belief is likely to be "I am completely helpless," or "I am all alone." Their *conditional* beliefs are "I can function only if I have access to somebody competent," "If I am abandoned, I will die," and "If I am not loved, I will always be unhappy." The *instrumental* level consists of imperatives such as "Don't offend the caretaker," "Stay close," "Cultivate as intimate a relationship as possible," and "Be subservient in order to bind him or her."

- *Threat:* The main threat or trauma is concerned with rejection or abandonment.

- *Strategy:* Their main strategy is to cultivate a dependent relationship. They will frequently do this by subordinating themselves to a "strong" figure and trying to placate or please this person.

- *Affect:* Their main affect is anxiety—the concern over possible disruption of the dependent relationship. They periodically experience heightened anxiety when they perceive that the relationship actually is strained. If the figure they depend on is removed, they may sink into a depression. On the other hand, they experience gratification or euphoria when their dependent wishes are granted.

Passive–Aggressive Personality Disorder

Even though this disorder is not included in DSM-5, we have found that a significant number of patients have behaviors and beliefs indicative of this disorder. A key word to describe this personality disorder is "stubborn." Individuals with passive–aggressive personality disorder have an oppositional style, which belies the fact that they do want to get recognition and support from authority figures. The chief problem is a conflict between their desire to get the benefits conferred by authorities on the one hand and their desire to maintain their autonomy on the other. Consequently, they try to maintain the relationship by being passive and submissive, but, as they sense a loss of autonomy, they are inclined to resist or even to subvert the authorities.

- *Self-view:* They may perceive themselves as self-sufficient but vulnerable to encroachment by others. (They are, however, drawn to strong figures and organizations because they crave social approval and support. Hence, they are frequently in a conflict between their desire for attachment and their fear of encroachment.)

- *View of others:* They see others—specifically, the authority figures—as intrusive, demanding, interfering, controlling, and dominating, but at the same time capable of being approving, accepting, and caring.

- *Beliefs:* Their *core* beliefs have to do with notions such as "Being controlled by others is intolerable," "I have to do things my own way," or "I deserve approval because of all I have done." Their conflicts are expressed in beliefs such as "I need authority to nurture and support me" versus "I need to protect my identity." (Borderline patients often express the same kinds of conflicts.) The *conditional* belief is expressed in terms such as "If I follow the rules, I lose my freedom of action." Their *instrumental* beliefs revolve around postponing action that is expected by an authority, or complying superficially but not substantively.

- *Threat:* The main threat or fears revolve around loss of approval and abridgement of autonomy.

- *Strategy:* Their main strategy is to fortify their autonomy through devious opposition to the authority figures while ostensibly courting the favor of the authorities. They try to evade or circumvent the rules in a spirit of covert defiance. They are often subversive in the sense of not getting work done on time, not attending classes, and so on—ultimately self-defeating behavior. Yet, on the surface, because of their need for approval, they may seem to be compliant and cultivate the goodwill of the authorities. They often have a strong passive streak. They tend to follow the line of least resistance; they often avoid competitive situations and are interested more in solitary pursuits.

- *Affect:* Their main affect is unexpressed anger, which is associated with rebellion against an authority's rules. This affect, which is conscious, alternates with anxiety when they anticipate reprisals and are threatened with cutting off of "supplies."

Obsessive–Compulsive Personality Disorder

The key words for obsessive–compulsive personality are "control," "should," and "perfectionist." These individuals make a virtue of justifying the means to achieve the end to such an extent that the means becomes an end in itself. To them, "orderliness is godliness."

- *Self-view:* They see themselves as responsible for themselves and others. They believe they have to depend on themselves to see that things get done. They are accountable to their own perfectionist conscience and driven by the "shoulds." Many of the people with this disorder have a core image of themselves as inept or helpless. The deep concern about being helpless is linked to a fear of being overwhelmed, unable to function. In these cases, their overemphasis on systems is a compensation for their perception of defectiveness and helplessness.

• *View of others:* They perceive others as too casual, often irresponsible, self-indulgent, or incompetent. They liberally apply the "shoulds" to others in an attempt to shore up their own weaknesses.

• *Beliefs:* In the serious obsessive–compulsive personality disorder, the *core* beliefs are "I could be overwhelmed," "I am basically disorganized or disoriented," and "I need order, systems, and rules in order to survive." Their *conditional* beliefs are "If I don't have systems, everything will fall apart," "Any flaw or defect in performance will produce a landslide," "If I or others don't perform at the highest standards, we will fail," "If I fail in this, I am a failure as a person," and "If I have a perfect system, I will be successful/happy." Their *instrumental* beliefs are imperative: "I must be in control," "I must do virtually anything just right," "I know what's best," "You have to do it my way," "Details are crucial," "People *should* do better and try harder," "I have to push myself (and others) all the time," and "People should be criticized in order to prevent future mistakes." Frequent automatic thoughts tinged with criticalness are "Why can't they do it right?" or "Why do I always slip up?"

• *Threats:* The main threats are flaws, mistakes, disorganization, or imperfections. They tend to "catastrophize" that "things will get out of control" or that they "won't be able to get things done."

• *Strategy:* Their strategy revolves around a system of rules, standards, and "shoulds." In applying rules, they evaluate and rate other people's performance as well as their own. In order to reach their goals, they try to exert maximum control over their own behavior and that of others involved in carrying out their goals. They attempt to assert control over their own behavior by "shoulds" and self-reproaches, and over other people's behavior by overly directing, or disapproving and punishing them. This instrumental behavior amounts to coercing and slave driving themselves or others.

• *Affect:* Because of their perfectionist standards, these individuals are particularly prone to experience regrets, disappointment, and anger toward themselves and others. The affective response to their anticipation of substandard performance is anxiety or anger. When serious "failure" does occur, they may become depressed.

Paranoid Personality Disorder

The key word for paranoid personality disorder is "mistrust." It is conceivable that, under certain circumstances, wariness, looking for hidden motives, or not trusting others may be adaptive—even lifesaving—but the paranoid personality adopts this stance in most situations, including the most benign.

- *Self-view:* The paranoid personalities see themselves as righteous and vulnerable to mistreatment by others.

- *View of others:* They see other people essentially as devious, deceptive, treacherous, and covertly manipulative. They believe that other people actively desire to interfere with them, put them down, discriminate against them—but in a hidden way in an innocent guise. Some patients may think that others form secret coalitions against them.

- *Beliefs:* The *core* beliefs consist of notions such as "I am vulnerable to other people," "Other people cannot be trusted," "They have bad intentions (toward me)," "They are deceptive," and "They're out to undermine me or depreciate me." The *conditional* beliefs are "If I am not careful, people will manipulate, abuse, or take advantage of me," "If people act friendly, they are trying to use me," and "If people seem distant, it proves they are unfriendly." The *instrumental* (or self-instructional) beliefs are "Be on guard," "Don't trust anybody," "Look for hidden motives," and "Don't get taken in."

- *Threats:* The main fears are concerned with being diminished or taken advantage of in some way: manipulated, controlled, demeaned, or discriminated against. They are readily threatened by any actions that represent encroachment on their territory, ideals, possessions, or key relationships.

- *Strategy:* With this notion that other people are against them, the paranoid personalities are driven to be hypervigilant and always on guard. They are wary, suspicious, and looking all the time for cues that will betray the "hidden motives" of their "adversaries." At times, they may confront these "adversaries" with allegations about being wronged and consequently provoke the kind of hostility that they believed had already existed.

- *Affects:* The main affect is anger over the presumed abuse or exploitation. Some paranoid personalities, however, may also experience constant anxiety over the perceived threats. This painful anxiety is often the prod for their seeking therapy.

Antisocial Personality Disorder

The antisocial personalities may assume a variety of forms: the expression of antisocial behavior may vary considerably (see DSM-5; American Psychiatric Association, 2013) from conniving, manipulating, and exploiting to direct attack. A key word across these variations is "irresponsible," as they are all persistently and extremely irresponsible in areas of work, finance, family, property or community, or impact of their actions on others.

• *Self-view:* In general, these personalities view themselves as loners, autonomous, and strong. Some of them see themselves as having been abused and mistreated by society and therefore justify victimizing others because they believe that they have been victimized. Other patients may simply cast themselves in the predatory role in a "dog-eat-dog" world in which breaking the rules of society is normal and even desirable.

• *View of others:* They see other people in two different ways, as exploitative and thus deserving of being exploited in retaliation, or as weak and vulnerable and thus deserving of being preyed upon. They will particularly focus on anyone perceived as both exploitative and weak.

• *Beliefs:* The *core* beliefs are "I need to look out for myself," and "I need to be the aggressor or I will be the victim." The antisocial personality also believes that "Other people are patsies or wimps," or "Others are exploitative, and therefore I'm entitled to exploit them back." This person believes that he or she *is* entitled to break rules: Rules are arbitrary and designed to protect the "haves" against the "have nots." This view is in contrast to that of people with narcissistic personalities, who believe that they are such special, unique individuals and that they are above the rules—a prerogative that they believe everybody should easily recognize and respect. The *conditional* belief is "If I don't push others around (or manipulate, exploit, or attack them), I will never get what I deserve." The *instrumental* or imperative beliefs are "Get the other guy before he gets you," "It's your turn now," and "Take it, you deserve it."

• *Strategy:* The main strategies fall into two classes. The overt antisocial personality will openly attack, rob, and defraud others. The more subtle type—the "con artist"—seeks to inveigle others and, through shrewd, subtle manipulations, to exploit or defraud them.

• *Affect:* When a particular affect is present, it is essentially anger—over the injustice that other people have possessions that they (the antisocial personalities) deserve, or having been caught or otherwise thwarted from their goals.

Narcissistic Personality Disorder

The key word for narcissistic personality disorder is "self-aggrandizement."

• *Self-view:* The narcissistic personalities view themselves as special and unique—almost as princes or princesses. They believe that they have a special status that places them above ordinary people. They consider themselves superior and entitled to special favors and favorable treatment; they are above the rules that govern other people.

- *View of others:* Although they may regard other people as inferior, they do not do this in the same sense as do the antisocial personalities. They simply see themselves as prestigious and as elevated above the average person; they see others as their vassals and potential admirers. They seek recognition from others primarily to document their own grandiosity and preserve their superior status. They tend to use others as a mirror, without sensitivity to the needs, feelings, or values of others.

- *Beliefs:* The *core* narcissistic beliefs are "Since I am special, I deserve special dispensations, privileges, and prerogatives," "I'm superior to others and they should acknowledge this," and "I'm above the rules." Many of these patients have covert beliefs of being unlovable or helpless. These beliefs emerge after a significant failure and form core elements in the patients' depression. The *conditional* beliefs are "If others don't recognize my special status, they should be punished," and "If I am to maintain my superior status, I should expect others' subservience." On the other hand, they have negatively framed beliefs such as "If I'm not on top, I'm a flop." Thus, when they experience a significant defeat, they are prone to a catastrophic drop in self-esteem. The *instrumental* belief is "Strive at all times to demonstrate your superiority."

- *Strategy:* Their main plans revolve around activities that can reinforce their superior status and expand their "personal domain." Thus, they may seek glory, wealth, position, power, and prestige as a way of continuously reinforcing their superior image. They tend to be highly competitive with others who claim an equally high status and will resort to manipulative strategies to gain their ends. Unlike the antisocial personality, they do not have a cynical view of the rules that govern human conduct; they simply consider themselves exempt from them. Similarly, they do regard themselves as part of society, but at the very top stratum.

- *Affect:* Their main affect is anger when other people do not accord them the admiration or respect to which they believe they are entitled, or otherwise thwart them in some way. They are prone to becoming depressed, however, if their strategies are foiled and their image becomes tarnished. For example, psychotherapists have treated several "inside traders" on Wall Street who became depressed after their manipulations were discovered and they were publicly disgraced. They believed that by tumbling from their high position, they had lost everything.

Histrionic Personality Disorder

The key word for histrionic personalities is "expressiveness," which embodies the tendency to dramatize or romanticize all situations and to try to impress and captivate others.

• *Self-view:* Because they fear being inadequate and vulnerable to neglect, they manifest a compensatory self-image as glamorous, impressive, and deserving of attention.

• *View of others:* They view others favorably as long as they can elicit their attention, amusement, and affection. They try to form strong alliances with others, but with the proviso that they are at the center of the group and that others play the role of attentive audience. In contrast to narcissistic personalities, they are very much involved in their minute-to-minute interactions with other people, and their self-esteem depends on their receiving continuous expressions of appreciation.

• *Beliefs:* The person with a histrionic disorder often has *core* beliefs such as "I am basically unattractive," or "I need other people to admire me in order to be happy." Among the compensatory beliefs are "I am very lovable, entertaining, and interesting," "I am entitled to admiration," "People are there to admire me and do my bidding," and "They have no right to, deny me my just deserts." The *conditional* beliefs include "If I entertain or impress people I am worthwhile," Unless I captivate people, I am nothing," "If I can't entertain people, they will abandon me," "If people don't respond, they are rotten," and "If I can't captivate people, I am helpless." Histrionic people tend to be global and impressionistic in their thinking, a factor that is reflected in their *instrumental* belief, "I can go by my feelings." If the obsessive–compulsives are guided by rationally or intellectually derived systems, then histrionics are guided primarily by feelings. Histrionics who feel angry may use this as sufficient justification for punishing another person. If they feel affection, they consider it a justification for pouring on affection (even though they may switch over to another type of expression a few minutes later). If they feel sad, this is sufficient rationale for them to cry. They tend to dramatize their ways of communicating their sense of frustration or despair, as in the "histrionic suicide attempt." These general patterns are reflected in imperatives such as "Express your feelings," "Be entertaining," and "Show people that they have hurt you."

• *Strategy:* They use dramatics and demonstrativeness to bind people to them. When they do not succeed, however, they believe they are being treated unfairly, and they try to coerce compliance through theatrical expressions of their pain and anger: crying, assaultive behavior, and impulsive suicidal acts.

• *Affect:* The most prominent positive affect is gaiety, often mixed with mirth and other high spirits when they are successfully engaging other people. They generally experience an undercurrent of anxiety and mild dysphoria, which reflects their fear of rejection. When thwarted, their affect can change rapidly to anger or sadness.

Schizoid Personality Disorder

The key word for schizoid personality disorder is "detached." These persons are the embodiment of the autonomous personality. They are willing to sacrifice intimacy to preserve their detachment and autonomy, and stay on the social periphery, even becoming quite isolated. They view themselves as vulnerable to being controlled, demeaned, or rejected.

- *Self-view:* They see themselves as oddballs who don't fit in socially and as loners. They seek freedom from the pressures of social expectations and prefer to avoid relationships altogether.

- *View of others:* They see other people as intrusive, demanding, and hostile.

- *Beliefs:* Their *core* beliefs consist of notions such as "I'm a misfit," "I need my space," "Relationships are too much trouble," and "I'm happier and better off alone." The *conditional* beliefs are "If I get too close to people, they will tease or impose on me," or "If I don't have anything to offer, there is no point in trying to connect with others." The *instrumental* beliefs are "Say no to their demands," "Slip away as soon as possible," and "Don't get involved."

- *Strategy:* Their main interpersonal strategy is to keep their distance from other people, insofar as this is feasible, and avoid contact when they are around others. They may get together with others for specific reasons, such as vocational activities or maybe sex, but usually avoid intimacy in any form.

- *Affect:* As long as schizoids keep their distance, they may experience a low level of sadness. If they are forced into a close encounter, they may become very anxious. In contrast to histrionic personalities, they are not inclined to show their feelings either verbally or through facial expressions; consequently they appear aloof and convey the impression that they do not have strong feelings.

Depressive Personality Disorder

Although depressive personality is not listed in DSM-5 personality disorders, this pattern of symptoms, beliefs, and behaviors is clinically relevant and helps to crystallize an important variant within the spectrum of both mood and personality disorders. Key words are "gloomy," "bitter," "cynical," "cheerless," and "pessimistic." People suffering from other depressive conditions temporarily manifest a negative view of themselves and the world, but still see human life as potentially valuable and rewarding, if only for other people. For the depressive personality, life itself is persistently viewed as a negative, pointless process.

- *Self-view:* The depressive personality is harshly self-critical much or all of the time. They see themselves as basically defective, and incapable of change.

- *View of others:* Depressive personalities are just as harsh on others as they are on themselves, even if they don't share or disclose this perspective. From their perspective, other people are uncaring, incompetent, punishing, deficient, and inevitably disappointing.

- *Beliefs:* The *core* beliefs are that "I'm incapable of happiness," "I'm pathetic," "I'm worthless," and "People are basically selfish and stupid." The *conditional* beliefs follow notions such as "If I get my hopes up, I'll only be disappointed," and "If something can go wrong, it probably will, and it will be my fault." Their *imperative* or self-instructional beliefs consistently reflect this pessimism as "Don't expect much out of others," "There is no point in trying," and "I should just give up."

- *Threat:* The main threat is a fear of deficiency and associated loss, which they attempt to control through a constant search for flaws, limitations, or other cues for impending devaluation or loss.

- *Strategy:* The main strategy seems to be a cycle of hypervigilance to real and potential failures and shortcomings in themselves, others, and the world in general such that they constantly critique and anticipate negativity, thereby habitually creating the very "letdown" feeling and sense of loss that they fear. They spend considerable time internally reviewing an inventory of wrongs, worrying and setting up avoidance goals in an attempt to deal with their inherent sense of worthlessness. They can vacillate among chronic complaining, giving and seeking negative feedback, or retreating into brooding isolation. When potentially solvable problems arise, their response is passive resignation. They are prone to procrastinate as a function of their avoidance orientation, although they may also cope by throwing themselves into work to avoid even deeper levels of failure.

- *Affect:* Affect is a distinguishing feature, in that these individuals are persistently dejected, cynical, bitter, and cheerless. Any overtly displayed affect is usually anger, most often at a level of irritability and sarcasm, tinged with disgust over perceived failings. They may be chronically angry and prone to latch on to a variety of dissatisfactions as a source of complaint. Their gloom and void of positive emotion is independent of circumstances or events, and they are prone to hopelessness. In the depressive personality's reality, *nothing* is ever good enough. Because positive emotions are so lacking, the relationships of the depressive personality are torn by ambivalence from hollow efforts to connect and guilt over the negative impact they often have on others.

THINKING STYLES

The personality disorders may also be characterized by their cognitive styles, which may be a reflection of the patients' behavioral strategies. These cognitive styles deal with the *manner* in which people process information, as opposed to the specific *content* of the processing. Several of the personality types have such distinctive cognitive styles that it is worthwhile to describe them.

People with histrionic personality disorder use the strategy of "display" to attract people and satisfy their own desires for support and closeness. When the strategy of impressing or entertaining people is unsuccessful, they show an open display of "dramatics" (weeping, rage, etc.) to punish the offenders and coerce them to comply. The processing of information shows the same global, impressionist quality. These individuals "miss the trees for the forest." They make stereotyped, broad, global interpretations of a situation at the expense of crucial details. They are likely to respond to their gestalt of the situation, based on inadequate information. People with histrionic disorder are also prone to attach a pattern to a situation even though it does not fit. For example, if other people seem unresponsive to their entertaining, they judge the situation in its entirety—"They are rejecting me"—rather than seeing the specifics that might account for other people's behavior. Thus, they are oblivious to the fact that the other people may be fatigued, bored, or preoccupied with other things. This impressionistic quality is also evident in the way they put a gloss on every experience: Events are romanticized into high drama or grand tragedy. Finally, because they are more attuned to the subjective rather than the objective measuring of events, they tend to use their feelings as the ultimate guide as to their interpretation. Thus, if they feel bad in an encounter with another person, this means the other person is bad. If they feel euphoric, the other person is wonderful.

People with obsessive–compulsive personality, in marked contrast to histrionics, "miss the forest for the trees." These persons focus so much on details that they miss the overall pattern; for example, a person with this disorder may decide on the basis of a few flaws in another person's performance that the other person has failed, even though the flaws may have simply represented some variations in an overall successful performance. Furthermore, in contrast to histrionics, people with obsessive–compulsive personality disorder tend to minimize subjective experiences. Thus, they deprive themselves of some of the richness of life and of access to feelings as a source of information that enhances the significance of important events.

The thinking style of people with avoidant personality disorder differs from that of the aforementioned individuals. Just as they tend to avoid situations that will make them feel bad, they also employ a mechanism of "internal avoidance." As soon as they start to have an unpleasant feeling, they try to damp it down by diverting their attention to something else or by taking a quick fix, such as having a drink. They also avoid thoughts that might produce unpleasant feelings.

The cognitive styles of the other personality disorders are not as sharply delineated as those of the disorders just described.

SUMMARY OF CHARACTERISTICS

Table 2.2 lists the characteristics of 12 personality disorders. The first two columns list the core view of the self and view of others, the next column gives the conditional and instrumental beliefs, and the last two columns list the specific strategies that are overdeveloped or hypertrophied and underdeveloped or absent. It can be seen from this table how the self-view, the view of others, and the beliefs mediate expression and predominance of the specific strategy. Although the strategy, or behavior, provides the basis for making the diagnosis of personality disorder, it is important for a full understanding of the nature of the disorder to clarify the self-concept, concept of others, and beliefs. These cognitive components are involved in information processing and, when activated, trigger the relevant strategy. In tying this back to our evolutionary model, the cognitive components can be thought of as the mechanisms by which individuals orient themselves toward resources (personal and social), and organize coordinated responses, based on prior learning history, that are intended to satisfy urges or cravings, and achieve primary goals in a way that is culturally adaptive.

An avoidant person, Jill, for example, *viewed herself* as socially inept and was vulnerable, therefore, to depreciation and rejection. Her view *of others* as critical and demeaning complemented this sense of vulnerability. Her *belief* that rejection was terrible added enormous valence to her sensitivity and tended to blow up the significance of any anticipated rejection or actual rejection. In fact, this particular belief tended to screen out positive feedback. Her anticipation of rejection made her feel chronically anxious around people, and her magnification of any signs of nonacceptance made her feel bad.

Two other beliefs contributed to her hanging back from involvements: namely, that (1) if she got close to people, they would recognize her as inferior and inadequate; and (2) she could not tolerate unpleasant feelings, which led her to try to avoid their arousal. Hence, as a result of the pressure of her various beliefs and attitudes, she was propelled toward the only strategy that would accommodate her serious concerns—namely, to avoid any situations in which she could be evaluated, and achieve her primary goal of protecting against devaluation by others. In addition, because of her low tolerance for unpleasant feelings or thoughts, she chronically turned off any thoughts that could evoke unpleasant feelings. In therapy she had difficulty in making decisions, identifying negative automatic thoughts, or examining her basic beliefs because these would lead to such feelings. In her anxious and depressed state, she was even more convinced of her core beliefs that she was socially inept, that others were critical, and that rejection was only a heartbeat away.

For case conceptualization, Figure 2.2 illustrates the basic flow of views of self, others, and thinking style as they lead to behavioral strategies. A similar individualized flowchart can be constructed in the clinical setting. The chart should incorporate the distinctive beliefs and the resultant behavior patterns. The person with dependent personality disorder, for example, differs from one with avoidant personality in that the former tends to idolize other potentially nurturing persons and believes that they will help and support him or her. Thus, he or she is drawn to people. Passive–aggressive individuals want approval but cannot tolerate any semblance of control, so they tend to thwart others' expectations of them, and thus defeat themselves.

Persons with obsessive–compulsive disorder idealize order and systems and are driven to control others (as well as themselves). The individual with paranoid disorder is extremely vigilant of other people because of a basic mistrust and suspiciousness and is inclined to accuse them (either overtly or mentally) of discrimination or exploitation. The antisocial personality asserts that he or she is entitled to manipulate or abuse others because of a belief that he or she has been wronged, or that others are wimps, or that we live in a "dog-eat-dog" society. Narcissists see themselves as above

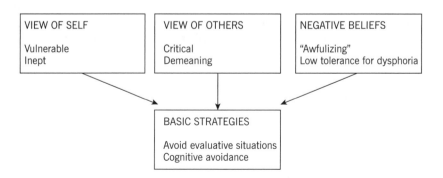

FIGURE 2.2. Relationship of views and beliefs to basic strategies.

ordinary mortals and seek glory through any methods that can safely be used. Individuals with histrionic disorder try to draw others to them by being entertaining but also through temper tantrums and dramatics to coerce closeness when their charm is ineffective. The person with schizoid disorder, with the belief that relationships are unrewarding, keeps his or her distance from other people.

CONCLUSION

Our cognitive model posits that personality is organized to fulfill the evolved mandates for survival and reproduction. Specific suborganizations of personality labeled "modes" are formed to implement these imperatives in a response to the opportunities, challenges, and obstacles in the environment, inclusive of culture. The modes are composed of strategies, beliefs, and motivation, and operate in proactive and reactive ways. Schemas are cognitive structures within the modes that contain beliefs, attitudes, and expectancies that mediate the selection of strategies. The evolved needs implemented by modes are experienced as cravings, urges, and drives. Individuals use personal and interpersonal resources to achieve the goal of satisfying or alleviating these urges and cravings, as directed by their belief system within the activated mode. Overactive modes and exaggerated beliefs lead to inappropriate, dysfunctional strategies. There is a continuum between adaptive and maladaptive for specific modes such that disorder occurs when normal strategies become exaggerated and inflexible. "Personality disorders" are labeled as such when certain modes become hypertrophied and inflexibly activated, causing problems in adaptation. Modes relevant to psychopathology can be labeled according to their diagnostic classification of personality disorders and their typical goals, beliefs, and strategies. The understanding of the typical beliefs, strategies, and modes of each personality disorder provides a road map for therapists. They should keep in mind, however, that most individuals with a specific personality disorder will manifest attitudes and behaviors that overlap other disorders. Consequently, it is important for therapists to expose these variations to make a complete evaluation.

ACKNOWLEDGMENTS

Thanks to several people who assisted in the preparation of this chapter by having typed and/or read my material to me. These include Kelly Devinney, Barbara Marinelli, and Susan Blassingham. I also appreciate the comments of Robert Leahy.

CHAPTER 3

Assessment of Personality Pathology

Jay C. Fournier

As is true in every other field of medicine, proper assessment of personality pathology is critical for accurate diagnoses and effective treatment. The last two decades have witnessed vigorous debate in the research literature regarding how best to conceptualize and assess for the presence of personality disorder. With the proliferation of multiple, often competing, systems, it may be difficult for clinicians to know which methods will be most useful in their practices. At the same time, the variety of tools currently available offers a rich set of resources with which clinicians can identify treatment targets and address core areas of distress and dysfunction in their patients' lives. In this chapter we describe the official diagnostic criteria for personality disorder and discuss some of the alternatives. We describe several different kinds of assessment tools that are currently available, and we close by discussing assessment instruments that may be particularly helpful for clinicians using the cognitive model of personality pathology for case conceptualization and treatment planning.

OFFICIAL DEFINITIONS

Diagnostic and Statistical Manual of Mental Disorders

Personality disorder has appeared in the official list of psychiatric illnesses since the first edition of the *Diagnostic and Statistical Manual of Mental Disorders* (DSM; American Psychiatric Association, 1952). Originally, personality disorders were not distinguished from other forms of mental illness, but beginning in 1980 with the third edition of the manual, a new multiaxial format was introduced to improve diagnostic accuracy. Personality disorders were separated and placed on the second axis of the new system. This was done to ease the burden on researchers and clinicians by allowing them to simultaneously diagnose clinical disorders and personality disorders when both were clearly present (American Psychiatric Association, 1980; Widiger, 2003). In response to several converging lines of research (see First et al., 2002; Krueger, 2005), the current edition of the system, DSM-5, has again removed the distinction between clinical and personality disorders (American Psychiatric Association, 2013). Although numerous criticisms of the DSM-IV system were published during the lead-up to the most recent revision (e.g., Costa, Patriciu, & McCrae, 2005; First et al., 2002; Livesley & Jang, 2000; Widiger & Clark, 2000), those responsible for DSM-5 decided to retain, with little modification, the diagnostic standards described in the previous edition. To this they added a separate, dimensional framework for understanding personality pathology to DSM-5: Section III "Emerging Measures and Models."

To assign a personality disorder diagnosis, the definition of personality disorder in DSM-5 requires that an individual display a pattern of behaviors and internal states (e.g., thoughts, feelings, motivations) that began relatively early in life (either during the teenage or young adult years), that remains consistent over time, is rigid across multiple settings, and causes notable problems for the individual, either with regard to his or her emotional state or functioning (American Psychiatric Association, 2013). Importantly, this pattern must fall outside the bounds of what is considered normative in the individual's culture. In addition, the individual must show this pattern in at least two of four possible areas, including interpretations of experience, feelings, relationship functioning, and management of impulses. As with all mental disorders, the pattern of symptoms cannot be better accounted for by another disorder.

DSM-5 recognizes 10 official personality disorder diagnoses, grouped into three clusters. Cluster A, the "odd or eccentric" cluster, includes paranoid, schizoid, and schizotypal personality disorders. Cluster B consists of antisocial, borderline, narcissistic, and histrionic personality disorders and is described as the "dramatic, emotional, or erratic" cluster. Cluster C is described as the "anxious or fearful" cluster and includes avoidant, dependent, and obsessive–compulsive personality disorders (American Psychiatric Association, 2013, p. 646). In DSM-5, the previous diagnostic category, "personality disorder not otherwise specified," has been replaced by two diagnostic entities: "other specified personality disorder" and "unspecified personality disorder." Both categories are designed to capture those individuals who meet the general criteria for personality disorder but who do not meet the technical criteria for any specific diagnosis. The primary difference between them is that the first is used when clinicians intend to provide additional information about why the patient did not meet criteria for any one category, for example, by adding the specifier "mixed personality features." The second is used when no such information is provided.

International Classification of Diseases, 10th Edition

The 10th edition of the *International Classification of Diseases* (ICD-10) is an alternative diagnostic system to the DSM. It was developed by the World Health Organization and captures diagnoses from across the fields of medicine (World Health Organization, 1992). ICD-10 is used in a variety of settings, including health care management systems and epidemiological studies of illness across countries. Although the definitions and diagnoses of personality disorder are not perfectly aligned between the DSM-5 and ICD-10 systems, there are several points of overlap. In fact, one of the appendices in DSM-5 provides the corresponding ICD-10 coding information for 9 of the 10 officially recognized personality disorders in DSM-5.

Like the official definition in DSM-5, ICD-10 conceptualizes personality disorder categorically, and the system acknowledges that the disorders are neither mutually exclusive nor entirely distinct. ICD-10 defines personality disorders as a "severe disturbance in the characterological constitution and behavioral tendencies of the individual, usually involving several areas of the personality, and nearly always associated with considerable personal and social disruption" (World Health Organization, 1992, p. 157). To meet general criteria for personality disorder in the ICD system, the individual must display "markedly disharmonious attitudes and behavior" (World Health Organization, 1992, p. 157), which typically occur in multiple areas of function. Like DSM, the pattern must be stable, pervasive, and long standing and cannot occur only within the confines of another mental illness. The pattern must have its onset in childhood or adolescence, and it must lead to distress.

The ICD-10 recognizes eight official personality disorder categories, but does not cluster them in the way that DSM does. Table 3.1 lists these disorders and their counterparts in the DSM-5 system. Two disorders, narcissistic and schizotypal personality disorders, appear in DSM-5 but not in ICD-10. Schizotypal pathology was recognized as a personality disorder in previous ICD editions, but has since been moved to the section describing "schizophrenia, schizotypal, and delusional disorders." Narcissistic personality disorder can only be diagnosed in the ICD-10 system as an "other specific personality disorder."

In addition to the eight recognized disorders of personality, ICD-10 also describes disorders characterized by enduring personality changes. These diagnoses require that the individual did not have a personality disorder prior to the change, and that the clinician can identify that the change occurred as a consequence of a "profound, existentially extreme experience" (World Health Organization, 1992, p. 163). Diagnoses of enduring

TABLE 3.1. Comparison of DSM-5 and ICD-10 Personality Disorder Categories

DSM-5	ICD-10
Paranoid	Paranoid
Schizoid	Schizoid
Schizotypal	—
Antisocial	Dissocial
Borderline	Emotionally unstable: borderline type
—	Emotionally unstable: impulsive type
Narcissistic	—
Histrionic	Histrionic
Obsessive–compulsive	Anakastic
Avoidant	Anxious
Dependent	Dependent

personality change are categorized by their causes. ICD-10 describes two specific causes, catastrophic experience and severe psychiatric illness, but also allows for diagnoses following other kinds of extreme experiences.

CONCEPTUAL ISSUES

Although there is little disagreement that personality can be disordered and that such pathology can profoundly impact several areas of functioning, the best way to conceptualize and capture personality dysfunction continues to be hotly debated in the research literature. In this section we briefly describe some of the challenges to the official systems and discuss other important issues that clinicians should keep in mind when assessing personality.

Categories versus Dimensions

A core unresolved issue regarding the proper assessment of personality disorders is whether they are best conceptualized as discrete categories of illness or whether personality is inherently continuous, such that individuals with and without personality disorder differ on a given trait only by a matter of degree. By setting categorical diagnostic thresholds, the official systems make strong claims that there are clear divisions, not only among disorders but also between normal and abnormal personality functioning (Clark, 1992; Livesley, 1998). The presence of a high degree of comorbidity among the personality disorder categories is frequently used to suggest that the current systems have failed to carve out distinct diagnostic entities (Bornstein, 1998; Livesley, 1998; Watson & Clark, 2006). Proponents of alternative models suggest that the high rates of comorbidity may be caused by shared, underlying dimensional traits (e.g., Clark, 2005c; Widiger & Samuel, 2005a).

An additional challenge to the validity of the current disorder categories focuses on the heterogeneity that exists among individuals with the same personality disorder diagnoses (Clark, 1992; Livesley, 1998; Saulsman & Page, 2004; Watson & Clark, 2006). Because no one criterion is either necessary or sufficient under the current system, there are multiple ways in which a patient could meet criteria for any given disorder. For example, criteria for borderline personality disorder and narcissistic personality disorder can each be met in 126 different ways. For antisocial and obsessive–compulsive personality disorders, it is possible for different patients to qualify for a diagnosis without sharing a single symptom in common. Such heterogeneity has likely made it difficult to identify the genetic and neurobiological underpinnings of the personality disorder categories (see Widiger, Simonsen, Krueger, Livesley, & Verheul, 2005, for a review).

Ultimately, the question of whether personality pathology is truly categorical or dimensional is an empirical one. Widiger and Costa (1994), for example, review research suggesting that individuals on either side of DSM's diagnostic thresholds experience similar levels of distress. Furthermore, measures of normal-range personality traits (e.g., the Five-Factor Model [FFM], reviewed below) account for a significant proportion of the variance in personality pathology (Clark, Vorhies, & McEwen, 2002). Although results like these are consistent with the conclusion that personality may be dimensional, evidence in support of the current system has also emerged. For example, correlations tend to be stronger among criteria within diagnostic categories than across categories (Grilo et al., 2001). Furthermore, new statistical techniques have been developed that try to empirically determine whether individuals with a given pathology differ in kind or merely in degree from those without the pathology (Ruscio & Ruscio, 2004). Although the evidence is mixed (Edens, Marcus, Lilienfeld, & Poythress, 2006; Harris, Rice, & Quinsey, 1994), at least some personality disorders seem to manifest as categorical entities (Fossati et al., 2005; Lenzenweger & Korfine, 1992).

Hierarchical Structure

Personality disorder no doubt represents a broad array of maladaptive cognitions, emotional response tendencies, behaviors, and motivations. Whether described and assessed as a collection of dimensional traits that lie on a continuum with healthy functioning or discrete, diagnostic cat-egories, one critical question is whether these entities group together in meaningful ways. The DSM system suggests that the 10 official personal-ity disorders can be described by three higher-order personality disorder clusters: A, odd; B, dramatic; and C, anxious. DSM-5 states that research in support of this clustering is inconsistent. While true, it should be noted that two independent groups have found at least moderate support for the three-cluster framework described in DSM (O'Connor & Dyce, 1998; Rodebaugh, Chambless, Renneberg, & Fydrich, 2005).

Several alternative higher-order structures have also been proposed. Perhaps the most well established is the FFM, which addresses dimensions of personality believed to exist on a continuum from healthy to pathological personality functioning (Costa & McCrae, 1992). The five components of this model are neuroticism, which reflects emotional instability and vulner-ability to psychological distress; extraversion, which represents the degree to which one is prone to social interaction, activity, excitement, sensation seeking, and optimism; openness to experience, which is characterized by active imagination, intellectual curiosity, and independence of thought and judgment; agreeableness, which represents altruism, trust, and helpfulness; and finally, conscientiousness, which reflects reliability, achievement striv-ing, and determination (Costa & McCrae, 1992). In addition to the five higher-order factors proposed by the original FFM, the model describes 30 lower-order trait facets thought to underlie the factors, with 6 trait facets for each factor. Several attempts have been made to translate the person-ality disorders recognized in DSM to patterns of elevations on the FFM's factors and facets (e.g., Morey, Gunderson, Quigley, & Lyons, 2000; Saulsman & Page, 2004), with mixed results. The relationships appear to be particularly strong for some disorders, such as schizoid and avoidant personality disorders, and less strong for others, such as narcissistic and obsessive–compulsive personality disorders (Bagby, Costa, Widiger, Ryder, & Marshall, 2005; Trull, Widiger, & Burr, 2001)

An alternative hierarchical organizing framework for understanding psychopathology turns the typical distinction between personality disor-ders and clinical psychiatric disorders on its head. This view suggests that clinical disorders (previously diagnosed on Axis I) can themselves be bet-ter understood by examining the broad domains of temperament that may underlie them (Widiger & Smith, 2008). Kendler, Prescott, Myers, and Neale (2003) observed that when examining the genetic contributions to psychopathology, psychiatric disorders largely divide into two broad cat-egories: internalizing disorders (e.g., anxiety and depression) and external-izing disorders (e.g., substance use disorders, conduct disorder, antisocial personality disorder). Theorists are beginning to suggest that dimensions of personality pathology may also fit nicely into this two-dimensional sys-tem (Krueger & Tackett, 2003; Widiger & Smith, 2008). For example,

Widiger and Smith (2008) suggest that neuroticism, from the FFM, might match well to the concept of internalization. By contrast, low conscientiousness might fit well into the concept of externalization. As Widiger and Smith note, the broad dimensions of internalization and externalization may be independent from one another, such that individuals may have high or low scores on one dimension, both dimensions, or neither dimension. The degree to which the 10 official personality disorders fit into such a system remains an open question. Some disorders, for example, antisocial and histrionic personality disorders, may turn out to be well characterized by externalization, whereas others, for example, avoidant and dependent personality disorders, may be better characterized by internalization. Some disorders, for example, borderline personality disorder, may involve high levels of both internalization and externalization, and some, for example, schizoid personality disorder, may be associated with low levels of each dimension. Certainly, more research will be needed to test hypotheses like these.

Stability and Change

Stability over time is frequently taken to be a core, defining feature of personality and personality pathology. Indeed, both of the official definitions of personality disorder from DSM-5 and ICD-10 include a requirement that the pattern of internal and external experiences associated with personality disorder be relatively stable over time and across situations. Despite the long-standing view that personality pathology represents an enduring pattern of dysfunction, more recent work has demonstrated that there can be substantial change over time in the symptoms of personality disorder. In a long-term study of personality disorders across 12–18 years, Nestadt and colleagues (2010) observed differences in stability among the 10 personality disorders represented in DSM. Specifically, antisocial, avoidant, borderline, histrionic, and schizotypal personality disorders demonstrated fair-to-moderate stability, and the remainder of the disorders demonstrated poor stability. Skodol (2008) reviewed four methodologically rigorous, large-scale, prospective studies of stability and change in personality pathology and concluded that "personality psychopathology improves over time at unexpectedly significant rates" (p. 501). Despite improvements in the symptoms of personality pathology, longer-term impairments in functional outcomes typically remain (Skodol et al., 2005). Furthermore, pathological personality dimensions appear to be more stable over time than are categorical diagnoses of personality disorder, perhaps owing to the arbitrary nature of the diagnostic systems' cutoff criteria (Clark, 2005b). Such patterns have led some (see Clark, 2005b) to suggest that personality disorder may be composed of both relatively stable trait-like elements, as well as acute symptoms that may be more amenable to change.

ALTERNATIVE DSM-5 TRAIT-BASED APPROACH

Although the official DSM-5 system explicitly assumes that the 10 recognized disorders are separate clinical entities, it acknowledges that they do not describe homogeneous groups and that no clear boundaries exist among them (American Psychiatric Association, 2013). The architects of DSM-5 further note that diagnoses are often comorbid within and across the three higher-order clusters (American Psychiatric Association, 2013). In part because of these considerations, DSM-5 offers an alternative dimensional conceptualization of personality pathology.

The new framework represents something of a synthesis of the multiple alternative systems that had been proposed in the years leading up to the DSM revision (Krueger, Derringer, Markon, Watson, & Skodol, 2012). Indeed, Widiger and Simonsen (2005) identified 18 plausible alternative dimensional models that could be used to assess personality pathology. The alternative system described in DSM-5 decomposes personality pathology into two core elements: personality functioning and personality traits. In the alternative system, a diagnosis of personality disorder can be given if the individual displays both a deficit in personality function (of at least moderate severity) and at least one pathological personality trait. As with the official criteria sets, these features must begin relatively early in life (either during the teenage or young adult years), must be relatively enduring over time and rigid across multiple settings, must fall outside the bounds of what is considered normative in the individual's culture, must not be better accounted for by another condition, and must cause notable problems for the individual, either with regard to his or her emotional state or functioning (American Psychiatric Association, 2013).

DSM-5 describes two areas of personality functioning that can be impaired in personality disorder: self-functioning and interpersonal functioning. Each of these two areas is further broken into two subelements. Poor self-functioning can be manifested in disturbances in identity or in self-direction. Impaired interpersonal functioning can be observed in impoverished empathy or intimacy. DSM provides a 5-point Level of Personality Functioning Scale on which each of these subcomponents can be rated from "little to no impairment" to "extreme impairment." Regarding the second general criteria for diagnosis in the proposed dimensional model, pathological personality traits, DSM-5 describes 25 personality trait facets that are organized into five higher-order trait dimensions: negative affectivity versus emotional stability, detachment versus extraversion, antagonism versus agreeableness, disinhibition versus conscientiousness, and psychoticism versus lucidity. These five dimensions are believed to be the pathological variants of the five traits described in the FFM of normal range-personality described above (American Psychiatric Association, 2013; Gore & Widiger, 2013).

In DSM-5's alternative model, there are two ways to reach a diagnosis of personality disorder. One can meet criteria for a specific personality disorder. Here, 6 of the original 10 personality disorders are retained: antisocial, avoidant, borderline, narcissistic, obsessive–compulsive, and schizotypal. For each, a collection of impaired personality functioning and pathological personality trait criteria are specified. Alternatively, one can be diagnosed with a "trait-specified" personality disorder. To meet criteria in this manner, the individual must present with at least moderate impairment in two of the four specific personality functioning areas: identity, self-direction, empathy, and intimacy. In addition, one must possess pathologically elevated levels on the higher-order personality dimensions or the lower-order trait facets. The alternative model recognizes that all of the dimensions it describes may exist on a continuum with healthy functioning. It instructs clinicians to use their judgment and/or formal assessment instruments to determine whether an individual's level on a particular trait is elevated compared with what is normative for that individual's age and culture.

ASSESSMENT TOOLS AND STRATEGIES

There are several different kinds of strategies that clinicians can use to evaluate the personality functioning of their patients. No doubt, this process starts during the clinician's first contact with a new patient. Much can be learned about the nature and the causes of a patient's current difficulties from unstructured, clinical interviews. These interviews are also important opportunities for rapport building between patient and therapist, a critical aspect of any therapeutic process, and one that may be particularly important when working with individuals who have personality disorder. Despite the importance of unstructured clinical interviews, several concerns must be considered when using this process as the primary (or only) method to assess and diagnose personality pathology. With unstructured interviews, the clinician has complete discretion to ask whichever questions he or she chooses. As such, the accuracy of the resulting diagnosis will depend in large measure on the clinician's level of familiarity with the diagnostic system, as well as his or her skill in posing questions that probe the appropriate patterns of behavior, emotion, cognition, and motivation. Across mental health disorders, unstructured clinical interviews tend to generate less accurate diagnoses compared with empirically supported, structured diagnostic interviews (Miller, 2001; Steiner, Tebes, Sledge, & Walker, 1995; Zimmerman, 1994). In addition to the difficulty involved in keeping all of the criteria sets in mind, there are several known cognitive biases that can interfere with accurate diagnoses during clinical encounters (see, e.g., Baron, 2000). For example, when making diagnoses, clinicians across the medical field tend to ignore what is known about the base rates of a particular diagnosis in a given population. Other potential sources of bias include the primacy effect, whereby information learned earlier in the interview tends to hold more weight than information learned later, and confirmation bias, whereby after preliminary diagnostic judgments are reached, clinicians tend to seek information that supports (as opposed to disconfirms) those initial judgments. Structured clinical interviews and other assessment strategies have been developed to try to mitigate these factors and lead to more accurate diagnoses.

Structured Interviews

Several structured clinical interviews have been developed to assess for the presence of personality disorder. Most of these tools focus on determining whether the categorical diagnostic criteria have been met for the disorders defined in DSM or ICD. Widely used examples include the Structured Clinical Interview for DSM-IV Axis II Personality Disorders (SCID-II; First, Gibbon, Spitzer, Williams, & Benjamin, 1997), the Structured Interview for DSM-IV Personality (SID-P: Pfohl, Blum, & Zimmerman, 1997), and the International Personality Disorder Examination (IPDE; Loranger, Sartorius, et al., 1994). These tools differ in their properties and format. For example, the SCID-II is typically administered as both a self-report tool and a structured interview. The self-report questionnaire is used to streamline the interview, such that the clinician can focus the interview on those criteria initially endorsed by the patient. By contrast, the SID-P does not use a self-report prescreener. Unlike the SCID-II, which organizes items by diagnosis, the SID-P interview is organized to flow more naturally from one domain of functioning to another. Unlike the other measures, the IPDE was designed to produce both categorical and dimensional personality disorder scores, although it is possible to derive dimensional scores from the other measures as well (see, e.g., Levenson, Wallace, Fournier, Rucci, & Frank, 2012).

The interrater reliability of assessments made using structured interviews is generally good. Agreement tends to be quite strong for the presence versus absence of any personality disorder (Tyrer et al., 2007), and agreement is also high for dimensional ratings of personality pathology (Maffei et al., 1997). Interrater reliability estimates can be high for most disorder diagnoses when the same structured interview is used (Farmer & Chapman, 2002), but agreement among different structured interviews tends to be rather poor (Clark, Livesley, & Morey, 1997).

Finally, the three instruments reviewed above differ from one another regarding the average length of administration, an important practical consideration for their use in clinical practice. Van Velzen and Emmelkamp (1996) reported that the SCID-II interview averages between 30 and 40 minutes, the SID-P 60 and 90 minutes, and the IPDE over 120 minutes to administer. Recognizing the need for shorter personality disorder screening instruments, Moran and colleagues (2003) examined the utility of the Standardized Assessment of Personality—Abbreviated Scale (SAPAS), an eight-item clinical interview, as a potential screening tool for the presence versus absence of personality disorder. The interview takes less than 2 minutes to administer, each item is rated as either present or absent, and a simple scoring algorithm generates screening scores ranging from 0 to 8. The authors reported that the measure has adequate internal consistency and test–retest reliability. Furthermore, using a cutoff score of 3 or above, they were accurately able to classify 90% of patients as personality disordered or not, when comparing the ratings against those made using the SCID-II. Subsequent work has generally supported the psychometric properties of the tool for use as a screening instrument, however, the percentage of correctly identified patients has tended not to be as high as was observed in the original report (Bukh, Bock, Vinberg, Gether, & Kessing, 2010; Hesse & Moran, 2010). There is no doubt that the longer clinical interviews provide more refined information about the nature of an individual's personality functioning, but in situations where such an assessment is not possible, the SAPAS may be an effective screening tool.

Self-Report Measures

Numerous self-report measures exist that assess for the presence of personality disorder. Unlike interview measures, most self-report devices were designed at the outset to result in dimensional ratings of personality pathology, although the conversion to categorical personality disorder diagnoses is typically possible.

Five-Factor Model

For the past several decades, the facets and factors of the FFM have typically been assessed using the Neuroticism, Extroversion, Openness to Experience Personality Inventory—Revised (NEO-PI-R; Costa & McCrae, 1992). A newer version of the measure, the NEO-PI-3 (Costa & McCrae, 2010), is also available to researchers and clinicians. In addition, there is a shorter version, the NEO Five Factor Inventory, which allows for the assessment of the higher-order factors without assessing the lower-order facets. The NEO measures have been extensively validated in multiple samples, and the psychometric properties of the instruments are strong (Costa & McCrae, 1992, 2010). Scores on the traits are believed to vary by degree between disordered and nondisordered individuals, and extreme scores in either direction could be used to indicate the presence of personality pathology (Widiger, Costa, & McCrae, 2002).

Dimensional Measures of Personality Pathology

The Schedule of Nonadaptive and Adaptive Personality (SNAP; Clark, 2005a) and the Dimensional Assessment of Pathological Personality (DAPP; Livesley, 1990) are two-dimensional personality pathology assessment devices that have garnered considerable research support (First et al., 2002; Widiger & Simonsen, 2005). Both measures were developed through a series of factor analytic studies, and both assess dimensions of pathological personality. The SNAP assesses 12 personality factors: mistrust, manipulativeness, aggression, self-harm, eccentric perceptions, dependency, exhibitionism, entitlement, detachment, impulsivity, propriety, and workaholism. To these, three temperament scales have been added: negative temperament, positive temperament, and disinhibition/constraint. By contrast, the DAPP is composed of the following 18 factors: compulsivity, conduct problems, diffidence, identity problems, insecure attachment, intimacy problems, narcissism, suspiciousness, affective lability, passive oppositionality, perceptual cognitive distortion, rejection, self-harming behaviors, restricted expression, social avoidance, stimulus seeking, interpersonal disesteem, and anxiousness. The SNAP the DAPP were constructed independently and contain no items in common. Still, the developers were able to match each scale on one inventory with a set of scales on the other (Clark & Livesley, 2002). Joint analyses of these instruments revealed that the two measures generally assess the same personality traits, with 92% of the hypothesized relations showing statistically significant correlations. Finally, the SNAP includes scales that assess the personality disorders recognized in DSM, and efforts have been made to translate patterns of elevation on the DAPP scales to represent DSM-defined disorders (Pukrop et al., 2009).

Personality Inventory for DSM-5

During the development of the alternative dimensional model of personality pathology that now appears in DSM-5, members of the DSM work group and their colleagues developed the Personality Inventory for DSM-5 (PID-5), a 220-item self-report instrument, to measure the higher- and lower-order dimensions and traits included in the model. The instrument has since been used by multiple research groups to examine its psychometric properties (see Bagby, 2013). The internal consistencies of the traits measured by the instrument are high (Quilty, Ayearst, Chmielewski, Pollock, & Bagby, 2013), and the instrument appears to measure well the five higher-order dimensions proposed in the alternative DSM-5 model (Quilty et al., 2013; Wright et al., 2012). The measure also appears to capture other higher-order configurations such as the two-factor internalizing and externalizing framework (Morey, Krueger, & Skodol, 2013; Wright et al., 2012). Methods have been described to utilize the dimensional trait ratings from the

PID-5 to diagnose the six personality disorder types described in the alternative system (Samuel, Hopwood, Krueger, Thomas, & Ruggero, 2013).

Informant Ratings

In addition to asking patients to report on their own cognitive, emotional, behavioral, and motivational experiences when assessing personality pathology, clinicians should consider gathering information from knowledgeable informants. Self-report instruments, whether interview or questionnaire based, depend on patients' ability and willingness to accurately reflect and report on their experiences. In the case of personality disorder, patients may not have an accurate understanding of key elements of their pathology, for example, the ways in which their behaviors affect others. Furthermore, given the potential for long-standing difficulties in the context of personality pathology, some patients may not realize that elements of their functioning are noteworthy or non-normative. As several researchers have pointed out (see Ready, Watson, & Clark, 2002), patients and informants tend to have access to different types of information. Whereas patients have unique access to their own internal states, informants may be better positioned to objectively report on the patient's behaviors and the consequences of those behaviors. It is perhaps not surprising, then, that patient- and informant-rated measures of personality functioning tend to be only minimally to moderately correlated (Oltmanns & Turkheimer, 2009; Ready et al., 2002; Zimmerman, Pfohl, Coryell, Stangl, & Corenthal, 1988). Because these two sources do not perfectly overlap, they each may contain useful and complementary information. Ready and colleagues (2002), for example, found that self and informant reports were each incrementally helpful in predicting patient behavior. Oltmanns and Turkheimer (2009) further point out that informant information may be particularly useful for predicting certain kinds of outcomes, such as the likelihood of experiencing future interpersonal problems. Some assessment tools can be used relatively easily to gather information from informants. The SID-P, for example, includes instructions for interviewing informants and notes which questions from the interview should be asked. Separate informant versions of other instruments, such as the PID-5 (Markon, Quilty, Bagby, & Krueger, 2013), have also been created.

COGNITIVE SYSTEMS

Personality Belief Questionnaire

In the first edition of this text, Beck, Freeman, and associates (1990) drafted a list of 14 beliefs hypothesized to underlie each of nine personality disorders: avoidant, dependent, obsessive–compulsive, histrionic, passive–aggressive, narcissistic, paranoid, schizoid, and antisocial personality disorder. Using this list, Beck and Beck (1991) developed the Personality Belief Questionnaire (PBQ), a 126-item self-report instrument, to assess these dysfunctional beliefs. Beck and colleagues did not specify beliefs associated with schizotypal or borderline personality disorders. They argued that patients with borderline personality disorder have several dysfunctional beliefs from many of the other categories, and individuals with schizotypal personality disorder suffer from dysfunction in the process of thinking as opposed to pathology in thought content.

Beck and colleagues (2001) demonstrated in a large sample of psychiatric outpatients that five of the original PBQ subscales (Avoidant, Dependent, Paranoid, Narcissistic, and Obsessive–Compulsive) showed adequate internal consistency and test–retest reliability, and they differentiated patients diagnosed with the relevant personality disorders from patients diagnosed with other personality disorders. Although their results were largely in the predicted direction, not all comparisons were significant. Narcissistic personality disorder, for example, was difficult to distinguish from obsessive–compulsive and paranoid personality disorders (Beck et al., 2001). In subsequent studies, the validity of several of the remaining PBQ scales has been examined (see Bhar, Beck, & Butler, 2012, for a comprehensive review). Jones, Burrell-Hodgson, and Tate (2007), for example, demonstrated that the presence of schizoid and passive–aggressive personality disorders were each predicted by scores on the associated PBQ subscales, and McMurran and Christopher (2008) found partial support for the validity of the Antisocial subscale. When compared with healthy controls, individuals diagnosed with antisocial personality disorder displayed elevated antisocial beliefs on the PBQ. But, individuals with antisocial personality disorder did not receive their highest scores on the Antisocial subscale. Rather, the Avoidant and Paranoid scales appeared to do a better job of indentifying individuals with antisocial personality disorder.

Since the first publication of the instrument, several efforts have been made to develop a Personality Belief scale for borderline personality disorder. Beck and Beck (1995a) developed a 19-item Borderline Personality Belief scale. Of these 19 items, 14 came from the other subscales of the full PBQ measure and five were new. Butler, Brown, Beck, and Grisham (2002) observed that patients diagnosed with borderline personality disorder endorsed that collection of 14 beliefs more than any other PBQ subscale. Arntz, Dietzel, and Dressen (1999) have demonstrated that a similar borderline personality disorder belief questionnaire could discriminate patients with borderline personality disorder from nonpatients and from patients diagnosed with Cluster C disorders.

Trull and colleagues (1993) conducted an independent investigation of the PBQ in a sample of healthy college students, and found that the internal consistency of the nine scales was acceptable. The authors then compared the PBQ with two other self-report personality disorder symptom measures and found that the correlation between the two personality disorder symptom measures was higher than that between either measure and the PBQ. In addition, they jointly factor analyzed the assessment instruments and, broadly speaking, found that the PBQ scale scores were weakly associated with corresponding scales on the two comparison measures. The fact that the PBQ is not strongly associated with other measures of personality dysfunction, particularly in a nonclinical sample, may not be surprising. The PBQ was designed specifically to examine the cognitive components of personality dysfunction, in part, because the other measures that were in existence did not adequately address cognitions.

Beck and Beck (1995b) developed a 65-item short-form version of the PBQ (PBQ-SF; see Appendix 3.1). As is true of the full measure, internal consistency and test–retest reliability are acceptable for many of the scales on the PBQ-SF (Butler, Beck, & Cohen, 2007). An added feature of the PBQ-SF is that unlike the original PBQ, items are presented in a random order. Fournier, DeRubeis, and Beck (2011) examined the factor structure of the PBQ-SF in a sample of 438 depressed outpatients, and they confirmed the resulting structure in a separate sample of 683 individuals seeking treatment for various psychiatric conditions. Fournier and colleagues observed that the PBQ items could be described by seven factors: avoidant/dependent, narcissistic/antisocial, obsessive–compulsive, paranoid, histrionic, schizoid, and autonomy. Whereas the first six factors were associated with personality disorders recognized in DSM, the seventh contained several beliefs reflecting self-reliance and the negative consequences of allowing oneself to be dominated by others. The authors suggested that this factor was consistent with the cognitive-personality construct autonomy (Beck, 1983), which represents placing a high degree of value on (1) individualistic achievement, (2) freedom from the control of others, and (3) maintaining a strong self-concept.

In addition to identifying and confirming the seven-factor structure in separate samples, Fournier and colleagues (2011) examined the validity of the PBQ-SF. They observed that for each of the seven PBQ factors, patients with personality disorders scored higher than did patients without personality disorders. Furthermore, they observed that for each of the five diagnostic categories for which they had data, patients with the personality disorder in question scored the highest on the factor representing the beliefs associated with that disorder.

A recent study examining the overlap between the PBQ and the alternative dimensional system described in DSM-5 suggests that the belief factors identified by Fournier and colleagues (2011) are associated with unique patterns of elevations across the higher-order personality dimensions and the lower-order pathological personality traits proposed in the new model

(Hopwood, Schade, Krueger, Wright, & Markon, 2013). For example, the avoidant/dependent belief factor was associated with particularly high elevations on emotional lability, anxiousness, insecurity, perseveration, withdrawal, anhedonia, depressivity, suspiciousness, and perceptual dysregulation. The authors suggest that their findings "indicate the potential for dysfunctional beliefs to elaborate the DSM-5 trait model" (Hopwood et al., 2013, p. 165).

Given that the PBQ was developed out of the cognitive theory of personality dysfunction, it may be uniquely suited for clinical use by cognitive therapists. As Bhar and colleagues (2012) note, the dysfunctional beliefs identified by the PBQ represent both targets for treatment as well as indicators of a core mechanism of change during therapy. It is expected that as beliefs begin to change, improvements in several areas of functioning will follow. Reflecting these considerations, the PBQ has been used in several treatment studies. There is some evidence that elevated scores on the Avoidant and Paranoid PBQ scales predict relatively poor outcomes for cognitive therapy for depression (Kuyken, Kurzer, DeRubeis, Beck, & Brown, 2001), and two studies have observed that scores on relevant PBQ scales are reduced by successful treatment of obsessive–compulsive (Ng, 2005) and borderline (Brown, Newman, Charlesworth, Crits-Christoph, & Beck, 2004) personality disorders. The primary clinical use of the PBQ-SF is to identify the most strongly endorsed beliefs, rather than to utilize any diagnostic scoring. As such, the items related to each personality are listed in Appendix 3.1, but there is no specific interpretive scoring system at this time (see Fournier et al., 2011, for an example of generating PBQ-SF scores for experimental purposes).

Personality Disorder Belief Questionnaire

Using a combination of clinical experience and the beliefs originally identified by Beck and colleagues (1990), Dreessen and Arntz (1995) developed the Personality Disorder Belief Questionnaire (PDBQ). The PDBQ is composed of 12 subscales, each consisting of 20 beliefs. Using a sample of 643 participants, some of whom were healthy volunteers and some were individuals with clinical and or personality disorder diagnoses, Arntz, Dreessen, Schouten, and Weertman (2004) demonstrated support for the proposed factor structure of the six belief subscales that they tested: Avoidant, Dependent, Obsessive–Compulsive, Paranoid, Histrionic, and Borderline. They also provide support for the validity of the measure. Scores on each of the six scales increased from healthy control individuals to patients with psychiatric diagnoses other than personality disorders to patients with any personality disorder diagnosis to patients diagnosed with the personality disorder most relevant for the scale in question.

Schema Questionnaire

Young and colleagues (Young, 1999; Young, Klosko, & Weishaar, 2003) offer a separate cognitive theory of personality pathology that does not take the disorders recognized in DSM or ICD as the starting point. Rather, Young (1999) developed the theory by describing developmental tasks that children must successfully complete to develop into psychologically healthy adults. He identified five broad domains that match these developmental tasks, and hypothesized that if a child fails to successfully complete a task, he or she will develop a maladaptive schema associated with the domain. In total, Young and colleagues (2003) have identified 18 maladaptive schemas. Young argues that one can respond to one's schemas in three ways: by behaving in a schema-congruent fashion, by attempting to avoid the schema by organizing one's life to minimize its activation, or by overcompensating for the schema. Individuals attempting to avoid their schemas might, for example, be more likely to abuse substances. Those who "overcompensate" might, on the other hand, behave as if the opposite of the schema were true. For example, in Young's conceptualization, patients with narcissistic personality disorder might adopt behaviors suggesting grandiosity and entitlement when their true underlying schema represents deep inferiority and self-doubt.

To assess for the presence and/or strength of these schemas, Young (1990) developed the Schema Questionnaire. The original long-form version of the instrument contained 205 items and assessed 16 schemas. Two factor-analytic examinations found support for 14 (Lee, Taylor, & Dunn, 1999) and 15 (Schmidt, Joiner, Young, & Telch, 1995) of the 16 constructs suggested by the measure. To reduce the burden on patients, Young (1998) developed the 75-item short-form version of the Schema Questionnaire to capture the 15 schemas identified by Schmidt and colleagues (1995). Early factor-analytic studies (e.g., Welburn, Coristine, Dagg, Pontefract, & Jordan, 2002) of the short form generally found support for several elements of its proposed structure (see Oei & Baranoff, 2007, for a critical review and discussion). In 2001, the Schema Questionnaire—Short Form was further revised to reduce response bias and lower the reading level required to complete the instrument. A recent analysis of the resulting measure (Samuel & Ball, 2013) failed to recover the 15 factors it aims to measure, and in fact, failed to identify any coherent lower-order factor structure for the measure. The authors conclude that the schemas identified in the scale may not be empirically separable. Despite difficulties identifying a lower-order structure, the authors subjected the 15 schema dimensions to a higher-order factor analysis. Here, they found support for four broad schema dimensions: interpersonal detachment, interpersonal dependency, perfectionism, and impulsive exploitation. No doubt more work is needed to further evaluate the construct validity of the Schema Questionnaire and its variants. These considerations aside, the measure has been used in clinical studies examining risk for bipolar disorder (Hawke, Provencher, & Arntz, 2011), change in schemas as a result of treatment for depression (Wegener, Alfter, Geiser, Liedtke, & Conrad, 2013), and prediction of response to exposure and response prevention treatment of obsessive–compulsive disorder (Haaland et al., 2011).

CONCLUSION

Clinicians have many choices to consider when deciding how best to think about and evaluate the presence of personality disorder in their patients. Perhaps the best approach is one that integrates a clinical interview, informant ratings, and a self-report questionnaire. Not only would multiple sources of information be more likely to fully describe the individual's pathology, but combining these approaches may also help to engage the client in the process of collaboratively generating a conceptualization for his or her unique set of difficulties. Of course, such an approach assumes that ample time and resources are available. When a multimethod approach is not possible, the next best option will depend on the purpose of the assessment, clinical efficiency of the methods relative to cost and time constraints, and level of patient cooperation. Certain circumstances and settings may prioritize categorical diagnoses. Categorical information can be helpful in communicating quickly with other clinicians, and it may be required for reimbursement and formal assessment purposes. In such cases, the use of one of the structured diagnostic interviews should be considered to protect against some of the challenges involved in rendering categorical diagnoses on the basis of unstructured clinical interviews alone. In settings in which time for assessments is scarce, clinicians might consider using a quick screening interview like the SAPAS. If a personality disorder appears likely given the patient's score, the clinician could follow up by probing positive responses. In other situations, dimensional approaches may be more appropriate, particularly when the goal is to capture the broad range of functional difficulties the patient is experiencing. Here, self-report instruments may be more useful. The most appropriate self-report measure will depend on which model of personality dysfunction is most appropriate for the task at hand. For cognitive therapists, the PBQ may be the most helpful for identifying the cognitive features of an individual's personality pathology, which could serve as targets for treatment. Regardless of which approach is adopted, clinicians should remember that personality pathology appears to be less stable than previously thought, particularly when it is adequately treated. As such, repeated assessments should be considered to monitor the patient's progress and identify areas for additional work.

Personality Belief Questionnaire—Short Form (PBQ-SF)

Please read the statements below and rate HOW MUCH YOU BELIEVE EACH ONE. Try to judge how you feel about each statement MOST OF THE TIME. Do not leave any statements blank.

4	3	2	1	0
I believe it totally	I believe it very much	I believe it moderately	I believe it slightly	I don't believe it at all

Example   How Much Do You Believe It?

1. The world is a dangerous place.   4   3   2   1   0
   (please circle)

	Totally	Very much	Moderately	Slightly	Not at all
1. Being exposed as inferior or inadequate will be intolerable.	4	3	2	1	0
2. I should avoid unpleasant situations at all costs.	4	3	2	1	0
3. If people act friendly, they may be trying to use or exploit me.	4	3	2	1	0
4. I have to resist the domination of authorities but at the same time maintain their approval and acceptance.	4	3	2	1	0
5. I cannot tolerate unpleasant feelings.	4	3	2	1	0
6. Flaws, defects, or mistakes are intolerable.	4	3	2	1	0
7. Other people are often too demanding.	4	3	2	1	0
8. I should be the center of attention.	4	3	2	1	0
9. If I don't have systems, everything will fall apart.	4	3	2	1	0
10. It's intolerable if I'm not accorded my due respect or don't get what I'm entitled to.	4	3	2	1	0
11. It is important to do a perfect job on everything.	4	3	2	1	0

Copyright 1995 by Aaron T. Beck and Judith S. Beck. Reprinted by permission.

	Totally	Very much	Moderately	Slightly	Not at all
12. I enjoy doing things more by myself than with other people.	4	3	2	1	0
13. Others will try to use me or manipulate me if I don't watch out.	4	3	2	1	0
14. Other people have hidden motives.	4	3	2	1	0
15. The worst possible thing would be to be abandoned.	4	3	2	1	0
16. Other people should recognize how special I am.	4	3	2	1	0
17. Other people will deliberately try to demean me.	4	3	2	1	0
18. I need others to help me make decisions or tell me what to do.	4	3	2	1	0
19. Details are extremely important.	4	3	2	1	0
20. If I regard people as too bossy, I have a right to disregard their demands.	4	3	2	1	0
21. Authority figures tend to be intrusive, demanding, interfering, and controlling.	4	3	2	1	0
22. The way to get what I want is to dazzle or amuse people.	4	3	2	1	0
23. I should do whatever I can get away with.	4	3	2	1	0
24. If other people find out things about me, they will use them against me.	4	3	2	1	0
25. Relationships are messy and interfere with freedom.	4	3	2	1	0
26. Only people as brilliant as I am understand me.	4	3	2	1	0
27. Since I am so superior, I am entitled to special treatment and privileges.	4	3	2	1	0
28. It is important for me to be free and independent of others.	4	3	2	1	0

	How Much Do You Believe It?				
	Totally	Very much	Moderately	Slightly	Not at all
29. In many situations, I am better off to be left alone.	4	3	2	1	0
30. It is necessary to stick to the highest standards at all times, or things will fall apart.	4	3	2	1	0
31. Unpleasant feelings will escalate and get out of control.	4	3	2	1	0
32. We live in a jungle and the strong person is the one who survives.	4	3	2	1	0
33. I should avoid situations in which I attract attention, or be as inconspicuous as possible.	4	3	2	1	0
34. If I don't keep others engaged with me, they won't like me.	4	3	2	1	0
35. If I want something, I should do whatever is necessary to get it.	4	3	2	1	0
36. It's better to be alone than to feel "stuck" with other people.	4	3	2	1	0
37. Unless I entertain or impress people, I am nothing.	4	3	2	1	0
38. People will get at me if I don't get them first.	4	3	2	1	0
39. Any signs of tension in a relationship indicate the relationship has gone bad; therefore, I should cut it off.	4	3	2	1	0
40. If I don't perform at the highest level, I will fail.	4	3	2	1	0
41. Making deadlines, complying with demands, and conforming are direct blows to my pride and self-sufficiency.	4	3	2	1	0
42. I have been unfairly treated and am entitled to get my fair share by whatever means I can.	4	3	2	1	0

	Totally	Very much	Moderately	Slightly	Not at all
43. If people get close to me, they will discover the "real" me and reject me.	4	3	2	1	0
44. I am needy and weak.	4	3	2	1	0
45. I am helpless when I'm left on my own.	4	3	2	1	0
46. Other people should satisfy my needs.	4	3	2	1	0
47. If I follow the rules the way people expect, it will inhibit my freedom of action.	4	3	2	1	0
48. People will take advantage of me if I give them the chance.	4	3	2	1	0
49. I have to be on guard at all times.	4	3	2	1	0
50. My privacy is much more important to me than closeness to people.	4	3	2	1	0
51. Rules are arbitrary and stifle me.	4	3	2	1	0
52. It is awful if people ignore me.	4	3	2	1	0
53. What other people think doesn't matter to me.	4	3	2	1	0
54. In order to be happy, I need other people to pay attention to me.	4	3	2	1	0
55. If I entertain people, they will not notice my weaknesses.	4	3	2	1	0
56. I need somebody around available at all times to help me to carry out what I need to do or in case something bad happens.	4	3	2	1	0
57. Any flaw or defect in performance may lead to a catastrophe.	4	3	2	1	0
58. Since I am so talented, people should go out of their way to promote my career.	4	3	2	1	0
59. If I don't push other people, I will get pushed around.	4	3	2	1	0
60. I don't have to be bound by the rules that apply to other people.	4	3	2	1	0

	How Much Do You Believe It?				
	Totally	Very much	Moderately	Slightly	Not at all
61. Force or cunning is the best way to get things done.	4	3	2	1	0
62. I must maintain access to my supporter or helper at all times.	4	3	2	1	0
63. I am basically alone—unless I can attach myself to a stronger person.	4	3	2	1	0
64. I cannot trust other people.	4	3	2	1	0
65. I can't cope as other people can.	4	3	2	1	0

Item key to personality profiles

Avoidant: 1, 2, 5, 31, 33, 39, 43

Dependent: 15, 18, 44, 45, 56, 62, 63

Passive–Aggressive: 4, 7, 20, 21, 41, 47, 51

Obsessive–Compulsive: 6, 9, 11, 19, 30, 40, 57

Antisocial: 23, 32, 35, 38, 42, 59, 61

Narcissistic: 10, 16, 26, 27, 46, 58, 60

Histrionic: 8, 22, 34, 37, 52, 54, 55

Schizoid: 12, 25, 28, 29, 36, 50, 53

Paranoid: 3, 13, 14, 17, 24, 48, 49

Borderline: 31, 44, 45, 49, 56, 64, 65

Neural Mechanisms of Maladaptive Schemas and Modes in Personality Disorders

Michael T. Treadway

Personality disorders describe a set of enduring patterns of perceiving and relating to oneself and others that are maladaptive, distressing, and functionally impairing. Many features of personality disorders can be viewed as extreme ends of personality traits, thereby reflecting a continuum of functioning rather than discrete categories. Like personality traits, personality disorders are relatively heritable, with heritability estimates ranging from 55 to 75% for most disorders (Kendler, Myers, Torgersen, Neale, & Reichborn-Kjennerud, 2007; Reichborn-Kjennerud et al., 2007; Torgersen et al., 2012). Additionally, personality disorders are developmental in nature, and early signs of their core symptoms are often identifiable at a young age (Weiner & Bardenstein, 2000).

These basic facts suggest that personality disorders may be usefully conceptualized as neurodevelopmental disorders. That is, disorders whose defining symptoms develop slowly through time, and reflect complex interactions between life experiences and neurobiological development. Among the various domains impacted by personality disorders, key processes include reactivity to emotional stimuli (internal or external), reward-seeking behavior, and social interactions. Of particular importance for cognitive approaches to treatment, all of these domains involve cognitions and schemas that are maladaptive when taken to extremes, and play a fundamental role in the self-expansive and self-protective modes (A. Beck, Chapter 2, this volume). A growing number of studies have sought to employ neuroimaging, neurophysiological, and experimental psychopathology techniques to understand the functional neural architecture of these processes. This chapter provides a brief overview of current knowledge regarding the basic neural architecture involved in each of these areas, and how they appear to be affected in personality disorders. It should be noted that to date, most neuroimaging studies in populations with personality disorders have focused on borderline personality disorder, psychopathy and antisocial personality disorder, and schizotypal personality disorder, with almost no studies examining Cluster C disorders.

There are several important caveats to note about neuroimaging approaches to the study of psychiatric disorders. When neuroimaging methods are used to compare groups of individuals with and without personality disorders, the resulting group differences in neural activity could represent any one of the "four Cs," as described by Lewis and colleagues: (1) cause of illness: for example, when an individual experiences sudden changes in personality or mood following a traumatic brain injury, information about changes to brain structure and function would likely be causal; (2) consequence: a change to brain function resulting from behaviors that emanate from personality disorders, such as the deleterious effects of excessive substance use; (3) compensation: individuals with personality disorders recruit different neural mechanisms to meet certain task demands in order to overcome limitations; or (4) confound: group differences in function that reflect the fact the individuals with personality disorders may process task demands differently (Lewis & Gonzalez-Burgos, 2008). Although researchers are often most interested in identifying patterns of activity associated with 1 (cause), the developmental nature of most personality disorders requires substantial longitudinal research to isolate this contribution, much of which has yet to be done.

A second caveat that applies broadly to all clinical or practical application of neuroimaging research is the problem of individual differences (Treadway & Buckholtz, 2011). In the vast majority of neuroimaging studies performed to date, researchers average across groups of different individuals to try and identify the brains that appear commonly engaged by a particular task or process "on average." However, such group-average patterns of neural activity are not necessarily useful as a diagnostic test, as the function and structure of specific individual brains can vary so widely. This is why the implementation of "neuromaging-based" tests for diagnosis or treatment effects remains far in the future (Kapur, Phillips, & Insel, 2012). Therefore, in the summaries of the neuroimaging findings that follow, it is important to remember that these results do not necessarily apply to all individuals.

FUNCTIONAL NEURAL NETWORK ABNORMALITIES
IN PERSONALITY DISORDERS: A SELECTIVE OVERVIEW

Processing Emotional Stimuli and States

One of the central issues in many forms of personality disorders is how individuals respond to emotional stimuli and experiences. It has increasingly been recognized that emotional signals play a crucial role in many of the decisions we make (Damasio, 2005). Feelings of uncertainty or anxiety may further activate beliefs in the self-protective mode that help us to be appropriately cautious in certain situations, or direct our attention to possible threats. A sense of guilt may energize beliefs related to social self-protection that are useful in helping us recognize our hurtful behavior toward someone we care about, and prompt us to take corrective actions. For individuals with personality disorders, however, this type of normative emotional input is often perceived as too painful to be tolerated, and they may go to great lengths to deny, dissociate from, compensate for, self-medicate, or otherwise avoid these feelings and thoughts. The efforts to avoid these experiences can manifest in abuse of substances, food, or sex; running away from relationships or responsibilities; or lashing out at others; and many of the problems that are so common among patients with personality disorders. To date, the field of clinical neuroscience has begun to uncover some of the circuitry that may be partially responsible for this behavior.

A number of studies have identified structures such as the anterior insula and the amygdala as key structures in emotional experiences, among others. The insula is believed to be involved in generating representations of interoceptive states—that is, a general sense of how the body is feeling (Craig, 2002, 2009). The amygdala is often described as an "early responder" to stimuli that helps shape the level of arousal we feel in response to them, thereby prompting us to reorient our attention and prepare to act, if necessary (Phelps & LeDoux, 2005). While initially believed to be primarily responsive to negatively valenced stimuli, more recent work suggests that the amygdala is relatively valence neutral, and that it primarily reacts to the novelty and salience of a stimulus, regardless of whether it is threatening, enticing, or simply new (Blackford, Buckholtz, Avery, & Zald, 2010).

When the amygdala is overly active, however, it may result in a tendency to respond to otherwise neutral or mild stimuli with an intense emotional response, as can often happen in cases of primary anxiety and mood disorders, or as part of personality pathology (Davidson, Pizzagalli, Nitschke, & Putnam, 2002). Supporting this hypothesis, a number of studies have identified elevated amygdala activity in response to emotional stimuli in patients with anxious and depressive symptoms (Beesdo et al.,

2009; Etkin & Schatzberg, 2011; Hamilton et al., 2012; Siegle, Steinhauer, Thase, Stenger, & Carter, 2002). Further work has also identified a similar phenomenon present in individuals who report personality traits associated with anxious or ruminative temperaments, such as trait neuroticism (Cremers et al., 2010; Haas, Omura, Constable, & Canli, 2007). Further emphasizing the trait-like nature of amygdala responses, individuals who were assessed as infants and found to show an anxious attachment style of responding (Kagan, Reznick, & Snidman, 1987) were also found to show elevated amygdala responses during a functional magnetic resonance imaging (fMRI) scanning session performed 18–20 years later (Schwartz, Wright, Shin, Kagan, & Rauch, 2003).

Emotional responses of patients diagnosed with borderline personality disorder also elicit greater responses in both the anterior insula and the amygdala relative to controls (Hazlett et al., 2012; Krause-Utz et al., 2011). Such increased activity may serve as a substrate for affective lability in borderline personality disorder, given the amygdala's role in generating rapid emotional arousal in response to stimuli. In contrast, individuals with psychopathy or antisocial personality disorder—a disorder associated with cold, callous, or unemotional responses to others—has been distinguished by a relative lack of amygdala responses to affective stimuli (Kiehl et al., 2001; Mueller et al., 2003). This pattern has also been detectable in earlier developmental stages of individuals with callous or unemotional traits (Jones, Laurens, Herba, Barker, & Viding, 2009; Marsh et al., 2008).

Taken together, these findings suggest that alterations in core affect-related regions such as the amygdala and insula may be partly responsible for exaggerated responses to affective stimuli observed in these populations. It may be useful for patients to understand that their responses are likely stronger than the average person's, and that this is not necessarily always a bad thing. Heightened emotional sensitivity is a useful for trait for developing deep, sustaining relationships. But it requires that individuals first learn to effectively regulate their strong initial responses. Understanding the biological basis of such reactions can be an initial step toward understanding, acceptance, and developing a plan for functionally adapting to this trait.

Salience, Addiction, and Impulsivity

In addition to altered responses to affect-laden stimuli, many personality disorders—especially Cluster B disorders—also involve impulsive and addictive patterns of poor self-regulation, connected to the self-expansive schema mode. For example, individuals with borderline personality disorder and antisocial personality disorder are often at much greater risk for substance abuse and dependence, and often exhibit impulsive tendencies around natural reinforcers, such as sex and food (Bandelow, Schmahl, Falkai, & Wedekind, 2010; Trull, Sher, Minks-Brown, Durbin, & Burr, 2000). Though often discussed as a singular phenomenon, such reward-seeking behaviors involves many subcomponents, including anticipation or craving, motivation or the willingness to exert effort to achieve the reward, and the experience of pleasure or relief when the reward is finally received. Over the last several decades, a large body of research has uncovered strong evidence to suggest that these aspects of reward processing rely on distinct neurobiological mechanisms, an observation that has significant implications for the development of addictive behavior patterns.

Specifically, this work has identified a critical role for the neurotransmitter dopamine in underlying the anticipatory and motivational aspects of reward processing, while opioid systems are most strongly implicated in the hedonic response to receiving a reward (Berridge, 2007). As a primary driver of approach and motivated behavior, the dopamine system was postulated as playing a key role in personality dimensions of extraversion and novelty seeking (Cloninger, 1986; Depue & Collins, 1999; Gray, 1987). More recent empirical work has supported this general conceptualization, with studies showing that individual differences in dopamine release in response to dopamine-releasing agents can predict personality traits related to novelty seeking, risk taking, and impulsivity (Buckholtz, Treadway, Cowan, Woodward, Benning, et al., 2010; Buckholtz, Treadway, Cowan, Woodward, Li, et al., 2010; Leyton et al., 2002; Treadway et al., 2012; Zald et al., 2008).

It has long been recognized that dopamine neurons have two general "states" that have very different function implications (Grace & Bunney, 1984). At baseline, they fire spontaneously and infrequently, creating a basal level of dopamine availability that is necessary for voluntary movement (it is the loss of these neurons and their baseline activity that results in Parkinsonian symptoms). However, these neurons also can enter into phases of so-called burst-firing patterns that lead to steep, rapid dopamine increases in the presence of a reward-predicting cue. For example, when you see an ad for your favorite food, receive a suggestive look from your partner, or get word that you are under consideration for a big promotion at work, the surge in craving, arousal, or excitement that you feel is partly mediated by rapid volleys of dopamine bursts (Schultz & Montague, 1997). However, it is important to underscore that dopamine's role is primarily circumscribed to the expectation of reward—and associated feelings of motivated anticipation—and not the pleasure of the reward once received. When you finally have a chance to consume the reward, dopamine neurons show little change from their normal baseline activity. As one researcher has described it, dopamine neurons are critical for "wanting" rewards, but are relatively uninvolved in "liking" them (Berridge, 2007).

This dissociation in the brain between wanting and liking can help explain the familiar experience of feeling craving something even though a part of you knows you won't enjoy it that much, or feeling let down by an event that didn't match your level of anticipatory excitement.

From a cognitive perspective, dopamine burst firing can be thought of as an energizing signal that is biased in favor of activating schemas and modes. In the context of personality disorders, individuals with antisocial personality disorder or psychopathy traits show greater dopamine bursts in response to reward-predicting cues (Bandelow et al., 2010; Buckholtz, Treadway, Cowan, Woodward, Benning, et al., 2010; Pujara, Motzkin, Newman, Kiehl, & Koenigs, 2014). This hypersensitivity within dopaminergic anticipation systems may help explain elevated risk for impulsive and abusive relationships to food, sex, and substances, as well tendencies for explosive anger or aggression toward others. Certain forms of personality disorders are associated with a stronger dopaminergic response to reward-predicting cues, which may rapidly overwhelm attempts at self-control or restraint. It may therefore be useful for such individuals to recognize early in treatment that their cravings are stronger than average, and they may be faster to develop bad habits.

Aberrant dopamine function has also been implicated in symptoms relating to Cluster A disorders, particularly schizotypal personality disorder. While excessive dopamine responses to reward cues may prompt impulsive, risky, or substance-seeking behavior as described above, more sustained dysregulation of dopamine functions may result in paranoid delusions and hallucinations. As an example of this phenomenon, when individuals consume moderate doses of dopamine-releasing agents such as amphetamine or cocaine, their behavior often becomes riskier, more impulsive, and in some cases more aggressive. As levels increase further, individuals may eventually experience full-blown psychotic symptoms, including delusions and hallucinations (Harris & Batki, 2000). As a result, dopamine dysregulation has been posited to play a critical role in the pathophysiology of positive symptoms in disorders such as schizophrenia as well as schizotypal personality disorder.

To date, relatively few studies have examined dopamine function in the context of schizotypal personality disorder, but some important hints have emerged. In cases of diagnosed schizotypal personality disorder, patients typically show greater dopamine release in response to dopaminergic drugs like amphetamines, possibly suggesting that they have a more sensitive dopamine system (Abi-Dargham et al., 2004), as well as a greater dopamine synthesis capacity (Howes et al., 2011). Emphasizing the dimensional relationship between dopamine function and schizotypal personality disorder, similar results have been observed in nonpatient samples of individuals with elevated levels of self-reported schizotypal traits (Woodward et al., 2011).

Taken together, these studies suggest that dopamine dysfunction and its attendant effects on motivation, risk, addiction, and paranoia may be an important component of personality disorders pathology.

Cognition and Social Processing

A final area of common difficulty in many personality disorders is assumptions about the actions and intentions of others. In particular, sensitivity to rejection is a common theme across Clusters B and C disorders, and can produce a range of potentially maladapative coping strategies including avoidance, idealization/devaluation, and preemptive rejection or lashing out. Social processing is also implicated in many Cluster A disorders in the form of cognitions related to paranoia and distrust, which can result in a poor reading of social cues or lack of interest in social connection.

To explore the biological basis of social processing, researchers have increasingly turned to two-player economic "games" that help model basic social interactions (King-Casas & Chiu, 2012). Games are particularly useful as an index of distortions in social cognition, as they can be designed in such a way as to require that individuals engage in a certain degree of trust or cooperativeness to reach an optimal solution. These paradigms usually involve various forms of monetary transaction or bargaining between two players, and can be used to uncover ways that different individuals initiate, build, or break cooperation and trust with strangers. For example, in so-called prisoner's dilemma paradigms, two individuals play multiple rounds where they can choose to "cooperate" or "defect." When both players cooperate, they both earn a medium-sized reward. If they both defect, they earn a lower reward. But if one defects and one cooperates, the defector earns the largest reward, while the cooperator gets nothing. Consequently, the optimal choice for a single player depends heavily on his or her beliefs about what the other will do, thereby providing a window into how each person thinks about others during a potentially competitive interaction. Games also reveal an individual's capacity to balance short-term versus long-term gain maximization in the context of interpersonal interactions. Over the course of multiple rounds, such games provide an opportunity to explore how people build trust, punish defection, and attempt to repair relationships. A central benefit of this approach also comes from the fact that game research is a transdisciplinary field that draws from economics, behavioral ecology, and computer science.

In the context of personality disorders and related traits, such games have been particularly revealing. Individuals with generalized social anxiety symptoms often show a willingness to be "taken advantage" of in such games, as evidenced by a willingness to tolerate unfair or predatory behavior on the part of their partner, despite having the option to make a retaliatory gesture (Grecucci, Giorgetta, Brambilla et al., 2013; Wu, Luo,

Broster, Gu, & Luo, 2013). Such actions can be viewed as representing a self-protective mode in which the desire to avoid conflict takes precedence over maximization of monetary gain. Similarly, individuals with borderline personality disorder often exhibit more distrusting patterns of choices during social economic tasks (Seres, Unoka, & Keri, 2009; Unoka, Seres, Aspan, Bodi, & Keri, 2009). In one study, the authors combined a social task with fMRI, and found that individuals with borderline personality disorder exhibit significant greater activity in the anterior insula—discussed above—and that such activity was predictive of less cooperative behavior (King-Casas et al., 2008). One possible interpretation of these findings is that heightened insula responses accounted for heightened emotional reactivity in patients with borderline personality disorder, creating a fear of possible noncooperation on the part of the confederate and leading to a preemptively uncooperative move. Finally, individuals with psychopathy have generally shown more noncooperative responses during such games, which have been accompanied by reduced amygdala reactivity to the uncooperativeness of others (Rilling et al., 2007).

It is worth highlighting that studies of social interactions in personality disorders correspond with studies of more basic affective processes. Just as individuals with borderline personality disorder and psychopathy show altered neural activity in insular and amygdalar regions in response to basic affective stimuli, these same patterns appear during social interactions, suggesting they may mediate some of the impairments in interpersonal dynamics that are common to personality disorders. Moreover, game-based models can be used to test hypothesized mechanisms of action for cognitive treatment. For example, instructed rumination or cognitive reappraisal has been shown to alter performance on economic two-player games, by helping people alter their affective reactions to the behavior of other players (Grecucci, Giorgetta, Van't Wout, Bonini, & Sanfey, 2013; van't Wout, Chang, & Sanfey, 2010). Consequently, these paradigms can be useful for understanding the mechanisms of cognitive mediation techniques.

INFORMING COGNITIVE-BEHAVIORAL TREATMENT: CURRENT UTILITY AND FUTURE DIRECTIONS

While clinical neuroscience has made great strides, it remains a science in its infancy. Indeed, as new powerful techniques provide ever-greater capacity to study the brain, they often reveal even greater complexity than we had previously imagined (Koch, 2012). This reality should temper expectations for a neuroscience-led revolution of clinical practice, but such restraint is not always present in much of our popular media (Satel & Lilienfeld, 2013). The following are several current ways that foundations of neuroscience support well-tested and emerging technology in clinical applications of cognitive-behavioral therapy for personality psychopathology.

Cultivating Nonjudgment

Many individuals who experience personality disorders suffer from a deep sense of inferiority, worthlessness, and unlovability. Indeed, some specific symptoms of different personality disorders can be viewed as an attempt to avoid contact with these core beliefs of low self-esteem. When the process of therapy brings attention to these beliefs, defensive avoidance can make it difficult to address certain cognitions directly, and hinder further progress. Discussing symptoms in terms of neurobiology can help diffuse this process by encouraging an "observer" stance toward one's emotional experiences. This introduces new information that can de-energize the schema for thoughts of self-recrimination and shame. In this sense, a neuroscience perspective may help augment the "observe and describe" exercises initially tested in the application of dialectical behavior therapy (Linehan, 1993).

Developing Narratives and Explanations

There is substantial evidence that narrative understanding of psychological symptoms can aid in their relief. Painful experiences are often less distressing when they are predictable and understood, even if the pain remains equally intense. Mechanistic explanations of specific symptoms can often be very powerful in this context—even relatively simple mechanisms such as amygdala reactivity. Such explanations can of course be offered without reference to neurobiology, as they have been in cognitive-behavioral therapy settings for decades. However, neurobiology may help buttress such explanations for certain patients. Additionally, it may help family members adopt an empathic perspective, as it provides an interpretive alternative that is less noxious than character motivations.

Combined Behavioral and Neurological Interventions

Finally, one of the most widely discussed ways that neuroscience may impact treatment is through the development of novel medications and medical devices. One of the greatest successes in this area has been the use of electrical stimulators implanted in the brain that have been shown to alleviate depressive symptoms (Mayberg et al., 2005). More recently, the possibility of using short-acting, targeted biological interventions to enhance the effects of behavioral therapy have begun to emerge. For example, D-cycloserine (DCS), a drug originally developed for the treatment of tuberculosis, was subsequently discovered to enhance memory-related synaptic plasticity through its actions on N-methyl-D-aspartate (NMDA) receptors in the brain. These receptors play a key role in the development of new memories, particularly during extinction learning of conditioned fear (Davis, Ressler, Rothbaum, & Richardson, 2006). Given that extinction learning plays a key role in exposure therapy for various forms of anxiety, researchers have found that DCS administration prior to exposure therapy sessions can augment the efficacy of exposure sessions alone (Hofmann, Meuret, et al., 2006; Hofmann, Pollack, & Otto, 2006). Importantly, this type of treatment is distinct from more traditional forms of combined behavioral and pharmacotherapy, in that the pharmacological agent is specifically designed to target and enhance the biological effects of the behavioral intervention (Hofmann, 2007).

Neuroplasticity

Last, it is worth highlighting that contrary to how neuroscience was taught in high school biology classes for many years, the neural networks of the adult brain are not fixed. Rather, they are constantly rearranging themselves in an experience-dependent way. The technical term for this is "neuroplasticity," and denotes the variety of epigenetic, synaptic, and network-level mechanisms that enable ensembles of neurons to adapt their inputs and outputs so as to learn new ideas, strengthen prior representations, or weaken habitual responding patterns. In simplest terms, it is the process through which a brain solves the difficult problem of deciding how much of its prior ideas about self, the world, and the future to hold on to, and how much should be updated in the face of new information. It's not hard to see how this is applicable to cognitive mediation strategies of change; the mere act of considering an alternative interpretation of a well-worn automatic negative thought can, over time, help reduce the power of that thought by reducing the strength of its representation in cognitive neural networks (DeRubeis, Siegle, & Hollon, 2008; Disner, Beevers, Haigh, & Beck, 2011). Studies in both humans and animal models suggest that neuroplastic mechanisms may be impaired in disorders such as major depression, and that interventions that target or enhance neuroplasticity may improve treatment (Duman & Aghajanian, 2012; Player et al., 2013). Future work will help to further uncover the applicability of neuroplasticity to treatment of personality disorders.

CONCLUSION

In sum, neuroimaging approaches to the study of personality disorders have begun to shed light on some of the basic biological mechanisms that may underlie specific disturbances in behavioral and cognitive domains. The self-expanding and protecting modes can be further understood by links to functional differences in the affect-related regions of the amygdala and insula as well as in dopamine sensitivity and synthesis. This conceptualization of personality disorder symptoms in terms of biological substrates may be therapeutic for some patients, in as much as it provides a way of describing symptoms that can avoid stimulating self-blaming cognitions. As the field of psychiatric neuroscience continues to mature, it is hoped that more powerful neuroscience-based treatments for personality disorders will be discovered.

CHAPTER 5

General Principles and Specialized Techniques in Cognitive Therapy of Personality Disorders

Aaron T. Beck
Arthur Freeman
Denise D. Davis

Patients with symptomatic disorders typically return to their premorbid cognitive mode as the disorder subsides. If this cognitive mode is well adapted, they will return to a baseline of relatively normal functioning. For example, most patients who have recovered from depression no longer blame themselves for every mishap, and are able to respond effectively to everyday stresses. They are less prone to think of themselves as inadequate and have positive anticipations about the future. Patients with personality disorders, however, frequently continue to perceive themselves or their experiences in problematic ways and may acknowledge that they have "always" thought this way, even though they no longer feel as depressed or anxious.

The personality disorder mode differs from the symptom disorder mode in a variety of ways. The frequency and intensity of dysfunctional automatic thoughts observed during the acute disorder level off when patients return to their regular cognitive functioning. Although the patients may have fewer dysfunctional automatic thoughts and feel less distressed overall, their exaggerated or distorted interpretations and the associated disruptive affect continue to occur in specific situations. A highly intelligent and competent woman, for example, would automatically have the thought "I can't do it" whenever she was asked to do something that involved intellectual skills. She would feel highly anxious, and tend to revert to her overdeveloped strategy of avoiding such tasks, despite knowing how to recognize and challenge her automatic thoughts and safety behaviors.

The most plausible explanation for the difference between the syndromes and the personality disorders is that the extreme faulty beliefs and interpretations characteristic of the symptomatic disorders are relatively plastic—and, indeed, become more moderate as the depression subsides even without any therapeutic intervention. However, the more persistent dysfunctional beliefs of the personality disorder are "structuralized"; that is, they are built into the "normal" cognitive organization, and embedded in primal schemas related to survival, health, goals, identity, and attachments to individuals and groups (Beck & Haigh, 2014). Hence, considerably more time and effort are required to produce the kind of structural change necessary to alter a personality disorder than to change the thinking of uncomplicated affective disorders.

The dysfunctional beliefs remain operative because they form the substrate for patients' orientation to reality. Because people rely on their beliefs to interpret events, they cannot relinquish these beliefs until they have incorporated new adaptive beliefs and strategies to take their place. When patients return to their premorbid level of functioning, they rely once again on their customary strategies, keeping the underlying beliefs activated through interconnected networks. Although underlying beliefs are generally less dysfunctional in this phase than during the depression or generalized anxiety disorder, they are also less amenable to further modification than during acute distress. Both patient and therapist need to acknowledge that these hard-core residual beliefs (schemas) are deeply ingrained and do not yield readily to the techniques used in the standard psychological treatment protocols. Even when patients are convinced that their basic beliefs are dysfunctional or even irrational, they cannot make them disappear simply by questioning them, doing a single exercise, or "wishing" them away.

In treatment, the therapist generally uses "standard" cognitive therapy techniques to relieve acute disorders such as depression (Beck, Rush, Shaw, & Emery, 1979) or generalized anxiety disorder (Beck & Emery, 1985). This approach is effective in dealing with the dysfunctional automatic thoughts and helps to produce the cognitive shift from the depressive (or generalized anxiety disorder) mode of processing back to the "normal" mode. The testing of automatic thoughts and beliefs during the depressive or anxious episode is good practice for dealing with these cognitive processes during the relatively quiescent period. Patients with comorbid personality problems observed during this quiescent period have been described in earlier psychiatric and colloquial terminology as "neurotic." The characteristics of the "neurotic personality" have generally been described in terms of labels such as "immature" or "childish": emotionally labile, with exaggerated responses to rejection or failure, unrealistically low or high concept of self, and—above all—intense egocentricity. This labeling, while descriptive, does not provide a common language that can be shared with patients or explain any mechanisms for the persistence of these difficulties.

A long, sometimes tedious process is necessary to effect change in these patients' character structure or personality. The "characterological phase" of treatment tends to be prolonged and much less punctuated by dramatic spurts of improvement, although steady effort based on a sound case conceptualization can produce valuable incremental gains in building more adaptive, strengths-based schemas and new behavioral strategies.

DATA-BASED CASE CONCEPTUALIZATION

Specific individual conceptualization that is data based and collaborative in nature is essential for understanding the patient's maladaptive behavior, selecting effective treatment strategies, and modifying dysfunctional attitudes. Consequently, the therapist should engage the patient early on, preferably during the evaluation process, in codeveloping a formulation to explain the nature and source of the patient's difficulties. Much of the data will come from discussions about the patient's current life situation, and the problems that precipitated treatment consultation, including treatment history. This may start with asking the patient to share his or her theory about what is wrong and how the problem developed. Second, the therapist gathers data about the patient's general developmental history, drawing out emotionally prominent memories and experiences, and asking the patient to consider how these might be connected. Indeed, a frequent sign of an underlying personality disorder is the patient's statement "I've always been this way; this is who I am." A third important source of data is direct interaction with and observation of the patient in the course of consultation.

A general "therapeutic triad" model for guiding the focus of attention in treatment over time is illustrated in Figure 8.2 (in Brauer & Reinecke, Chapter 8, this volume). Using this model, the therapist simultaneously integrates attention to the developmental narrative, current life problems, and the treatment relationship. Because patients with various personality disorders present with unique cognitive profiles, have individual learning styles, and may be confronting different life issues, specific techniques will vary with the goals specific to the disorder and the person. At the same time, the therapist can approach the work of conceptualization and intervention as a fluid movement among these spheres to assist the patient in identifying and modifying core schema.

The basic data needed for a cognitive conceptualization includes typical core beliefs about the self and others, one or two conditional assumptions and imperative beliefs, observations of underdeveloped and overdeveloped strategies (behavior), and if relevant, any treatment-interfering beliefs and behaviors. Of course, as new data are collected, the therapist modifies the formulation accordingly. Some hypotheses are confirmed, others are modified or dropped, and still others are entered into the formulation.

When therapists engage the patient in ongoing data gathering, they are providing a guide for the patient to learn how to isolate problem situations and to identify relevant thoughts and behaviors for a preliminary conceptualization. Patient and therapist can test new information for "fit" into the preliminary conceptualization, and make adjustments as needed. They can add in mediating strengths, including cultural strengths, and work together to "cocreate" the conceptualization (Kuyken, Padesky, & Dudley, 2009, p. 307). Early on, the therapist carries much of the responsibility for advancing this work; as treatment progresses, the patient acquires tools for sorting out complaints in terms of psychological and behavioral constructs, and applying various strategies for change. Drawing diagrams for patients can show them how to fit subsequent experiences into the overall formulation. It often helps for the patients to take the diagrams home with them. Some therapists use a blackboard or flip cards to demonstrate to the patients how their misconstruction of reality is derived from their beliefs. There are a number of ways to sketch out such conceptualizations, which are illustrated in the clinical applications chapters that follow in this volume (see also Kuyken et al., 2009).

For example, a patient with dependent personality who is confronting a new challenge and tells the therapist "I can't do it; I'm lost; I need directions," might be helped via a "downward-arrow" exercise to identify a link between this reaction and the conditional belief "If I don't feel competent, I should find someone to lean on," and the core belief "I am weak." The therapist and patient might then devise a behavioral experiment for gathering some new information, perhaps something involving a challenge where the patient is willing to experiment with resisting the urge to seek assistance. This new information can then be integrated with the model sketched up to that point. Ongoing intervention might involve further behavioral experiments to retest the dysfunctional beliefs and lay the groundwork for more adaptive attitudes. New attitudes might include "I can carry out a wide range of tasks without help" and "I am competent in many ways." The believability of these attitudes will depend on active experimentation and explicitly linking it to the patient's core beliefs.

Such explorations can be highly emotionally charged, so the progression toward explicit mapping of core beliefs about self and others must be sensitive to the patient's trust and ability to collaborate effectively. Usually, the therapeutic alliance should be well established and the patient should have a general grasp of the cognitive approach before hypotheses about core beliefs are explored in depth.

IDENTIFICATION OF SCHEMAS

The therapist can use the data that he or she is collecting to extract patients' self-concept, view of others, and the rules and formulas by which they live. Often, the therapist has to determine the patients' self-concept from its manifestations in their descriptions across a variety of situations. Listening carefully is a primary method for gathering this information, along with asking appropriate follow-up questions, and observing patient behavior, both in direct interaction and from patient self-report. It is very important to collect enough information in this manner to develop a working hypothesis about the meaning attached to the patient's statements, as very similar statements can be linked to vastly different assumptions and core meaning. In addition, schemas can overlap, so their characteristic beliefs and assumptions may reflect more than one of the typical cognitive profiles associated with different personality disorders.

For example, a patient makes statements such as the following: "I made a fool of myself when I gave the driver the wrong change," "I don't know how I got through college. I always seem to be fouling up," and "I don't think that I can describe situations properly to you." The therapist can pick up a thread that suggests that at a basic level the patient perceives him- or herself as inadequate or defective. However, the meaning attached to these self-appraisals ("I made a fool of myself," "I can't do things properly") could be very different depending on the core self-concept (e.g., "I'm awkward and can't take their ridicule," "I'm helpless and need their assistance," "I'm totally responsible and will be punished for mistakes," "I'm weird and can't deal with people," "I'm a target and might get exploited," "I'm perfect and shouldn't have to do these things," "I'm on display and surrounded by drama," or "I'm bad and overwhelmed by everything"). Many times it is the follow-up questions about meaning connected to the patient's thoughts and self-appraisals that reveal a more precise understanding of their schematic profile. The therapist might use any of several different probes to tap this information, such as "What do you think made this so upsetting to you?" or "When things go this way, what do you think it might mean about you?" or "What did you fear might be true in this situation?"

To further understand this meaning, the therapist can elicit the *conditional* assumptions through statements that specify the context under which the particular self-concept will express itself. For example, if the person has thoughts such as "Bob doesn't like me anymore" when another individual shows less than the usual friendly response, the therapist can derive the underlying formula: "If other people do not show a strong expression of affection or interest, it means they don't care for me." Most people would feel a twinge of discomfort at being the object of social ambivalence or rejection, as some striving for social attachment is genetically embedded in our core schema. Under normal conditions, individuals develop more nuanced expectations for relationships and are able to place them in situational context and understand their fluid nature. Individuals with personality problems, however, tend to apply the formula arbitrarily, in an all-or-nothing fashion across all situations, even when there are alternative explanations or compelling evidence that is contradictory to this belief. They may fail to adapt their broad expectations to the considerations of reality, applying irrational conditions such as "My well-being depends on strong affection from everyone, at all times," and they show overdeveloped, inflexible behaviors that are driven by this assumption.

Similarly, the therapist tries to elicit the patient's views of other people. Certain statements of a paranoid personality, for example, may indicate a basic schema that other people are devious, manipulative, prejudiced, and the like. The perception of dislike from Bob might be interpreted as malevolence and trigger imperative beliefs about the need for self-protection, as in "I had better be careful because Bob must be out to get me." The patient then becomes hyperalert to Bob's actions, ruminating about his possible motives and feeling compelled to hide or be secretive as a defense against impending harm. Other examples of this schema would be manifested in statements such as "The doctor smiled at me. I know it's a phony professional smile that he uses with everybody because he is anxious to have a lot of patients," or "The clerk counted my change very slowly because he doesn't trust me," or "My wife is acting extra nice to me tonight. I wonder what she wants to get out of me." Patients may reach these conclusions without any evidence to support them or even when there is strong contradictory evidence. When such persons are in an acute paranoid state, global thoughts run through their minds, such as "He's trying to put something over on me" or "They are all out to get me." The core schemas are "I'm vulnerable to harm," and "People are deceitful and abusive." A consequent pattern of arbitrary conclusions reflects a cognitive bias and is said to be "schema driven." These arbitrary conclusions trigger overdeveloped strategies or behaviors to cope with the emotions aroused by these beliefs. Overdeveloped strategies then become more rigid over time, and function as safety behaviors, avoiding potentially disconfirming information and reinforcing the basic schema.

Table 5.1 presents a structural formulation of the problems of a couple who had somewhat similar sets of beliefs but who differed in crucial ways. The presenting problems of this couple have been presented in detail elsewhere (Beck, 1988b). In brief, Gary, who had a narcissistic personality disorder, had periodic violent outbursts against Beverly, whom he accused of needling him all the time for not attending to specific chores. Gary believed the only way he could control Beverly, who had a dependent personality disorder, was to strike out at her to make her "shut up." Beverly, on the other hand, believed that she had to control Gary's continuous defaulting

TABLE 5.1. Cognitive Processing from Core Schemas: An Example

Automatic thought	Beverly's beliefs: "Gary isn't helping me enough."	Gary's beliefs: "Beverly is nagging me."
Should	"Gary should help when I ask."	"Beverly should show more respect."
Must	"I must control others' behavior."	"I must control others' behavior."
Special conditional belief	"If Gary doesn't help, I won't be able to function."	"If I give them a chance, people will dump on me."
Fear	"I will be abandoned."	"I will lose status and be henpecked."
Core schema	"I am a helpless baby."	"I am a wimp."
Overdeveloped strategy	Prod and remind Gary of her needs Show distress and helplessness	Bully Beverly into backing off Exploit status as head of house
Underdeveloped strategy	Self-reliance and problem solving Assertive negotiation of roles and tasks	Empathy for Beverly's anxiety Active participation in domestic tasks

on his role as husband and father by "reminding" him in a reproachful way of his derelictions. She believed that this was the only way she could carry out her responsibility as housewife and mother. Beneath this view was her firm belief that she could not function at all unless she had somebody to lean on, and that she needed to get him to fulfill this role.

Gary had been brought up in a household in which "might makes right." His father and older brother had intimidated him into believing he was a "wimp." He compensated for this image of himself by adopting their interpersonal strategy: In essence, the best way to control other people's inclination to dominate or demean one is to intimidate them—if necessary, through threat of force. The initial formulation, which was borne out by subsequent conjoint and individual interviews, was as follows: Gary's core schema was "I am a wimp." This self-concept threatened to surface whenever he regarded himself as vulnerable to being demeaned. To protect himself, he consolidated the belief "I have to win the argument" that was inherent in his father's behavior. Later, we return to the methods used to deal with these beliefs. In essence, the therapist was able to trace Gary's behavior to these beliefs.

Beverly similarly believed that "I need to get Gary involved." Her imperative was derived from a fear of being incapable of performing her duties without help. Her core schema was "I am a helpless child." Note that Beverly's schema ("I'm helpless without support") processed Gary's behavior ("not helping") as a threat, further activating core identity schema (I am weak) leading to a limp feeling in Beverly. She reacted to this debilitating feeling as a threat to her very being, blaming Gary and becoming enraged.

Through imagery and reliving past experiences of helplessness, the therapist was able to activate the core schema and help Beverly to recognize that her profound involvement in getting Gary to help out was derived from her image of herself as a helpless child. Consequently, her nonadaptive "nagging" was an attempt to stave off her profound sense of incompetence. The interaction of Gary and Beverly demonstrates how partners' personality structures can aggravate each other's problems and illustrates the importance of viewing personality problems as they are expressed in a particular context, such as a marital situation.

SPECIFICATION OF UNDERLYING GOALS

People generally have broad goals that are very important to them but may not be completely in their awareness. The therapist has the job of translating the patient's stated aspirations and ambitions into the underlying goal, using the clues provided by patient statements, along with overt patterns of behavior. Observable patterns that are prominent and repetitive (overdeveloped), as well as certain expected behaviors that are conspicuously absent or weak (underdeveloped), are both important. For instance, a patient may say, "When I got to the party, I felt bad because only a few people came up to say hello to me," or "I had a great time because a lot of people crowded around me and wanted to know how my trip went." From a wide range of descriptions across a number of diverse situations, the therapist can infer that the underlying goal is something like "It is very important for me to receive attention and acceptance." Goals are derived from the core schema; in this case it would be to enhance the sense of social value, thus expressing a basic drive that is adaptive for survival, and suggestive of specific personality modes that may, when overdeveloped, become problematic. Probing further to ask the patient how he or she reacted at the party can provide important detail as to the typical behavioral pattern. The patient who reports, "I stayed for 30 minutes and then had to get out of there," will likely have a very different goal than the patient who says "I got on a roll and had quite a night."

Another patient, for example, stated that he felt bad because he did not get a perfect grade on an exam. He also felt a little put out when he was unable to recall the name of a particular artist during a conversation with a friend. In addition, he became so excited that he had a sleepless night after being told that he was going to get a full scholarship into graduate school.

His goal, which he did not articulate until he was questioned about his experiences, was "to be famous." Associated with this goal was this conditional assumption: "If I do not become famous, then my whole life will be wasted." Descriptions of his typical behavior gave further indication of the underlying goal of achieving self-worth through fame. He was very boastful, and seemed to be lacking in sensitivity toward his peers, expecting their admiration of his graduate scholarship while he showed no reciprocal interest in their achievements or challenges.

Other kinds of goals may be inferred in much the same way. Take an individual who rejects any offer of help, insists on having complete freedom to move around, and is reluctant to become involved in any type of "relationship." Once the therapist extracts the common theme, "I need to have space," he or she can test this striving by observing the patient's reaction in therapy and in other situations. If the patient, for example, tends to seek physical distance during the interview, terminates the interview promptly, and expresses the desire to work on his or her problems alone, these are indicators of an underdeveloped strategy of tolerating some social exchange and an underlying goal of self-protection. The conditional assumption may be "If I let people in, they will make demands and waste my time." Associated with this notion is the belief that "I am happier and more effective on my own" and the goal of preserving autonomy and freedom from social obligations.

When the therapeutic alliance has been established and sufficient data gathered on the core assumptions, conditional beliefs, behavioral strategies, and goals, the therapist can then sketch out a case formulation according to the cognitive model (e.g., the formulation of Gary and Beverly's case previously discussed), and discuss it with the patient, explaining the idea of core beliefs, and modifying or adjusting the formulation as needed.

EMPHASIS ON THE THERAPIST–PATIENT RELATIONSHIP

Collaboration

One of the cardinal principles of cognitive therapy is instilling a sense of collaboration and trust in the patient. The building of the relationship is probably more important when addressing personality disorders than in treating symptomatic problems. With acute distress (usually depression and/or anxiety), the patient can usually be motivated to try out the therapist's suggestions and is rewarded by the fairly prompt reduction of suffering. In dealing with the scope of personality disorder, the changes take place much more slowly and the payoff is much less perceptible. Hence, therapist and patient have considerable work to do on the long-term project of personality change, and agreement to work together on these intrapersonal and interpersonal objectives is critical.

Beginnings are very important for setting expectations in the working relationship. Patients with personality disorders often show difficulties in trust or collaboration as an early indicator of the scope of their problems. In response, therapists can review their use of the basic tools for fostering treatment engagement to ensure that they are providing an optimal framework (see also J. Beck, 2005; Kuyken et al., 2009). First, proposing and securing the patient's agreement to work on specific goals that are personally meaningful can enhance motivation. Second, brief psychoeducation on the cognitive model can help the patient become oriented and interested in the work, and perhaps reduce uncertainty concerning what will be asked of him or her. Third, outlining and following a general structure within sessions from the start creates familiarity and predictability, and sets the tone for how the time will be used. This involves describing the agenda-setting process, and then actively engaging the patient in discussing what to put on the agenda at the beginning. Therapists then seek input from the patient on decisions and choice points throughout the sessions, such as how much time to allot to a topic, when to shift topics, and when to schedule the next meeting. Explaining at the outset that there is a structure to sessions and to the direction of therapy helps to build a sense of safety. Explaining what to expect and what is expected of the patient demystifies the experience and makes it more concrete and understandable.

Fourth, during each session, the therapist checks on the patient's understanding of information shared, concepts explained, or the purpose of activities suggested in session. This typically includes offering capsule summaries to assess the patient's thoughts and reactions, and verify the therapist's accuracy of understanding. Fifth, they brainstorm or create homework together as much as possible. Sixth, therapists offer positive feedback about patient strengths. They support the patient's efforts, show concern for the patient's preferences, and demonstrate respect for the patient's challenges. Finally and perhaps most important, the therapist seeks the patient's feedback on the impact of the session and perceived usefulness of the therapist's effort. Asking for feedback can be very difficult for both therapist and patient, so it is important to do so in an artful and reinforcing way. The tone of the session and nature of the patient's personality should be kept in mind, as there are times when a lighthearted approach will set the patient at ease, and other times when it might come across as dismissive or confusing. Likewise, being overly serious can trigger negative schema or put the patient off in other ways. The therapist's job is to model receptiveness to both positive and negative feedback, in the interest of best serving the patient's needs.

Patients with personality disorders frequently have problems collaborating on homework assignments, which is a form of therapy-interfering behavior. They may feel anxious about completing activities, or underestimate the potential usefulness. Beliefs that are characteristic of the personality disorder itself frequently interfere with carrying out assignments. The avoidant personality may think, "Writing down my thoughts is too painful"; the narcissistic, "I'm too good for this sort of thing"; the paranoid, "My notes can be used against me" or "The therapist is trying to manipulate me."

The therapist should regard these forms of "resistance" as "grist for the mill" and should subject them to the same kind of analysis as that used for other forms of material or data, without giving up on the collaboration. Structure, persistence, and creativity are tools that therapists might find especially useful in working with these challenges. A certain therapeutic leverage is possible if concrete goals that are meaningful to the patient can be established. Examples provided in the clinical applications chapters later in this book include gaining access to housing, finding relief from pain, overcoming employment probation, avoiding divorce, attaining more emotionally satisfying relationships, and so forth. Engaging the patient in adapting or creatively designing homework is also valuable. For example, patients who are averse to written exercises might be more open to recording thoughts on their phone or using a mobile application, and they are more apt to follow through if they come up with the idea. Case consultation is another important fundamental tool that therapists can use for getting fresh ideas to help with homework or other challenges.

Therapists who use a schema-focused approach often use a method of explicitly labeling the therapeutic stance as one of "limited reparenting," in which the caring relationship is intended to partially repair what was wrong or missing from the patient's developmental experiences. The therapist explicitly deepens the level of expressed emotional involvement and availability and provides feedback to support the patient's skill development and awareness of his or her interpersonal impact, all in the context of healthy or adaptive limits (see Behary & Davis, Chapter 14, and Arntz, Chapter 17, this volume, for more detail). Some or all of these elements may also be present in other variations of the cognitive model, without necessarily labeling the stance as reparenting.

Guided Discovery

Part of the artistry of cognitive therapy consists of conveying a sense of adventure—in unraveling and ferreting out the origins of patients' beliefs, exploring the meanings of traumatic events, and tapping into the rich imagery. Otherwise, therapy can decline into a repetitive process that becomes increasingly tedious over time. In fact, varying the way hypotheses are presented, using different phrases and words, and illustrating points with metaphors and anecdotes all help to make the relationship into a human educational experience. A certain lightness and judicious use of humor can also add spice to the experience.

Throughout treatment of personality disorders, the therapist spends more time with patients on unraveling the *meaning* of experiences, to determine the patients' specific sensitivities and vulnerabilities and ascertain what triggers them to overreact to specific situations. As indicated by A. Beck (Chapter 2, this volume), the meanings are determined to a large extent by the underlying assumptions and beliefs ("If somebody criticizes me, it means that person doesn't like me"). To determine the meaning, the therapist may have to proceed gradually through a number of steps. This includes looking back through the patient's narrative history of his or her personal and psychological development, identifying key emotional experiences that support the believability of his or her maladaptive conclusions.

Use of "Transference" Reactions

The patient's emotional reactions to therapy and the therapist are of central concern. Always alert but not provoking, the therapist is ready to explore these reactions for more information about the patient's system of thoughts and beliefs. If not explored, possible distorted interpretations will persist and likely interfere with collaboration and progress in treatment. If brought out into the open, they often provide rich material for understanding the meanings and beliefs behind the patient's idiosyncratic or repetitious reactions. Empathically delivered interpersonal observations and feedback may be among the most powerful interventions that the therapist provides, especially when focused on interactions that occur within the therapeutic relationship, including on-the-spot interactions as they happen in session. This must always be done in a supportive and honest way, inviting further exploration rather than delivering an expert interpretation. Taking the role of interpretive expert will have the impact of flattening collaboration and distancing the patient, but providing honest personal feedback can make key schema more available in the moment and increase the patient's involvement.

In terms of countertransference, it is extremely important to remain nonjudgmental, compassionate, and warm, yet objective in responding to the patient's maladaptive patterns. Work with personality disorders typically requires significant effort, planning, and stress management on the part of the therapist. Davis and J. Beck (Chapter 6, this volume) details more fully the general strategies for conceptualizing therapy-interfering beliefs and behaviors and managing emotional reactions to therapy by both patient and therapist. Subsequent chapters on clinical applications each address this matter in greater detail within the context of specific personality modes.

SPECIALIZED TECHNIQUES

The specific pathology of the patient's personality can be addressed with a flexible and creative use of cognitive and behavioral strategies and techniques, selecting from the wide variety available, including experiential methods that integrate affect with cognitive and behavioral processes. Therapists can use standard methods or improvise new ones to meet specific patient needs. A certain amount of trial and error may be necessary. At times, introspection may be most successful; at other times, role plays or skills training may be the appropriate choice. Skillful evoking of the patient's internal motivation through guided conversations about ambivalence and change using motivational interviewing (Miller & Rollnick, 2013) may be needed periodically along the way.

The most effective application of techniques depends not only on a clear conceptualization of the case and the formation of a friendly working relationship but also on the artistry of the therapist. The *art of therapy* involves the judicious use of humor, anecdotes, metaphors, and therapeutic self-disclosure of the therapist's experiences, as well as the standard cognitive and behavioral techniques. Skillful therapists know when to draw out sensitive material, draw back when necessary, and confront avoidances. They can heat up a monotonous rendition or cool off an overly heated flow. They vary their words, style, and mode of expression while remaining relaxed, attentive, professional, and focused on goals of therapy. *Flexibility* within a given session is important. The therapist may vary his or her approach from active listening to focusing and probing to modeling new behavioral styles. It is expected that therapists reading this volume understand the basic techniques of cognitive-behavioral psychotherapy (e.g., Beck et al., 1979; J. Beck, 2005, 2011; Greenberger & Padesky, 1995; Wright, Basco, & Thase, 2006), as well as emerging technology such as mindfulness practices (Germer, Siegel, & Fulton, 2013), values clarification (Hayes & Strosahl, 2004; Strosahl, Hayes, Wilson, & Gifford, 2004), and strengths conceptualization (Kuyken et al., 2009).

We have arbitrarily divided techniques into those that are primarily "cognitive," "behavioral," or "experiential." We need to keep in mind that techniques are not really purely cognitive, behavioral, or experiential, and changes in one domain may precipitate changes in another. Cognitive strategies can produce behavioral change, and behavioral methods generally instigate some cognitive restructuring. Among the most effective tools in treating personality disorders are the so-called *experiential techniques*, such as reliving childhood events, imagery, dialogues among modes, or expressive exercises (see Freeman, Felgoise, & Davis, 2008, for more clinical examples). Such dramatic techniques seem to open up the sluices for new learning—or unlearning. A general heuristic is that cognitive change depends on a certain level of affective arousal. Other experiential interventions focus on altering attention or the focus of attention in key situations, and can incorporate training in various mindfulness practices, defusion of thought and meaning, or clarification of values.

Thus, cognitive, behavioral, and experiential techniques all interact in the treatment of personality disorders. The main thrust is to develop new schemas and modify old ones, decreasing the valence of maladaptive modes and increasing the strength and availability of more adaptive modes. Ultimately, of course, the cognitive techniques probably account for most of the change that occurs. The cognitive work, like the behavioral, requires more precision and persistence than usual when patients have personality disorders. Because specific cognitive schemas of these patients continue to be dysfunctional, even after more adaptive modes have been developed, a larger variety and longer duration of cognitive reworking is typically required.

COGNITIVE STRATEGIES AND TECHNIQUES

The following list details some of the primary cognitive techniques that may be helpful in dealing with personality disorders.

1. Guided discovery, which enables the patient to recognize stereotyped dysfunctional patterns of interpretation. This may take the form of a Socratic dialogue where the therapist uses cognitive probes to gather data and help the patient to observe deeper levels of meaning.

2. Psychoeducation about cognitive processes and modes of thoughts, feelings, and behavior, and normal goals and needs. Selected self-help bibliotherapy can be very useful as an adjunct to in-session discussion and may include books (e.g., Greenberger & Padesky, 1995; Leahy, 2006, 2010), selected handouts, or references to blogs or Internet-based resources.

3. Thought records, worksheets, and/or in-session graphic depiction of cognitive connections, often including situations, automatic thoughts, emotions, evidence, and alternative thoughts. Diagrams that map out relevant patterns also help patients to observe and understand the links among triggers, thoughts, feelings, actions, and consequences. Various written tools can be selected or modified to meet the needs of the patient. Applications for electronic devices can also be used for tracking thoughts and moods and other cognitive exercises.

4. Labeling of inaccurate inferences or distortions, to make the patient aware of bias or unreasonableness of particular automatic patterns of thought. Reviewing the pros and cons, or advantages and disadvantages, is another way to increase awareness of bias.

5. Collaborative discovery—applying curiosity in the form of behavioral tests to help the patient assess the validity or practicality of his or her beliefs, interpretations, and expectations.

6. Examining possible explanations for other people's behavior.

7. Scaling experiences on a continuum to translate extreme interpretations into dimensional terms and counteract typical dichotomous or catastrophic thinking.

8. Constructing pie charts of responsibility for actions and outcomes to reduce attributions of overcontrol.

9. Brainstorming and articulating positive beliefs and options, as patients with personality disorders often have difficulty in constructing ideas in the positive or adaptive frame. This can include identifying and appreciating strengths and sources of resilience, as well as discussing goals in terms of approach versus avoidance and recognizing various types and degrees of positive emotions.

10. Examining data from schema diaries. These diary entries are targeted to gather specific schema-related information to address one or more functions: (a) to store new observations that counter old schema; (b) to compare reality to schema-related predictions; or (c) to compare old and new schema when responding to critical incidents and accumulate data that supports the substance and availability of new, more adaptive schema for strengths.

11. Defining ideas or constructs relevant to the patient's self-concept or current situation to increase self-understanding, appreciation of multidimensionality, and self-acceptance. Collecting data with assessment tools such as the Personality Beliefs Questionnaire, the Schema Questionnaire, or other psychological inventories such as symptom measures, stress inventories, self-esteem/self-compassion inventories, or other psychological checklists can be very helpful in adding structure and flexibility to the patient's cognitive construct.

12. Constructing coping cards to provide a memory prompt and "on-the-spot" coaching of alternative interpretations when emotional distress occurs or in other targeted situations.

Implementing "Cognitive Probes"

Cognitive probes are primary tools used in therapeutic discussion to bring attention to the cognitive underpinnings of emotionally arousing incidents. For example, Lois, a patient with avoidant personality disorder, reported an upsetting event when other workers at her job appeared to ignore her. The first cognitive probe would attempt to recover her automatic thoughts (Beck, 1967) by asking, "What went through your mind when this happened?" If the patient is well trained at identifying automatic thoughts, she might say, "I thought 'They don't like me.'"

If the patient fails to recover the automatic thought, she might then be encouraged to *imagine* the experience "as though it is happening right now." As the experience is brought to life, as it were, she is likely to experience the automatic thoughts just as she would in the actual situation. Of course, she would have many opportunities in future encounters to ascertain the automatic thoughts as they occur without priming. If a patient can anticipate a particular "traumatic" experience, it is useful to prepare in advance by starting to tune in to the train of thought prior to entering the aversive situation ("I wonder whether Linda will snub me at lunch today"). Our patient, Lois, thus is primed to catch the relevant thought of rejection. Noting that Linda seems to be aloof, she can pick up the negative thoughts: "She doesn't like me," and "There is something wrong with me." Of course, automatic thoughts are not necessarily dysfunctional or unrealistic and, as we shall see, need to be tested.

Of most importance is the ultimate meaning of the event. For example, Lois could shrug off Linda's seeming rejection with the thought, "So what? She's not one of my closest friends," or "I could just relax over lunch and let the socializing be spontaneous." However, when the patient has a specific vulnerability to rejection, a chain reaction is started that may culminate in a prolonged feeling of sadness, related to the underlying belief.

Sometimes the patient is able to discern the chain reaction through introspection. Often, through skillful questioning, the therapist can arrive at the salient starting point (core schema). He or she can also use this exercise as a way of demonstrating the particular fallacy or flaw in the patient's process of making inferences and drawing conclusions. Take the following interchange between the therapist and Lois, who has become upset because Linda, her friend, has been absorbed in a conversation with a fellow worker at lunch:

THERAPIST: What thought went through your mind at lunch?
LOIS: Linda is ignoring me. [Selective focus, personalization]
THERAPIST: What did that mean?
LOIS: I must be boring. [Self-attribution, overgeneralization]
THERAPIST: What does that mean?
LOIS: I will never have any friends. [Absolute prediction]
THERAPIST: What does it mean "not to have friends"?
LOIS: I am all alone. [Core schema]
THERAPIST: What does it mean to be "all alone"?
LOIS: I don't count; I'm defective and will always be unhappy. (*Starts to cry.*)

Because the patient starts to cry, the therapist stops the line of questioning because he believes he has come to the bedrock, the core schema ("I'm defective"). The arousal of a strong feeling suggests not only that a core schema has been exposed but also that the dysfunctional thinking is more accessible to modification. This type of questioning, attempting to probe for deeper meanings and access to the core schema, has been called the downward-arrow technique (Beck et al., 1985). At a later date, therapist and patient will want to explore further to ascertain whether there are other core schemas.

In this particular case, Lois's problem stems from her beliefs: "If people are not responsive to me, it means they don't like me" and "If one person doesn't like me, it means I'm unlikable." When she goes into the cafeteria in the office building in which she works, she is very sensitive to how receptive the other workers are—whether they seem eager to have her sit next to them, whether they include her in the conversation, whether they are responsive to her remarks. Because she has an avoidant personality disorder and tends to avoid entering situations of possible rejection, she is inclined not to sit at a table with people she knows, particularly Linda. One way to deal with this is to confront the issue head on, as illustrated in the following dialogue about entering a group of women engaged in animated conversation:

THERAPIST: Suppose the people don't welcome you with open arms, then what?

LOIS: I don't know. I suppose I would feel they don't like me.

THERAPIST: If they showed they liked you, then what?

LOIS: I'm not sure. I really don't have much in common with them.

THERAPIST: Would you choose to have any of them as your close friends?

LOIS: I guess not.

THERAPIST: So it's the meaning, the importance you attach to "being liked" or "not liked" rather than the practical importance that throws you. Is that right?

LOIS: I guess it is.

Because of her core schemas revolving around the issue of being likable, almost every encounter Lois has with other people involves a test of her acceptability, becoming almost a matter of life and death. By exposing the core schema through the downward-arrow technique, the therapist is able to bring the underlying meanings of "being ignored" to the surface and demonstrate that the belief about the necessity of being liked by everyone is dysfunctional.

Once the underlying beliefs are made accessible (conscious), the patient can then apply realistic, logical reasoning to modify them. Thus, Lois is able to counter the automatic thought, "They don't care for me," with the rational response, "These are casual workplace interactions with people who know only a little about me; I'm a moderately introverted person and not really motivated to seek a lot of friends, which is okay." Patients tend to attach absolutistic meanings to events and to view them in all-or-nothing terms. The therapist's role is to help the patient see the importance of events or connections in shades of gray, and to find a functional level of self-acceptance. Of course, in most situations casual acquaintances usually are neutral rather than rejecting, but because patients with avoidant presonality disorder are prone to interpret neutrality as rejection, they need to articulate the core beliefs and experience the associated affect to change this dysfunctional way of thinking.

Labeling and Modifying the Schemas

In discussing or elucidating the schemas with the patient, the diagnostic labels of paranoid, histrionic, narcissistic, schizoid, or borderline may induce a bias in the therapist's view of the patient. Instead, the patient's style can be translated into operational terms. The schizoid style, for example, can be described and discussed as the patient's being "very individualistic" or being "low on social dependence." The dependent personality disorder can be discussed in terms of "having a strong belief in the value of attachment to others," or "being a 'people' person." In every case, a nonjudgmental description modified to fit the particular belief system can be offered to the patient. Therapists will need to use their judgment as to when and if to share the specific diagnostic category beyond establishing the specific problems in self-concept or relationships that are the focus of treatment. Key treatment goals and options for determining treatment success with particular disorders are discussed in each of the clinical applications chapters later in this volume.

The objective of cognitive therapy for personality disorders is schema modification and adaptive adjustment rather than striving for personality transformation. An overarching goal is to decrease the valence of the dysfunctional schemas, and strengthen the availability of benevolent schemas. Related to improving adaptive functioning is the option of "schematic reinterpretation." This involves helping patients to understand and reinterpret their schemas and strategies in more functional ways. For example, a person with histrionic personality disorder could recognize the dysfunctionality of compulsively seeking attention and admiration in inappropriate situations and still find adaptive ways to obtain this gratification—for example, by participating in community theater productions, or doing volunteer work with a highly appreciative population. Anxiety is likely to be aroused as schemas are challenged and changed, so it is helpful to apprise patients of this possible occurrence, and provide support for anxiety management.

Mary, a 23-year-old technology worker who attempted to achieve perfection in virtually all tasks, was experiencing great difficulty at work due to problems in meeting expected deadlines. She thought it was essential to keep her "high standards." Attempts to alter these hypervalent schemas were met with great resistance. She wanted relief from the stress but did not want to alter her rules and standards. One choice discussed in therapy was seeking a new position that would emphasize "high standards." After a brief job search, she found a position where she was expected to work "slowly and carefully" without regard to time, to produce carefully detailed results. Mary's coworkers found her style compatible with the aims of their project. Continued therapy worked toward modification of her rules in social situations and in personal matters such as taxes, bills, and home management.

Making Decisions

One of the areas in which therapists often enter into the "outside lives" of patients with personality disorders is helping them to make decisions. While the personality problems are being treated, joint work is required to help patients learn how to make certain important decisions that have been postponed initially. During the acute phase of depressive or anxiety disorders, the therapist focuses on getting patients mobilized and back into the pattern of confronting *immediate problems*, which may seem insoluble during the depression (indeed, this feeling may be a byproduct of the depression): "Should I get out of bed today?" "How can I get the children off to school?" "What should I buy at the supermarket?" A depressed attorney, for instance, could not decide which cases she should attend to first when she got to the office. She needed help in setting priorities and then listing what needed to be done for each case. The symptoms of depression may interfere with making even the simplest routine decisions. Important long-range decisions—for example, regarding marital problems, childrearing, or career changes—may need to be put off until the depression has subsided.

When the acute symptoms have subsided, therapy can focus on the more chronic or long-range problems regarding marriage, career, and so on. Decisions that seem to tie patients in knots—especially in the area of interpersonal relations—need to be tackled. Some patients are paralyzed into inaction, and others make impulsive decisions when faced with questions regarding choice of career, dating, marriage or divorce, and having children (as well as more mundane issues). The calculated procedures involved in making decisions are often blocked by the patients' personality problems. People with avoidant and passive–aggressive personalities tend to procrastinate; the person who is histrionic is more likely to be impulsive; the person who is obsessive–compulsive gets caught up in perfectionism; the person who is dependent looks for somebody else to make the decision; the person who is narcissistic focuses on how the decision will make him or her look; the person who is antisocial focuses on immediate personal gain.

It is clear that the therapist cannot treat the personality problems in a vacuum. The cognitive problems encroach on the way the individual is able to cope with "real-life situations." Conversely, by helping the patient to learn and integrate new coping strategies, the therapist is able to neutralize some of the maladaptive strategies that are manifestations of the personality disorder. Incorporating a new strategy of decision making can increase the self-reliance of the person who is dependent, improve interpersonal risk-taking of the person who is avoidant, make the person who is histrionic more reflective, and increase the flexibility of the person who is obsessive–compulsive. Thus, new decision-making patterns can modify the personality styles of each disorder.

A method that helps people sort out their feelings about a key decision is to list the pros and cons for each option in separate columns. With the therapist's assistance, the patient lists the advantages and disadvantages of each alternative and attempts to assign weights to each of these items. For example, Tom, who tended to obsess about decisions and performance in general, had decided to drop out of law school because of the discomfort he felt in taking exams and his fear of not living up to expectations. He was prompted to consider dropping out by his belief that this was the only way he could relieve the stress. As a way of helping him to make an objective decision, the therapist and Tom set up four columns and filled them in together as shown in Table 5.2. The first column listed the reasons for dropping out or staying. In the second column, he gauged the importance of these reasons. The third column contained rebuttals and the fourth the value or importance of the rebuttals.

After Tom went down the list with his therapist, he was able to view the question of dropping out more objectively. He experienced some relief when he realized that his perfectionism and obsessing were the real sources of distress rather than the difficulties of law school per se and that he could get help from his therapist with this distressing personality problem that had plagued him most of his life. It should be noted that decisions that may be relatively simple for one patient become momentous for another because they touch on specific personality sensitivities. Thus, Agnes, who had a dependent personality, had no difficulty in deciding to have a dinner party but agonized over making a decision whether to take a trip alone. On the other hand, Phil had a schizoid personality and was able to plan trips alone but was stymied when he needed help due to car trouble.

TABLE 5.2. Tom's Decision-Making Process

	Value	Rebuttal	Value
In favor of dropping out			
"I won't have to worry so much."	60%	"I'm in therapy to get me over my *perfectionism*, which is what's making me miserable."	40%
"I can find out whether I want to be a lawyer."	10%	"I don't need to make an irreversible decision to find this out . . . I can play it by ear as I continue in school."	30%
"It will be a big relief. I can take time out and knock around for a while."	40%	"I will feel relieved at first, but I may feel really sad about it later."	30%
In favor of staying			
"I've prepared myself for going to law school and have only 1½ more years to go."	40%	None	—
"I might really like the practice of law (it's the exams that are getting me down)."	30%	None	—
"Even if I don't like the practice of law, it's a good jumping-off point for a number of different jobs (even a college presidency!)."	30%	None	—
"Some of the courses turn me on."	20%	None	—
"My perfectionism might work well for me in the law."	20%	None	—

BEHAVIORAL TECHNIQUES

The goals of using behavioral techniques are threefold. First, the patient may need to work directly to alter self-defeating behaviors. Second, the patient may need support in building specific skills. Third, behavioral assignments can be used as homework to gather new data for evaluating cognitions. Behavioral techniques that can be helpful (although we do not discuss all of them in detail here) include the following:

1. Activity logs, which permit retrospective identification and prospective planning of changes, including assessment of basic levels of activation and goal direction, and satisfaction with daily productivity.

2. Scheduling activities, to enhance personal efficacy in targeted areas such as positive emotions (mastery and pleasure), independence (skill building), social relations (intentional, reciprocal), or purpose (personal values or meaning).

3. Behavioral rehearsal, modeling, and assertiveness training for skill development to respond more effectively in challenging or stressful situations. This typically involves thinking through the specific behavioral skills needed and talking through the sequence of enactment, rehearsing a cognitive map of procedure for how to effectively implement the actions to achieve a desired outcome, such as obtaining cooperation from another person, and troubleshooting for points of difficulty.

4. Relaxation training and behavioral redirection techniques, for use when anxiety or worry increases during efforts to change.

5. *In vivo* exposure, by arranging for the therapist to assist the patient in confronting a stimulus likely to trigger a problematic schema, and support the effort to experience and respond effectively to problematic cognitions. Alternatively, imaginal exposure may be useful if specific situations are difficult to arrange *in vivo*.

6. Graded task assignment, so that the patient can experience changes as an incremental step-by-step process, during which the difficulty of each component can be adjusted and mastery achieved in stages.

7. Behavioral chain analysis to assist the patient in breaking down problem sequences and developing ideas for response alternatives at each stage in the sequence. Competing responses (doing the opposite) can be introduced as a means of redirection and increasing behavioral control.

8. Time and routine management, to assist the patient in setting priorities for use of his or her time, organizing effective routines for activities of daily living, and in allocating a realistic portion of time for various tasks and events. Often this includes discussion of sleep and wake schedules, and stabilizing routines after disruptive times or events.

9. Stimulus control, or the purposeful alteration of cues to prompt desired responses or behaviors, and create conditions that will discourage maladaptive behaviors.

10. Contingency management, to systematically link rewards or positive reinforcement with desired efforts, and decrease the benefits associated with maladaptive responses.

EXPERIENTIAL METHODS

A variety of activities can be used in session to create an experience that blends emotional components of schema with thoughts and behavior, to assist in building skills, altering particularly resistant schema, or building practices that the patient can continue at home to identify and regulate emotions. Patients with different cognitive profiles will vary significantly in their willingness to engage in experiential exercises, and in specific needs for altering cognitions and overdeveloped or underdeveloped strategies. Generally, patients who tend to be inhibited and constricted, who believe it is risky or inappropriate to let their feelings show, benefit from a gradual approach that supports greater flexibility in these inhibitory barriers. Those who tend to be more disinhibited, who believe it is important to express themselves and get their message across at any cost, may need expressive exercises that help them to contain and effectively direct their messages. For the inhibited, constructive expression typically means giving a little louder message, and for the disinhibited, it means going a little softer in tone, volume, and intensity. In addition to the experiential use of interpersonal feedback in the therapeutic relationship already noted above, the following types of activities are extremely useful in working with deeply embedded schemas.

Role Play

Role play may be used for skill development in interpersonal communications, as in "assertiveness training." When the role play involves an emotionally charged topic, dysfunctional schemas usually are activated and available for modification.

In reverse role playing, the therapist can "model" appropriate behavior, and assist the patient in reflecting on the impact of their schemas and behavioral strategies. Such reverse role playing is a crucial component of empathy training. For example, Alana, an 18-year-old student, was in a continuous state of anger toward her father, whom she regarded as "critical, mean, and controlling." She claimed, "He tries to run my life for me and disapproves of everything I do." After proper briefing, the therapist played the father role in a recent scenario in which the father had questioned her about spending money and the patient had flared up. During the role play, she had these thoughts: "You're always criticizing me!" "You don't understand me!" and "I deserve more credit!" Subsequently, they reversed roles. The patient made a strong effort to do a good job—to see the situation through her father's eyes. She was moved to tears during the role play and explained, "I can see that he wants the best for me and that includes being more accountable." She had been so locked into her own perspective that she had been unable to see his.

Schema Origins

Use of childhood material is not crucial in treating the acute phase of depression or anxiety but is often important in treating personality disorders.

Recalling experiences and reviewing childhood material opens up windows for understanding the origins of maladaptive patterns. This approach can increase perspective and objectivity. For example, a patient who kept criticizing herself, despite consistent demonstration of the unreasonableness and dysfunctionality of her beliefs, was able to attenuate her self-criticisms when she reexperienced childhood scenes of criticism. "I criticize myself now not because it's right to do so, but because my mother always criticized me and I took this over from her." Another patient realized the source of his high standards for accountability came from internalized messages about this being a primary source of worth and pride in his family. The main objective is to identify a pattern in the schema and to activate the potential for changing the pattern. Patients may feel guilty about locating blame on their family or others, which is not the point of the exercise, so they should be encouraged to place the experience in a context of understanding.

Schema Dialogues

Role-play dialogues between different schema modes such as vulnerable child and healthy adult can be a very effective way to mobilize affect and produce "mutation" of the schemas or core beliefs. Recreating "pathogenic" situations or key interactions of the developmental period often provides an opportunity to restructure attitudes that were formed during this period. Cases like this are similar to "combat neurosis": The patients need to experience an emotional catharsis in order to change their strong beliefs (Beck et al., 1985).

By role-playing a figure from the past, patients can see a "bad" parent (or sibling) in more benign terms. They can start to feel empathy or compassion for the parents who traumatized them. They might see that they themselves were not and are not "bad," but that they developed a fixed image of badness because their parents were upset and vented their anger on them. They may also see that their parents had rigid unrealistic standards that they arbitrarily imposed. Consequently, the patients can soften their own attitudes toward themselves. Or they may be able to speak more assertively to the unreasonable parent and defend their right to protection and reasonable care as a vulnerable child.

The rationale for "reliving" specific episodes from childhood may be fitted into the more general concept of state-dependent learning. To "reality test" the validity of childhood-originated schemas, these beliefs have to be brought to the surface. A schema dialogue can help patients to see that their core views of themselves were not based on logic or reasoning but were products of the parents' unreasoning reactions. A parent's statement, "You are a bother," is taken as valid and incorporated into a patient's system of beliefs—even though the patient him- or herself may not actually believe the label is justified. Reexperiencing the episode facilitates the emergence of the dominant structures (the "hot schemas") and makes them more accessible to modification.

Imagery

Another way to activate emotional components of schema is through the use of imagery. This may be particularly useful for salient memories, perhaps combined with schema dialogues. The rationale for this procedure requires some consideration: Simply talking about a traumatic event may give intellectual insight about why the patient has a negative self-image, for instance, but it does not actually change the image. To modify the image, it is necessary to go back in time, as it were, and re-create the situation. When the interactions are brought to life, the misconstruction is activated—along with the affect—and cognitive restructuring can occur.

A young woman with panic disorder and avoidant personality reported feeling particularly upset over not having done her therapy homework. The therapist asked her where the feeling was localized, and the patient said she felt it somewhere in her "stomach." The therapist then asked if she had an image in reference to what was upsetting her, and she said, "I see myself entering your office. You are larger than life; you are critical and demeaning; you are like a big authority, and will be very mad at me." The therapist then inquired when this might have occurred in the past. The patient had experienced this many times during childhood during unpleasant encounters with her mother. Her mother drank a good deal and was frequently irritable toward the child when she had been drinking. One day the child came home from school early, and her mother "blasted" her for waking her up.

The therapist asked her to re-create this experience in image form. The patient described the following image: "I came home and rang the doorbell. My mother came to the door. She looked at me. She was larger than life. She looked down and screamed at me for waking her up. She said, 'How dare you interrupt my sleep!' She said I was bad, wrong." The patient extracted from this experience (and many other similar experiences) the following: "I am a bad kid" and "I am wrong because I upset my mother." After exploring possible explanations for the mother's behavior other than the patient being a bad kid, the therapist focused on the patient's "adult mode" in dealing with this powerful memory. She "modeled" for the patient what would be an appropriate response to the mother if the child had all the maturity and skills of an adult. The patient practiced these rejoinders, with the therapist playing the role of the mother. Each time that she practiced, she became less uncertain about it until she was finally able to say it with some degree of conviction: "It's not my fault—you are being unreasonable, picking on me for no good reason. I haven't done anything wrong."

Expressing Emotions

Individuals who believe that mistakes are intolerable, that self-control is imperative, and that revealing or expressing emotions is inappropriate or dangerous may develop personality disorders where a pervasive masking of affect in social situations exacerbates loneliness, isolation and a lack of connection with others, and may contribute to a sense of self-alienation. There is some emerging evidence that behavioral exposures might be more effective for highly inhibited individuals when facilitated by practice in altering the physiology of their temperamental bias toward inhibition prior to exposure (Lynch et al., 2013). This can be accomplished by activating the parasympathetic or safety system through various soothing and expressive exercises such as deliberately exaggerating positive facial expressions, practicing expressive gestures with open hands, listening to calm music, stretching the body, and others. The effect of such exercises is to reduce physiological signals of distress and defensive mood that tend to automatically provoke negative responses from others, thus setting more optimal conditions for new learning and success in social interactions.

In addition, emotionally inhibited, overcontrolled patients may benefit from assistance in breaking through their inhibitory barriers with behavioral rehearsal of emotional expressions in sessions (Lynch, 2014). This can involve a nondemanding "practice" of exaggerated emotions, perhaps contrasting with more subtle expressions, as well as practice in expressing emotions as they might be manifested in a variety of contexts. It is important to set a rationale for such practice that explains the notion of decreasing inhibition and defensive modes, and conduct a debriefing of the patient's thoughts and self-appraisals after the exercise. Homework versions of expressive exercises might include practicing expressions in front of a mirror or with a trusted partner, for example, showing excitement upon greeting a friend. This may help patients who are anhedonic or highly negativistic become more aware of positive emotions that are simply not an active part of their emotional, cognitive, or behavioral vocabulary.

Values Clarification

Beliefs about meaning and purpose in life can be brought to conscious awareness in an emotionally charged way through personal values exercises. The most dynamic of these exercises use imagery about end-of-life events (imagining one's tombstone or eulogy) or milestone celebrations (e.g., tributes at one's 50th or 80th birthday), and may include dramatically expressive statements (e.g., stand and declare). This clarification of "what's important"—virtues or priorities in major life domains that the patient wants their actions to represent—is then tied to behavioral strategies and goals (see Strosahl et al., 2004). Exercises of this sort can help strengthen adaptive modes, as well as provide a point of entry for loosening maladaptive schemas, as in the patient who is antisocial with criminogenic values (see Mitchell, Tafrate, & Freeman, Chapter 16, this volume). Patients activate schema for prosocial values (e.g., "I value being kind and honest"), and gain perspective on how they can choose to shape their personality by expressing and "living" those values. Identified values can be used as salient cognitive reference points that are helpful in making decisions and handling challenging situations. Another popularized method of values clarification is the creation of a personal or family mission statement, which provides an alternative approach to working with these beliefs.

Attention Focus

Personality disorders also involve an inordinate amount of self-focused attention, often fixated on urges or needs, which is experienced as compelling and difficult to control, and creates a self-schema bias in information processing. Attention-based exercises that broaden awareness of detail and context facilitate a more reflective cognitive process, which helps the patient alter the defensive, self-focused thinking associated with personality problems. Activities can include monitoring and redirecting attention in specific situations (e.g., looking up and toward people instead of away from them, signaling interest over disinterest), or noticing repetitive themes such as attending to negative subjects and complaints, and then deliberately changing subjects.

Various mindfulness practices (e.g., Germer et al., 2013) can help the patient learn to disengage from the "pull" of a train of thought, and become more adept in the skill of shifting attention to different or new stimuli. Mindfulness meditations can also be used to draw attention to positive emotional experiences such as warmth and loving-kindness, or to build tolerance for more difficult emotions by taking a wider, more reflective and less reactive stance toward these internal states (Hofmann, Glombiewski, Asnaani, & Sawyer, 2011). These practices need to be selected with the patient's core schema in mind, and offered with a clinical rationale that meets with the patient's agreement. For example, a patient with dependent personality might practice being mindfully aware of uncertainty as a way to build tolerance and self-support, without immediately escaping these feelings by seeking help. A patient with narcissistic personality might benefit from loving-kindness meditation to increase his or her ability to respond with empathy toward others. The patient with paranoid personality would likely benefit from practice in relaxing his or her outward vigilance and instead noting internal body sensations, but first he or she must be engaged enough in the process of therapy to willingly do the exercise. Highly critical (of self or others) patients such as those with avoidant, obsessive–compulsive, or depressive personality disorders might also strengthen new adaptive schema through compassion-focused mindfulness practices.

CONCLUSION

The dysfunctional beliefs involved in personality disorders are thought to be deeply embedded in the person's schema for life direction, identity, and relationship attachments, and therefore extended time and effort will likely be needed for substantial change to occur. These maladaptive beliefs form a substrate for a basic orientation to reality and will continue to operate until they are modified and new, more adaptive beliefs are developed and strengthened. Cognitive treatment of the personality disorders rests on a data-based case conceptualization, where information is drawn from three main sources: the patient's current life problems, his or her developmental history, and his or her reactions to the treatment relationship. Essential data for the case conceptualization includes a sketch of the core beliefs about self and others, key assumptions and imperative beliefs, behavioral strategies, and any treatment-interfering beliefs and behaviors. Data gathering is an ongoing collaborative process that therapists lead at first, with the patient's active involvement increasing over time. Key therapist skills for managing this process include listening and following up with appropriate questions, carefully observing the patient, using cognitive probes for meaning at relevant junctures, testing hypotheses about the patient's objectives, sensitively guiding discovery in a way that keeps the patient involved and motivated to continue, and maintaining attention to the therapeutic relationship. With a sound case conceptualization, therapists can draw on a variety of techniques to alter the cognitive schema, directly build skills, or alter maladaptive behaviors, as well as identify and improve self-efficacy in emotional expression and regulation. The strategies described throughout this chapter may be used flexibly and interchangeably, and would typically be combined as the best available means for promoting adaptive and enduring change.

CHAPTER 6

The Therapeutic Alliance with Patients with Personality Disorders

Denise D. Davis
Judith S. Beck

Therapists generally need to spend significantly more time and effort developing and maintaining the therapeutic alliance with patients with personality disorders than they do with patients who have an acute disorder such as anxiety or depression with stable and adaptive premorbid personality adjustment. When treating patients with uncomplicated acute disorders, therapists need to display solid counseling skills (including empathy, genuineness, accurate understanding, and positive regard), foster a collaborative relationship, adapt their style to suit the patient, elicit and sensitively respond to patients' feedback, alleviate distress, and generally treat patients in the humane, respectful way that they themselves would like to be treated.

Patients with acute disorders often enter treatment with positive expectations of the therapist, for example, "The therapist is likely to be understanding, caring, and competent" and of treatment, "Therapy will help me feel better." These patients usually accept and welcome the therapist's guidance, without undue authority conflicts or anxiety. They trust their therapist and do not have strong doubts or concerns about how their therapist views or behaves toward them. They understand and accept responsibility for working in and between sessions and make appropriate efforts toward improvement. In response to the therapist's guidance, the patient often feels

125

warmth and gratitude, first in anticipation of relief and then in recognition of improvement. This interpersonal exchange reflects functional expectations and skills of both parties.

When therapists treat patients who have the more complex personality disorders, they need to use these same skills to enhance the alliance—but difficulties in the relationship invariably ensue. These patients often enter treatment with a different set of expectations, for example, "My therapist may hurt or criticize or try to control me" and "Therapy could make me feel worse." They bring the same entrenched, negative, overgeneralized, long-standing dysfunctional beliefs they hold about themselves and others, and the same dysfunctional interpersonal coping strategies, to the therapy setting. Because patients with personality disorders typically use their over-developed strategies in a maladaptive way with therapists, there is ample opportunity for patients and therapists to experience a range of emotional reactions to each other.

Adequately developing the therapeutic alliance requires more than just additional time. Therapists also need to be acutely attuned to patients' emotional reactions in sessions so they can quickly identify and repair ruptures in the alliance. When therapists successfully work through difficulties in the therapeutic relationship, they can help patients generalize what they have learned to improve relationships outside of treatment.

The quality of the therapeutic alliance is important. Specifically, therapists seek to build a warm and trusting relationship with patients. To do so, they must show genuine interest in patients and in their lives and a commitment to working with them to improve their well-being. They may need to help patients with personality disorders understand how to evaluate their own best interests, and do so without being pushy, dogmatic, or disrespecting the patient's autonomy. They must also especially attend to negative emotional reactions that they or their patients have, so they can identify and modify maladaptive cognitions that lead to unproductive ways of responding to each other. Therapists may need to expend considerable effort to foster trust and acceptance of the therapist's influence and to understand the how the patients' negative cognitions and coping strategies interfere with their ability or willingness to work toward therapeutic goals.

Therapists generally devote more time to asking patients who have personality disorders about their lives, inquiring, for example, about their children, spouse, job, friends, family of origin, personal history, and leisure pursuits—for several reasons. One, showing such interest demonstrates to patients that the therapist cares about them and understands the realities of the patient's life. This helps the patient build a sense of emotional involvement and trust within the therapeutic relationship, encouraging him or her to overcome avoidance and delve more fully into highly emotionally charged areas of difficulty. Two, therapist and patient may be able to detect important patterns of difficulties (in cognition, mood, and behavior) that cut across various aspects of the patient's life. Three, discussion of such topics can reveal important data (such as positive experiences and healthier relationships) and patient strengths, the identification of which is important in treatment.

Developmental history as it pertains to the patient's key problems is sometimes a recurring focus of discussion, as it may help both therapists and patients understand how the patient's dysfunctional beliefs and coping strategies originated and became maintained throughout the years, and how these beliefs and coping strategies currently interfere with the ability of patients to achieve their desired goals. Figure 8.2 (in Brauer & Reinecke, Chapter 8, this volume) illustrates a model that can be generalized to all of the personality disorders, in which the therapy discussion may fluidly shift among developmental history, current life situation, and direct personal interaction with the therapist. The process of education, skill building, and emotional support is particularly important in treating patients with personality disorders, whose negative experiences may have been associated with difficulty in acquiring and consolidating basic emotional regulation and interpersonal skills and functional beliefs concerning self-control, stress tolerance, and trust in others.

In preparing to work with patients who have personality disorders, therapists need to be especially mindful of judgmental thoughts. The very terms that are used to describe these disorders (e.g., "narcissistic," "compulsive," "dependent") carry a pejorative taint. It is difficult to take the "personal" out of "personality" when we refer to the nature of the disorder, yet very important to remain sympathetic and sensitive to how painful it is to patients when core beliefs about themselves become activated. By trying to put themselves in patients' shoes—perhaps imagining themselves with the same set of acute sensitivities and vulnerabilities—therapists can better understand their patients. At the same time, therapists need to be on guard to maintain their objectivity and remain realistically optimistic. Patient, persistent, and problem focused in a nonjudgmental context describe the desired therapist demeanor.

In schema-focused therapy, the therapist might explicitly frame the therapist's role as one of limited reparenting that provides, within professional limits, elements of the emotional nurturance and guidance that was insufficient in their developmental experience. Even when not explicitly framed in this way, it is important for therapists to maintain and communicate a benign view of patients, and continually seek to identify patient data that supports this view. Therapists may function as limited attachment figures in patients' lives, stimulating strong (positive or negative) emotions for both in their evolving relationship. Traditionally, these reactions have been termed "transference," and "countertransference." To avoid confusion with psychodynamic assumptions, we refer to these simply as patients' reactions to therapists and therapists' reactions to patients.

It is important for both therapists and patients to have realistic expectations about treatment to avoid disappointment, frustration, or discouragement. Improvement in long-standing problems may be slow and treatment may be lengthy. The optimal duration of treatment is difficult to estimate at the outset, and the rate of acute symptom remission may vary considerably. When discussing treatment, it is usually beneficial to label a patient's acute disorder. It may, however, be counterproductive to do so for a personality disorder diagnosis, as the patient may feel demeaned, helpless, or hopeless.

Although the role of the therapist may expand in treating the patient with a personality disorder, basic therapeutic boundaries should be maintained at all times. Therapists strive to remain objective and responsible for ensuring that protective limits are kept intact, especially when the patient's skill deficits are taxed or impaired beliefs are highly activated (Newman, 1997). As in any professional psychotherapy, sexual involvements are explicitly prohibited (American Psychological Association, 2002; Koocher & Keith-Spiegel, 1998). Multiple relationships, while not always unethical, carry a greater risk of harm for patients with personality disorders due to potential for confusion, misunderstanding, or interfering with therapy and thus should generally be avoided.

DIFFICULTIES IN THE THERAPEUTIC RELATIONSHIP

It is helpful for therapists to recognize that difficulties in the alliance are common when treating patients with personality disorders. Personality disorders are clinically complex and typically include impaired interpersonal functioning and limited insight or self-awareness, in addition to the acute symptoms or situational problems that may have sparked the referral for therapy. Working with these challenges is a substantial component of treatment, necessary not only to gain collaboration but also helpful in providing important learning opportunities for the patient. Armed with the theoretical skills of case conceptualization, the therapist can thoughtfully respond to the unique needs of different patient personalities. We consider it essential that therapists master the conceptual model of cognitive therapy and consistently follow the general and specific treatment guidelines offered in the other chapters of this volume.

It is difficult for many patients with personality disorders to establish a collaborative relationship with the therapist, although individual patient strengths and weaknesses can also mediate the prominence or disruptiveness of such problems. Therapists should be alert to patterns of interpersonal difficulties in session and look for common themes, such as an overpowering desire for emotional validation, a fear of emotional intensity, a pull toward self-consistency, or a moral dilemma (Leahy, 2001).

Before assuming that a problem is related to the therapeutic alliance, however, therapists should rule out other factors. Patients who miss sessions, for example, might have the dysfunctional belief "If I fully engage in treatment, I'll be letting my therapist control me." Or they may hold benign views of the therapist and of therapy, but have disorganized and chaotic lives and their therapy-interfering behavior may not be related to the therapeutic relationship at all.

Collaboration can also break down, not in relation to patients' psychopathology, but because of mistakes therapists themselves make. Therapists may, for example, be overbearing or overcontrolling. They can push patients too hard, too early in treatment. They can fail to respond to changes in patients' affect during the session. They can interrupt too much or too little. They can be too empathic or not empathic enough. They can fail to accurately understand the patient. They can act in noncollaborative ways. Review of therapy session recordings, preferably with a colleague or supervisor, is often needed to identify errors that therapists unwittingly make (J. Beck, 2005).

CONCEPTUALIZING PATIENTS' MALADAPTIVE BELIEFS AND BEHAVIORS

When problems arise, it is important to avoid broad descriptions of patients (e.g., the patient is resistant, lazy, unmotivated) but instead to specify patients' behavior (e.g., the patient has harshly criticized the therapist, insisted therapy cannot help, refused to answer questions, lied to the therapist, or demanded entitlements) and then conceptualize how the patients' core beliefs and assumptions are related to the problematic behavior.

Patients who continually say "I don't know," when their therapist tries to do collaborative problem solving, for example, may believe "If I try to find solutions to my problems in treatment, I'll fail (because I'm incompetent) but if I depend on my therapist to solve my problems, I'll be okay." This belief is usually a subset of a broader assumption: "If I rely on myself, I'll fail, but if I rely on others, I'll be okay."

Patients may fail to disclose important information because of their belief "If my therapist knows something negative about me, he will judge me harshly (because he'll find out I'm defective) but if I keep quiet about it, he'll accept me." Their broad assumption is "If people know the real me, they will hurt or reject me, but if I hide my true self, they'll accept me, at least for a time."

When patients criticize their therapist or dismiss their ideas out of hand, they may hold the belief "If I denigrate my therapist, I'll be the superior one (at least for the time being), but if I listen to him and show I value his ideas, it will mean I'm inferior." Their broad assumption is "If I act in a superior way and subordinate others, I'll be superior, but if I don't, they'll be superior and I'll be inferior." A list of therapy-interfering beliefs and behaviors for each personality disorder can be found in J. Beck (2005).

Thus many collaborative challenges are consistent with patients' particular cognitive profiles. When patients enter treatment, their negative core schemas have often been activated, and they are apt to view themselves in predictable ways, as well as to perceive their therapist through the lens of their characteristic view of others. Table 6.1 summarizes a profile-specific list of cognitions and assumptions that are apt to impact the therapeutic relationship and interaction at different points in treatment.

As can be seen in the summary, characteristic beliefs of patients with avoidant, paranoid, schizoid, and schizotypal personality disorders suggest a potential for difficulty in initial engagement and a tendency for premature termination. These individuals are highly threat sensitive and may view treatment as too threatening, for various reasons, such as "I'll be judged, hurt, humiliated, manipulated, exploited, homogenized, made to look foolish, thought weird, or locked up."

Obsessive–compulsive, passive–aggressive, dependent, and also avoidant personalities may tend to see therapists as sovereign figures and overly rely on them. These individuals also tend to be overcontrolled and can be easily threatened by perceived criticism or disappointment, resulting in premature termination after what seemed to be a promising start. On the other hand, when the relationship is successfully established, they may prolong treatment, believing that improvement is due solely to the therapist. They may catastrophize, fearing "I might fail and wreck my life," "I'll be alone and overwhelmed by feelings," "What will I do if I can't rely on my therapist?" To avoid termination, they may drift toward discussion of peripheral issues.

Patients with antisocial, borderline, narcissistic, and histrionic cognitive profiles hold expectations of others that lead to more overtly expressed conflict in the therapeutic relationship. They respond to arousal of their core self-schema in defensive ways, and attempt to engage the therapist in their overdeveloped pattern. For example, the patient who is passive–aggressive may believe "I'll be manipulated and controlled," and thus passively resist collaboration. The patient who is narcissistic is vigilant for (and often misreads) signs that the therapist will diminish him or her in some way, and may try to gain the upper hand by expecting or even demanding special considerations or favors from the therapist, becoming angry when the therapist sets reasonable limits.

The patient with depressive personality disorder might throw negative barbs at the therapist about the futility and stupidity of treatment, and then

TABLE 6.1. Cognitive Profiles and the Therapy Relationship

Personality disorder	Fearful view of others/therapist	Overdeveloped strategy	Suggested therapist stance
Paranoid	"Their scheme is to make money off me"; "They want to use me for their experiments."	Protects self by terminating early; questions motives; trusts no one	Offer short-term plan; discuss purpose, goals, and charges openly; emphasize transparency in your recommendations; use caution with the word "experiments"
Schizoid	"They want to pull me in against my wishes and will waste my time."	Passive detachment; fails to schedule, return calls; no-show	Set agenda together; emphasize efficiency; comment on respect for autonomy; space out timing of appointments; soft follow-up with calls
Schizotypal	"They are hostile to my special gifts"; "They want to make me fit in"; "They might lock me up for being crazy."	Anxiously avoids direct contact; very tentative and evasive; dissociates; exhibits hostility; pursues counterculture or unusual ways of coping	Demonstrate calm interest in patient's unusual topics; speak supportively of individuality; offer bits of self-disclosure to aid trust; provide reassurance as appropriate about nonintrusive nature of therapy
Avoidant	"They will judge and criticize me, and think I'm not worth the effort."	Anxiously discusses peripheral topics; self-deprecation; tries to hide negative emotions	Signal safety with relaxed posture; use collaborative agenda to add more central topics; ask for personal feedback; gently inquire about emotions
Dependent	"They are smarter than me and have it figured out"; "I should rely on them and do as they say."	Expresses distress; acts deferential and needy; passively depends on therapist	Shape the patient's agenda setting skills; ask for patient's ideas and provide encouragement for active problem solving; provide support in limit setting, especially if entangled in abusive relationships
Obsessive–compulsive	"They might not do things the right way"; "They need all the information to sort out the right answer."	Extremely thorough; gives overdetailed reports; trouble summarizing and shifting topics	Ask for input on setting time allotments for agenda items; provide rationale for limiting overdetailed description of problems; offer capsule summaries; ask for evaluative feedback

(continued)

TABLE 6.1. *(continued)*

Personality disorder	Fearful view of others/therapist	Overdeveloped strategy	Suggested therapist stance
Passive–aggressive	"They are trying to control me and dump all the work on me."	Surface agreement and suppressed emotions; indifferent to tasks or results; talks in circles	Empathically negotiate treatment goals; Brainstorm or cocreate homework; ask about emotions; designate a task for yourself in homework
Narcissistic	"They might not recognize how special and superior I am."	Brags and puts therapist down; focuses on self-aggrandizement; avoids taking responsibility for interpersonal problems; may have "blowups" and focus on blaming others; may terminate early	Allow patient to feel superior, especially initially; empathize with interpersonal difficulties; help patient see why it is to his or her advantage to improve his or her relationships; carefully provide rationale when setting limits; provide complimentary attention to ordinary, prosocial behaviors
Antisocial	"They might stand in my way."	Projects an image to manipulate or intimidate the therapist, either for gain or amusement; may disappear and be unresponsive to follow-up	Resist attempts to conspire in a "special" relationship; keep realistic, self-protective limits and confront intimidating behavior at low levels; consider termination if manipulation escalates
Histrionic	"They might find me boring and dull and not pay enough attention to me, or care about my feelings."	Tells dramatic stories; may escalate with complaints or demands if feeling neglected; tantrums and/or abrupt termination a possibility	Validate concern for the patient's feelings; reduce risk of abrupt termination by affirming therapist's commitment to care without the patient having to "capture" attention; try experiential methods
Borderline	"They will draw me in and then turn on me or fail to be there when I need them."	Masked emotion alternates with emotional crisis; unable to manage tension	Establish agreement on how to handle conflicts and access the therapist's support; use consultation for self-care
Depressive	"They will turn out to be idealistic, unrealistically optimistic, and disappointing."	Remains emotionally detached and skeptical of everything; critical or demeaning of therapy or therapist; gives up as effort is perceived as futile	Project curiosity and interest in possible options; use therapeutic self-disclosure to model skills for mood repair and persistence

withdraw and shut down, consumed by negative rumination. Ruptures in the alliance can result in an oblique termination where the patient simply fails to return to treatment without notice or in a complex termination where the patient storms out only to return later, threaten the therapist, or continue in a highly ambivalent state (Davis, 2008). These types of terminations and alliance ruptures are especially stressful for therapists and are best handled with attention to reflection, consultation, and self-care (Davis, 2008; Davis & Younggren, 2009).

Difficulties in the alliance can arise in the first session or in any session in which patients have negative cognitions about the therapist. Patients may, at any point, employ therapy-interfering behaviors. Occasionally, patients with personality disorders may show extreme forms of problematic behaviors that cross the line into harassment, emotional abuse, or potential physical abuse of the therapist. In such cases, therapists should conceptualize the patient's assumptions, asking themselves "What positive outcome might there be or what positive meaning does engaging in this behavior have for the patient?" For example, a patient might believe "If I harass my therapist, she won't try to make me change," or "If I make my therapist upset, it will show that I'm strong and he's weak." At the same time, the therapist should clearly label the behavior as a therapy-interfering process that cannot be allowed if treatment is to proceed (see Newman, 1997) and which may indicate a need for termination (see Davis, 2008; Davis & Younggren, 2009). Consultation with colleagues in instances of extreme patient behaviors is typically helpful for developing one's conceptualization of the collaboration challenge, generating ideas for effective contingencies that may redirect the therapy into a productive direction, and obtaining emotional support, appropriate self-protection, and plans for risk management.

IDENTIFYING AND RESOLVING
THERAPEUTIC RELATIONSHIP PROBLEMS

Difficulties in collaboration can be quite useful when their successful resolution serves as a model for patients to improve other relationships that are important to them. A difficulty in the alliance is usually apparent when patients use therapy-interfering behaviors. There are many such possible behaviors, including but not limited to persistently avoiding certain homework assignments, or avoiding homework altogether. Other therapy-interfering behaviors might involve going to great lengths to please, impress, or entertain the therapist, or insisting on relating every detail of a problem. Difficulty accepting input from others can also become therapy-interfering behavior if the patient consistently dismisses new information the therapist offers, or repeatedly questions the therapist's motives. Engaging in self-harm is also a therapy-interfering behavior that requires direct and specific attention before proceeding further.

Other therapeutic relationship problems can be identified by careful attention to patients' emotions during the session as possible indications of a reaction to something the therapist has said, done, or failed to do. Therapists should be continually alert for changes in patients' affect, facial expressions, behavior, body language, tone of voice, and choice of words that might signal that patients are feeling dysphoric, anxious, angry, disappointed, hopeless, or frustrated. Therapists might then ask patients how they are feeling and what they are thinking or reflect on the change they have observed and elicit the patient's automatic thoughts ("You're looking more distressed. What was just going through your mind?").

It is important for therapists to positively reinforce patients for expressing negative feedback, whether or not they think the patient has an accurate view. Therapists might first say "It's good you told me that," when the patient makes a negative comment or reveals negative thoughts about the therapist. Left unaddressed, patients' negative reactions can seriously undermine progress in the session. Next, therapists should, overtly or covertly, conceptualize the problem in cognitive terms and plan a strategy to ameliorate the difficulty and repair the alliance. When therapists believe they have made a mistake (e.g., they have overestimated the patient's tolerance for interruption), they can model apologizing. ("I'm sorry, I think you're right, I have interrupted you too much) and do problem solving ("How would it be, if for the next 10 minutes or so, I don't interrupt you at all? And at the end of that time, what I'd like to do, if it's okay with you, is to summarize what I heard you say so I can make sure I understood you correctly—and then we can figure out one problem you'd like to work on.")

If therapists believe that patients' negative feedback is based on misperceptions (e.g., a patient erroneously believes that the therapist is frustrated with him or her), they should still provide positive reinforcement but plan a different strategy. For example, therapists can provide direct corrective feedback ("It's so good you told me that. I'm actually not feeling frustrated at all. I know this problem with your neighbor is really complicated."). Or, through Socratic questioning, they can help patients' evaluate their thinking. ("That's an interesting idea. What evidence do you have that I'm frustrated with you? How could you find out for sure?")

When therapists do not believe they have made a mistake, they can express regret for the patient's distress, but only if they genuinely feel regretful ("I'm sorry talking about your sister made you so upset") and then collaboratively decide what to do next. They might ask for the patient's preferences on how to handle the upsetting issue ("Do you want us to leave the subject of your sister off the agenda until you want to bring it up?"), or they might offer alternatives ("Would it be better if we talked about the work problem instead in the time we have remaining?").

Some patients with personality disorders are highly reluctant to express negative feedback. When patients cannot or will not identify their automatic thoughts, therapists should gently encourage them, and normalize potential concerns: "I wonder if you were thinking that I . . ." or "Sometimes patients feel I don't understand or I'm being too directive. Do you think if you were having any thoughts like that, you'd be able to let me know so I can fix the problem?"

Finally, it is important to recognize that patients' change of affect may not be associated with negative cognitions about the therapist but instead may be about the process of therapy (e.g., "This isn't suited to me") or about themselves ("I'm too far gone for this [treatment] to help"). Interrupting the session to elicit patients' cognitions when they are having a negative emotional reaction and problem solving or responding to their cognitions may be essential before patients are able to refocus their attention on the original problem under discussion.

THERAPISTS' BELIEFS AND REACTIONS TO PATIENTS

Establishing and maintaining a friendly working relationship can be difficult and emotionally challenging, especially when therapists have unrealistic expectations for themselves or their patients. Some interpersonal behaviors of patients with personality disorders can be aversive and may trigger negative cognitions and associated uncomfortable emotions in the therapist. Although it often takes time to fully conceptualize the patient's difficulties, negative schemas and interpersonal psychopathology may impact treatment from the first meeting forward. Therapists may need to adjust their expectations if they expect that patients with personality disorders should have the same attitudes and behaviors toward them as do patients without personality disorders.

Therapists need to be alert for changes in their own affect before, during, and after therapy sessions by assessing their physical sensations, mood, body language, tone of voice, choice of words, and behavior. They may find, for example, that their body feels tense, that they avoid looking at the patient, that they skirt important issues, or talk in a commanding or hesitant tone of voice. They should monitor their emotional reactions toward patients outside of therapy, too, and address cognitions that may lead to distress or dysfunctional behavior such as avoidance of returning patients' phone calls, or unhelpful rumination.

It is useful for therapists to look each morning at the list of patients who have appointments that day and to ask themselves who they wish would not come in. These are the patients to whom they are undoubtedly having a negative reaction and it is important for therapists to address their negative cognitions before the patients enter their office. The transition time between sessions is also an important window for therapists to check their feelings about the session they have just concluded, note their sense of anticipation for the next patient, and implement any needed coping or preparation strategies. Because treating patients with personality disorders is apt to be more emotionally arousing and the relationship requires more careful attention, it is important for therapists to explicitly think about how to address their needs.

When experiencing a negative reaction toward a patient, it is helpful for therapists to ask themselves what their expectations are for the patient and also for themselves. Unrealistic expectations are bound to lead therapists to think, feel, and/or behave in unhelpful ways. As mentioned previously, if patients characteristically display interpersonal patterns such as manipulation, avoidance, suspicion, hypersensitivity, dramatic behavior, or aggression toward others, it should be expected that they may employ these same strategies with the therapist. If therapists do not expect patients to behave in this fashion, they themselves may become distressed, view the patient in a negative light, and perhaps behave maladaptively.

The alliance may also become impaired if therapists unrealistically expect that they should be able to make better progress with patients than they are able to achieve. Therapists may blame themselves, if beliefs about incompetence become activated, or they may blame their patients for a lack of improvement. Expectations for themselves may stem from a number of sources, including therapists' views of their professional role, cultural or value-related beliefs, and unique learning history, as well as from the interactions with the patient's problematic behaviors (Kimmerling, Zeiss, & Zeiss, 2000). Consultations with colleagues can help therapists develop reasonable expectations for themselves and their patients as well as improve their competence so they can be more effective with this difficult group of patients.

As working with patients with personality disorders can be especially demanding and stressful, therapists need to be aware of their own vulnerabilities and sensitivities and recognize when they may be having an overreaction due to the activation of their own dysfunctional beliefs. It is useful to recognize that these patients do not have the free choice to act in functional ways at times, given their genetic makeup, early and current experiences, distorted beliefs about themselves and others, overdeveloped coping strategies, and lack of more functional behavioral strategies. In other words, they should be difficult and pose challenges in treatment. Recognizing the emotional pain that patients experience can increase empathy and focusing on their strengths can increase hopefulness.

In addition, therapists should continually strive to increase their competence in working with patients with personality disorders. Gaining therapeutic skill in conceptualization, application of techniques, and relationship-building strategies are important. Various forms of self-care and coping skills for stress management can be useful as well. It is important to take breaks during the workday, even if they are short, for eating, relaxation, and physical activity. Outside the therapy setting, it is important to make regular opportunities for pleasant activities, exercise, social interaction, and other nurturing experiences. Many therapists find the regular practice of mindfulness to be especially helpful.

USING THE THERAPEUTIC RELATIONSHIP TO ACHIEVE THERAPEUTIC GOALS

Therapists can use a variety of strategies in the service not only of strengthening a collaborative alliance but also in achieving other therapeutic goals. They can supply data and viewpoints that are counter to patients' negative beliefs about themselves and others, provide positive relationship experiences, serve as a positive role model, and demonstrate how to solve interpersonal problems (J. Beck, 2005).

It is important for therapists to provide positive reinforcement when they uncover patients' positive qualities and when patients make changes in their thinking, mood, and behavior: "It's wonderful that you offered to help your neighbor," "I'm glad you were able to confront your coworker," "Did you give yourself credit for holding your temper?" "It's great you were able to calm yourself down," "I wish everyone would be as kind to people with disabilities as you are."

Using judicious self-disclosure can strengthen the alliance when patients feel honored that their therapist chose to share a relevant personal example. The therapist might, for example, disclose a problem and describe how he or she couldn't solve the problem until he or she gained a more realistic perspective.

Therapists can also provide a different perspective about the patient: "Well, no wonder you felt so upset. I suppose I would have felt that way, too, if I had labeled myself as 'bad' for yelling at my child and scaring him when he got too close to the street. When I did something like that, I saw myself as being a good mother for impressing on him what's dangerous and what he can't do. I certainly don't see you as bad. In fact, I'd say that's evidence that you're a good mom. . What do you think of that?"

When patients express a wish that they could have a closer, more social or familial relationship with therapists, it is important to be empathic and kind, while recognizing the limits of the therapeutic relationship. A helpful response (but only if it is genuine) might be along the lines of "I'm sorry I can't be your therapist and your friend but if I had to be one or the other, I think I'd like to be your therapist because I couldn't help you the way I have if you were my friend." Truthful statements such as "I was thinking about you this week and I realized it might help if we . . " can demonstrate that therapists still think about and feel connected to the patient even when the patient is not in their office.

In the course of time, a therapist can become a role model for patients—someone patients can emulate in showing consideration, tact, gratitude, and understanding toward their own circle of intimates and friends, and someone who cares about their best interests. Many patients have remarked how they have learned to be cool and relaxed under stress, not overreact to disappointment, think before talking or acting, or respond in a caring manner on the basis of observing the therapist's example.

As mentioned previously, therapists uncover patients' negative reactions toward them and help them evaluate their cognitions. Correcting their misappraisals of the therapist can greatly improve the alliance. Therapists can then explore whether patients have made a similar misappraisal of another person. Generalizing what they learned from correcting misperceptions and solving problems in the therapeutic relationship can help patients significantly improve interpersonal interactions and relationships outside of therapy. Patients often enter treatment believing that interpersonal problems are insoluble. Working through difficulties in the therapeutic relationship can help patients learn that interpersonal problems can be solved, given good will on both parts, and a willingness to examine one's assumptions and modify one's behavior, when indicated.

When patients display therapy-interfering behaviors in session, carefully expressed feedback by the therapist can be valuable. A therapist might say to an angry patient, for example, "It's important that you're telling me I'm not helping you enough, but it's difficult for me to think about how I might be more helpful to you when you raise your voice like this." Once the problem has been resolved, during this session or a subsequent session, the therapist might inquire whether the patient has had experiences with other people in which the patient's anger prevented him or her from getting the help he or she needed.

It is important that feedback be expressed in a calm, supportive, and useful way and that therapists carefully choose the timing of this feedback. It may be important, for example, to allow patients to self-aggrandize at the beginning of treatment. Later on, when the alliance is strong, therapists might self-disclose about the impact of the patient's aggrandizement and inquire about the impact this coping strategy has on other people who are important to the patient. Examples of empathic feedback can be found in Behary and Davis (Chapter 14, this volume) and Arntz (Chapter 17, this volume). As Arntz notes, it is important to focus such feedback on behavior, not character.

CONCLUSION

Therapists who work with patients with personality disorders need to use the same good counseling skills as they use with patients with acute disorders. But engaging these patients in treatment, gaining their collaboration, and motivating them to make difficult changes that are necessary to achieve their goals can be challenging. Spending more time gaining an overall knowledge of the patient helps foster a good alliance and provides the therapist with important information to pinpoint interpersonal difficulties and strengths. Persistence, patience, problem focus, and a nonjudgmental stance toward the patient are essential. At the same time, therapists need to maintain sufficient boundaries. When patients have difficulty collaborating, the therapist conceptualizes why the problem has arisen. If the therapist has not made a mistake, such difficulties are often related to the patient's core beliefs and assumptions about him- or herself and others, his or her ideas of what he or she must or must not do to be safe or "okay," and the patient's characteristic behavioral coping strategies. Recognizing that patients with personality disorders do not generally have much choice about how they view their interpersonal experiences and how they react can increase empathy. Helping them modify their distorted cognitions about the therapist can not only improve the relationship but can also serve as important learning experiences when identifying and evaluating their beliefs and emotional and behavioral reactions to people outside of therapy.

CHAPTER 7

Diversity, Culture, and Personality Disorders

James L. Rebeta

Personality and its disorder must be considered in light of relevant cultural perspectives if we wish to ensure that treatment is ethically framed and effectively delivered. Ascoli and colleagues (2011) aptly state that "the diagnosis of a Personality Disorder, as well as the very definition of what constitutes a 'normal personality' is entirely a cultural and social construct" (p. 53). They further contend, "Culture plays a role in the definition of the self, in the expectations on the orientation of the person (towards the individual or the social group) and in the definition of how a normal personality is constructed and expresses itself. The very difference between what is considered a normal or an abnormal personality depends on culture" (p. 53). This contextualization for anyone considered to have a personality disorder poses an even greater challenge than mere recommendation to attend to aspects of "diversity" in the patient–therapist relationship. Treatment for various symptoms or diagnoses of personality disorder is rarely discussed with emphasis on, or explanation of, any cultural limitations or influence. This chapter attempts to address these issues with further discussion of the assessment of culture and its meaning, how it can be used to inform the diagnosis of personality disorders and treatment planning, and ways to apply cognitive-behavioral interventions within a cultural framework.

CULTURE AND DIAGNOSTIC ACCURACY

The American Psychiatric Association defines personality disorders within the context of culture. This group of mental illnesses entails rigid patterns of thinking, behaving, and functioning that are long-standing and pervasive across settings. By definition, individuals with any mental disorder depart from the norms, conventions, and values of their particular family, community, and broader social network (cf. *Diagnostic and Statistical Manual of Mental Disorders, Fourth Edition: Text Revision* [DSM-IV-TR], American Psychiatric Association, 2000; *Diagnostic and Statistical Manual of Mental Disorders, Fifth Edition* [DSM-5], American Psychiatric Association, 2013). Those with personality disorders are perceived as experiencing significant distress and having difficulty with or limitations in relationships, social encounters, school setting, and the workplace. Thus, clinicians define mental disorders relative to the individual's cultural frame of reference that fundamentally mediates how the person may be experiencing and giving expression to those elements necessary for diagnosis (American Psychiatric Association, 2013).

To frame any intervention, DSM-5 provides specific guidance to address how clinicians might review an individual's cultural context, how one's background might frame the expression of symptoms, and the potential impact of cultural differences upon the therapeutic relationship. The suggested Cultural Formulation Interview (CFI) attempts to address the cultural identity of the individual—the explanatory function of culture vis-à-vis the patient's illness; the combination of facets of culture that represent both protective factors as well as sources of potential stress; real or perceived differences in culture and social status within the professional relationship that might facilitate or limit the communication of information needed to appropriately assess, diagnose, and frame possible interventions being considered; and some indication of how understanding the culture might alter the course of the evaluation and treatment (American Psychiatric Association, 2000, 2013). More pointedly, cultural considerations inform the treatment such that any behavioral changes made would be acceptable within the patient's cultural context. Although clinicians may find that the CFI provides a useful context for understanding the presentation of symptoms and the appropriate avenue for treatment, critics find its application problematic (cf. Aggarwal, Nicasio, DeSilva, Boiler, & Lewis-Fernández, 2013).

Aggarwal and colleagues (2013) conducted a DSM-5 multisite international field trial to assess perceived barriers to CFI implementation in clinical practice reported by patients and clinicians, and their findings were used to refine it. The finalized CFI purportedly represented an improvement over DSM-IV-TR's incorporation of anthropological concepts in cultural formulation into psychiatric practice. Nonetheless, Aggarwal and colleagues showed "that concepts of culture among clinicians differ markedly from concepts of culture among researchers in medical anthropology and health services" (p. 527). Arguably, any application of a cultural framework across researchers and clinicians in their respective settings would first require an understanding of what is meant by culture. Yet research to date on this subject has utilized too narrow a definition of "culture," failing to explore the true cultural context with a predominant focus on race and/or socioeconomic status. Even in this context, studies have revealed a gender and racial bias in the diagnosis of certain psychological disorders.

Moreover, "ethnicity, rather than culture, appears to be the decisive factor in defining whether patients receive traditional or cross-cultural psychotherapy" (La Roche, 2005, p. 170). Referencing Betancourt and Lopez (1993), ethnicity typically refers "to an identifiable group of people who share common nationality, language, and/or set of beliefs or values, whereas culture (citing Rohner, 1984) is understood as a variable set of meanings learned and shared by a group of people that is often transmitted from one generation to another" (La Roche, 2005, p. 170).

To put this into perspective, although the American Psychological Association defined evidence-based practice in psychology (EBPP) as "the integration of the best available research with clinical expertise in the context of patient characteristics, culture, and preferences" (APA Presidential Task Force on Evidence-Based Practice, 2006, p. 273), the inclusion of cultural considerations in any treatment intervention, especially for personality disorders, is at best a challenge. Terms—diversity, multiculturalism, and so on—are used interchangeably and often are too narrowly defined. There remains a tendency to compartmentalize populations into seemingly distinct groups and overlook the range of diversity within each one of them. And there is a paucity of research on the impact of culture and ethnicity on the diagnosis or assessment of personality disorders (Widiger & Samuel, 2005). To illustrate, DSM-5 (American Psychiatric Association, 2013) makes repeated reference to "culture-related" and "gender-related" diagnostic issues across the 10 personality disorders discussed. However, it extracts prevalence rates for three disorders from both Part II of the National Comorbidity Survey Replication (NCS-R; cf. Kessler, Chiu, Demler, & Walters, 2005) and the National Epidemiologic Survey on Alcohol and Related Conditions (NESARC; cf. Grant et al., 2004). DSM-5 then cites NESARC data alone for three additional disorders. Prevalence rates for the remaining four, including the most common (i.e., obsessive–compulsive personality disorder), are estimated from community samples or extrapolated from alcohol-related samples and the prison population. Of note, the sociodemographic NCS-R data include age, sex, race/ethnicity, education, marital status, family income, and county urbanicity. NESARC demographics include similar broad categories but, likewise, give rise to serious complications. They so stratify individuals that clinicians might interpret the data as conveying the meaning of someone's personal experience being a part of any of these groups. Any combination of these dimensions alone cannot fully capture how any individual might actually identify with and/or be seen as a member of a particular racial or ethnic group with whatever level of education, employment or employability, relational skills, and the like.

To illustrate, Tomko, Trull, Wood, and Sher (2013) suggest that presumptively different algorithms used in diagnostic rules for analyzing NESARC data by prior investigators resulted in discrepant prevalence rates for borderline personality disorder. Grant and colleagues (2004) reported a community prevalence rate of 5.9% that exceeds estimates found in other community samples (e.g., Lenzenweger, Lane, Loranger, & Kessler, 2007). In their reanalysis of NESARC data, Tomko and colleagues (2013) found that women and men met borderline personality disorder diagnostic criteria at approximately equal rates, and suggest that the previously reported, wide gender disparity may reflect the nature of the sampling—that is, clinical patients in treatment. Furthermore, they found borderline personality disorder prevalence rates to be higher for Native Americans and for blacks than for whites or Hispanics; Asian Americans reported the lowest rate of this disorder. These investigators place this finding within a key context. They note that "there are no previous epidemiological studies on BPD that allow for prevalence estimates in White, Black, Native American, Asian American, *and* Hispanic populations in the United States" (p. 12).

CULTURE AND TREATMENT EFFECTIVENESS

Research emphasizing race/ethnicity in the target clinical populations, while attempting to demonstrate intervention effectiveness, risks oversimplifying results. The clinician is significantly challenged to incorporate cultural sensitivity within a framework that must transcend the narrow definitions of "culture" available, especially if one embraces Falicov's (1995) definition:

> those sets of shared world views, meanings and adaptive behaviors derived from simultaneous membership and participation in a multiplicity of contexts, such as rural, urban or suburban setting; language, age, gender, cohort, family configuration, race, ethnicity, religion, nationality, socioeconomic status [SES], employment, education, occupation, sexual orientation, political ideology; migration and stage of acculturation (p. 5).

To these cultural diversity considerations, Muroff (2007) adds physical disability. One might also consider how individuals group themselves by social interests or standing, or reflect diverse aspects of a professional culture, such as the military or law enforcement. There are several key issues to keep in mind when applying a cultural lens to treatment conceptualization. These include the risk of misdiagnosis due to biases in ascribing clinical signs or interpreting culturally normative behavior as pathological, and the correlative tendency of certain populations to underutilize mental health services. Such attention is key for a culturally informed case conceptualization.

MISDIAGNOSIS IN SELECT CLINICAL GROUPS OF PERSONALITY DISORDERS

As one strives to diagnose within a culturally informed framework, Iwamasa, Larrabee, and Merritt (2000) provide a cautionary note, citing the considerable literature that has focused on possible sex bias of certain personality disorders. They attempt to address the confusion that may account for the seeming discrepant results in prevalence rates, citing assessment bias *versus* criterion bias. Clinicians' consistent application of certain diagnoses by sex is distinct from whether the actual criteria for each diagnosis are biased against men and/or women. Prevalence rate differences, some contend, result from assessment bias, while others assert that clinicians may apply diagnostic criteria appropriately, but differences in prevalence rates by sex derive from biased criteria. Iwamasa and colleagues proceeded to address the absence of empirical data on possible ethnicity assessment or criterion bias of personality disorders. They postulated that attitudes influence behavior, that covert prejudicial attitudes toward women and minorities persist despite reduced overt prejudice and discrimination, and that discrepant information does not alter stereotypes automatically. These investigators assessed possible ethnicity criterion bias of personality disorders using 193 Midwestern university undergraduates naive to psychological disorders. A card-sort analysis disclosed a disproportional attribution of all personality disorder criteria by ethnicity. Particular ethnic groups were systematically diagnosed as having specific personality disorders—that is, antisocial and paranoid for African Americans, schizoid for Asian Americans, and schizotypal for Native Americans. Criteria for all other personality disorders were assigned to European Americans and, for Latinos, no criteria sort resulted in any personality disorder. These authors acknowledge the limitations of this study, but the heuristic question remains: Do such perceptions reflect that certain ethnic groups are more likely to possess characteristics of select personality disorders, or do clinicians tend to attribute criteria for select personality disorders more readily to certain ethnic groups?

The importance of resolving this dilemma is illustrated by Adeponle, Thombs, Groleau, Jarvis, and Kirmayer (2012) in a Canadian study. Using

DSM-IV cultural formulation, their 10-year retrospective review of 323 patients' medical records found misdiagnosis of psychotic disorders occurring with patients of all ethnocultural backgrounds. Overdiagnosis was frequent such that, of the 70 patients initially diagnosed with a psychotic disorder, 34 patients (49%) were rediagnosed with illnesses that were nonpsychotic when clinicians with cultural expertise used DSM-IV cultural formulation. Of the 253 patients identified initially as nonpsychotic, only 12 (5%) were rediagnosed as having a psychotic disorder. Those in the former group—that is, those rediagnosed from psychotic to nonpsychotic—were more likely to be female, not black, had been referred by nonmedical professionals (social work, occupational therapy), and were more recent arrivals in Canada (residents for 10 or fewer years). Moreover, 20% of these were found to have posttraumatic stress disorder. The authors note that one-third of their sample were refugees, many from South Asia, and cite others who have noted the tendency to misidentify posttraumatic stress disorder for psychosis in migrant populations. Arguably, misdiagnosing symptomatic disorders due to inattention to cultural issues does not predict that personality disorders are subject to the same fate. However, McGilloway, Hall, Lee, and Bhui (2010) reviewed 15 studies of personality disorder and culture, race, and ethnicity. Their findings suggest that differences by race or ethnicity exist in treatment choices for personality disorders, or a personality disorder even being considered in the diagnosis, if comorbidities are present. In combination with clinical stereotype, the stage is set for inappropriate diagnosis, miscalibrated intervention, and inadequate treatment.

Paris and Lis (2012) theorize that sociocultural and historical mechanisms may influence the development of select personality disorders. They examine three mechanisms of historical changes in a culture that may inform and shape: how symptoms of distress are expressed, how social stressors impact the threshold for developing psychopathology, and how the divergence between individual temperament and social demands at different points of time and place may result in behavior construed as appropriate in one culture and as pathologic in another (cf. Alarcón et al., 2009). Paris and Lis acknowledge that data are not yet available to support their hypothesis that modernity and the rise of individualistic values provide the context for vulnerable individuals' developing—in their example—borderline personality disorder. They do provide compelling arguments for its symptom constellation and how those might be addressed in treatment. Their contentions also have key implications for a culturally informed case conceptualization.

Alarcón and Foulks (1995a, 1995b) review key concepts pertaining to culture and personality disorders and contend that culture informs the construction of self-concept and self-image, the egocentric/sociocentric dichotomy, and the determination of biases in the clinical study of personality disorders. The context of culture differentiates between the normal and abnormal, and they identify three roles that culture has in the development of psychopathology—"as an interpretive/explanatory tool; . . . as a pathogenic/pathoplastic agent; and . . . as a diagnostic/nosological factor" (1995a, p. 3). These authors highlight a basic element linked to personality—style—that is, in how the individual reacts to internal and environmental stimuli, views one's self, others, and the world, and copes with stress, problem solves, or otherwise responds. Culture can depathologize others' behavior if understood. Some behaviors determined by sociocultural contexts or specific life circumstances may be erroneously mislabeled and diagnosed as aberrant. Child-rearing practices, family based experiences, and societal influences may result in protective factors, for example, tight-knit networks of familial support, *versus* those that may leave the individual ill equipped to contend with life's demands in an age-appropriate and culturally acceptable manner.

Lewis-Fernández and Kleinman (1994) contend that anthropological concepts of culture, while able to address the cross- and intracultural complexity of human personality development and psychopathology, have yet to impact the individualistic assumptions of largely unexamined North American and Western European thinking that tends to de-emphasize the complex influence of social categories and relationships on experience. They assert that clinicians would be less prone to diagnose the adaptational strategies of inner-city minority youth to highly dangerous predatory environments as antisocial personality. Rather, clinicians might construe this situation to be the adaptive product of a different class, ethnic, and historical context.

UNDERUTILIZATION OF MENTAL HEALTH SERVICES BY SELECT POPULATIONS

Bender and colleagues (2007) have noted the lacunae in our understanding of the etiology and treatment of select personality disorders with severe manifestations. Drawing from their own and others' work, they note that patients with select personality disorders utilize more mental health treatment than do those with major depression without personality disorder, require more inpatient and medication interventions over time, but may tend to discontinue treatment prematurely with minimal functional improvement. Alluding to the disproportionately greater unmet needs among those with personality disorders, for example, risk of harm to self and others, these authors question the adequacy of their treatment and whether barriers exist to appropriate care. Their naturalistic, longitudinal study of over 500 participants with personality disorders (white [n = 396], African American [n = 78], Hispanic [n = 73]) disclosed that white subjects were significantly more likely to receive a range of inpatient and outpatient psychosocial treatments and medications than minority participants, especially Hispanics. This result may underestimate the actual discrepancy because these participants were either treatment seeking or had some prior treatment. These authors raise a host of questions prompted by such findings, for example, the experience with the mental health system that may prompt select minorities—that is, African Americans—to seek treatment in primary care settings; attitudes toward medications among diverse cultural groups that, in turn, may have different metabolic effects within and across groups; and culturally shaped attitudes about relationships such as the importance of trust that would impact the nature of the therapeutic relationship in different ways within ethnic groups, such as Hispanics or Caucasians.

IMPORTANCE OF CULTURALLY INFORMED CASE CONCEPTUALIZATION

Increasingly many contend that cultural competence represents one of "the most important initiatives in health care in the United States and throughout most of the world" (Purnell, 2013, p. 3). Clinicians who endeavor to provide care that is both culturally competent and empirically supported may find that this aspiration poses a thicket of significant clinical challenges. The clinical utility of empirically supported psychological interventions presupposes the clear identification, definition, and feasibility of the treatment. Moreover, patient acceptance and compliance impact any extent to which an intervention may benefit (Chambless & Hollon, 1998). Bernal, Jiménez-Chafey, and Domenech Rodríguez (2009) focused on the dilemma of providing greater evidence-based uniformity of care through research on treatment development, efficacy, or effectiveness, although cautioned against the potential unintended consequence of promoting a systematized one-size-fits-all approach to interventions. Attending sufficiently to the case conceptualization from initial session and throughout treatment to surface those diverse cultural dimensions that are present uniquely in a patient is one important way that this dilemma might be resolved. Thus, cultural considerations can be integrated within the cognitive model through adaptations based on specific cultural dimensions that are assessed and in collaboration viewed as most relevant. There are many ways this can be achieved, and this is a developing literature. To illustrate, this discussion highlights only a few of these possibilities applied in symptomatic disorders.

For anxiety and depression in geriatric patients, Paukert and associates (2009) recommend integrating religious beliefs and behaviors into cognitive-behavioral therapy (CBT), based on empirical literature concerning which aspects of religion affect mental health.

In the case of a depressed fundamentalist Christian client, Hathaway and Tan (2009) applied a religiously oriented mindfulness-based CBT. At one point in the therapy, the patient was encouraged to be mindful of "inviting" God into dialogue with her about the distressing thoughts and feelings she had through meditating on God's presence during the mindfulness activity and communicating with God during that time. This did not detract from the core elements of CBT but, rather, refined the particular techniques being used to be more relevant, meaningful, and culturally appropriate to this particular individual in this specific context.

Similarly, a culturally sensitive manualized CBT for individuals in Pakistan was effective in reducing symptoms of depression and anxiety, using folk stories and examples from the life of the Prophet Muhammad and Quran to clarify teachings (Naeem, Waheed, Gobbi, Ayub, & Kingdon, 2011). Hinton, Rivera, Hofmann, Barlow, and Otto (2012) describe how relaxation imagery and exposure were adapted for posttraumatic stress disorder in different groups of traumatized refugees and ethnic-minority patients. CBT has also been adapted to the Kenyan culture for alcohol treatment (Papas et al., 2010).

Culturally informed CBT adaptations have also been advocated to address psychotic symptoms. From a qualitative study of ethnic-minority groups (African Caribbean, Black African, Black British, and South Asian Muslims) including patients with schizophrenia, and therapists, using semistructured interviews and focus groups, Rathod, Kingdon, Phiri, and Gobbi (2010) concluded that CBT would be an acceptable treatment if culturally adapted—that is, by incorporating culturally based patient health beliefs and attributions concerning psychosis. A recent quantitative study with a small sample of participants with a schizophrenia-group diagnosis ($n = 33$) showed that subjects in the group using culturally adapted CBT for psychosis achieved statistically significant results posttreatment compared with the group receiving treatment as usual, with a select sample maintaining gains at 6-month follow-up, and reported high levels of satisfaction (Rathod et al., 2013).

CULTURALLY INFORMED COGNITIVE THERAPY FOR PERSONALITY DISORDERS

Case examples of culturally informed treatment might indicate the complexity and challenge for the clinician. Amy is a 34-year-old female who, born and raised in the mountains of West Virginia, has been married for 18 years. She, her husband, 41, and their four children, ages 18, 17, 15, and 9 years, now live in a small Midwestern city. Urged by her elder daughter, who works and lives outside the family home, and her own physician, Amy presented at a community mental health clinic somewhat befuddled as she insisted from the outset that her problem was "migraines." None-theless Amy proceeded with the evaluation. She disclosed that marriage was "the solution" to her first pregnancy at which time she dropped out of school. Her husband worked, and preferred that Amy stay home to raise the children, and she agreed because she perceived herself to be lacking in employable skills. Amy recalled that migraine headaches began to occur after the birth of her third child. So, too, did the marital conflict. Her husband repeatedly complained about her not controlling the children, not having meals on the table when he returned from work, and running up the telephone bill due to daily, long-distance calls to her older sister for advice. She denied physical abuse, but feared that someday, when he finished yelling, he would lose control. She felt "stupid." The clinician might interpret such a clinical picture as warranting consideration of dependent personality disorder.

However, to put this into a cultural context, the collaborative empiricism entailed in generating a case conceptualization might elicit Amy's sense of neediness, weakness, and incompetence in any of the roles she has—wife, mother, let alone potential employee. Her core beliefs—for example, "I'm stupid"—seem to dictate her insatiable need for reassurance, for instance, in reaching out daily to her sister. She is content to have her husband handle all finances. She may disclose her fantasy of working outside the home, but cites her husband's caustic and biting response when she once attempted to broach the subject by alluding to school "extras" that their youngest wanted, but she could not afford with the household money provided. She voices frustration in the marriage, but reflects fatalism that nothing better is possible for her. Their limited socializing gives her scant evidence for even considering such an alternative. The passivity that she displays may be coupled with the clinician's sense that Amy is looking for an immediate cure for migraine headaches, as she came to treatment only after having spoken with her mother and then her sister about herbal cures, then resorting to television-advertised over-the-counter symptom remedies, and only then approaching a pharmacist—the first "medical" professional to be contacted for a recommendation. Her episodic dash to an urgent care center for "something to ease the pain" tended to reinforce her belief that only someone else has the "cure" she desperately needs. The clinician might reasonably anticipate that engaging this patient will require persistent attention to the meaning of her Appalachian heritage—for example, the patriarchal structure within families and a woman's role therein, a rugged individualism and valued self-sufficiency, reliance upon folk medicine practices, a dour sense of fatalism and reluctance to seek medical help until one is in dire straits, and even then expecting immediate relief (cf. Huttlinger, 2013). Otherwise, reframing her reliance upon others' decision making, striving toward more realistic self-expression, and developing her own skills and interests may pose a seeming challenge to Appalachian values of individualism and nonassertiveness. One might anticipate that key treatment goals may alternate between more independent functioning through the acquisition of skills that increase her social contacts and interdependent support and more limited, but healthier dependence. The latter is likely to be experienced in her therapy that, nonetheless, focuses on increased self-reliance.

On the other hand, a different scenario might unfold if the prospective patient were Kyle, a 24-year-old, German American Nebraska farm boy who only finished high school to have the requisite diploma to enlist in the U.S. Marine Corps. Kyle's immediate and extended family at home is multigenerational and numerous. Only higher education dictated anyone's relocating for any length of time. Community and order are valued, as is "being in control" of oneself. Further aided by the proximity of family members in any time of crisis, individualism, self-reliance, and initiative are not fostered (cf. Steckler, 2013). Kyle adaptively acculturated to the prescribed order, emphasis upon honor and duty, and the value placed on work in the Corps. He received laudatory marks in proficiency and conduct, with few negatives. His friends are relatively few and from those to whom he keeps close, he seems to seek repeated assurances and takes little initiative. He follows orders and, in the opinion of superior officers, does so with precision. However, in one, then another, combat situation that required his immediate initiative, he "froze" as he reported later when confronted. A psychiatric evaluation was ordered. From the outset, Kyle's responses were concrete and unelaborated. The evaluator noted Kyle's almost excessive consciousness of military rank in their interaction.

In this instance, the eagerness to please may pose conflicts as self-disclosure of any negative or critical associated thoughts and beliefs may be perceived as leading to catastrophic consequences—that is, discharge from the Corps. Culturally and temperamentally, Kyle is not likely to tolerate well confrontations and interpretations of his dependency needs and behaviors. Time spent validating the institutions key to him—family and the Marines—is necessary. Such effort would support a therapeutic alliance sufficient to prompt more than passive compliance in his collaborative work. This will entail his exploring the various triggers of thought, affect, and behavior patterns that result in radically increased stress and immobilization, when more independent, self-reliant action is required. As such patterns begin to change with increased autonomy and interdependency, he may ultimately be able to engage the incompetence and failure-to-achieve schemas that he manifests. Replacing fears of abandonment with improved social interaction, self-mastery, and increased interdependence may engender more realistic hopes within the military, including possible advancement and opportunity within his scope of interests and expertise.

CONCLUSION

Understanding the long-standing and pervasive inflexible patterns of thought and behavior that represent significant departures from what is acceptable within the individual's cultural context (American Psychiatric Association, 2013) requires consummate patience and restraint. The clinician might note the essence of the question that Paul (1967) had pressed psychotherapy outcome researchers to adopt—that is, "*What* treatment, by *whom*, is most effective for *this* individual, with *that* specific problem, and under *which* set of circumstances?" (p. 111). Evidence-based clinical practice focuses great attention on the case conceptualization at the beginning of treatment to surface those diverse cultural dimensions that are present in a unique constellation in each patient.

Given the complexity and subtlety entailed in culturally informed treatment, however, the clinician must forgo all assumptions and premature interpretations to facilitate this individual's communicating the content of the stress as it is experienced and within what contexts it emerges. To provide culturally acceptable interventions, the clinician must remain conscious of the powerful influence of clinical stereotypes and therapist–patient perceptions as they impact the therapeutic alliance. To fail to do so risks misunderstanding the patient and overlooking potential supports to treatment within the person's cultural world and, conversely, the overt threats to its acceptance. The importance of such clinical attunement cannot be understated.

As we have seen, the disproportionately greater unmet needs among those with personality disorders and risks to which they are subject have prompted many to question the adequacy of their treatment. Providing culturally appropriate care means that giving even serious attention to any CFI alone is insufficient. It cannot supplant the clinical acumen, sensitivity, and informed thoroughness of the clinician who strives to understand and treat that culturally unique individual patient in need of assistance.

PART II

CLINICAL APPLICATIONS

CHAPTER 8

Dependent Personality Disorder

Lindsay Brauer
Mark A. Reinecke

Sara was a 26-year-old single woman with 16 years of education. She was employed as a secretary at a physician's office, and sought treatment due to recurrent, moderately severe feelings of depression, anxiety, and loneliness. She complained that her boss didn't give her enough direction to do the work that was expected of her, and this made her constantly worry about her performance and the possibility of losing her job. At the same time, she perceived herself as "completely dedicated" and knew that her boss appreciated all the little things she did for him that were "above and beyond" what was expected. But her feelings of depression and anxiety were long-standing in nature, dating back to her early childhood. As she stated, "I never felt really happy growing up." The results of a diagnostic interview indicated that Sara met criteria for major depression—recurrent, dysthymic disorder, and dependent personality disorder (DPD). Although she stated that she felt tense and anxious much of the time, she had no history of specific phobias, obsessive–compulsive disorder, panic, or posttraumatic stress disorder. Rather, she described herself as "a real worrier," noting that she "was always afraid of something . . . I'm just anxious all through the day, a lot of times for no reason."

Sara was the youngest of five children, and recalled having felt "lost and forgotten" as a child. When asked to elaborate, she noted that she was a "shy girl," and that she frequently played alone in her room. She reported that her mother was "just depressed and stressed . . . she was worn out," and that "I never thought she really loved me." Sara had little to say about her father, other than to note that he "worked hard to support us all" and

155

"always came home late." She characterized him as authoritarian, noting that he "wanted things done the right way . . . we had to follow the rules." Her family was highly religious, and structured their life around the dictates of their church and needs of their church community. Her statements are interesting in that they are congruent with recent research on cognitive, biological, and social factors contributing to risk for DPD. Sara's comments suggest, for example, that she may have manifested characteristics of inhibited temperament, and that her mother may have been depressed or anxious. Her parents may, in some ways, have been emotionally unavailable to her, which she experienced as an insecure attachment. Moreover, the possibility exists that her parents did not serve as effective models of affect regulation, and that their home environment was characterized by a more controlling parenting style. In this context, strict adherence to cultural rules for dependence on religious authority further contributed to the risk of DPD. Sara's descriptions of her life not only illuminate factors contributing to her distress, they suggest a path forward.

CLINICAL SIGNS AND SYMPTOMS

Dependency may be defined as an excessive need to rely on others for support, guidance, nurturance, and protection (Bornstein, 2012b). Individuals with DPD report significant levels of anxiety, triggered by making everyday decisions, initiating and completing tasks, and perceived rejection by others (American Psychiatric Association, 2013). To regulate this distress, they seek guidance, reassurance, and support. They often relinquish control over daily aspects of their lives, as seen by asking for advice on what to have for breakfast, what to wear, or what time to schedule an appointment. They often feel helpless on their own. Thus, seeking support is a means of reducing anxiety related to the perceived immensity of caring for one's self. In other instances, support-seeking behaviors may be motivated by a desire to attain approval from others (Bornstein, 2005; Bornstein, Riggs, Hill, & Calabrese, 1996). Social approval is rewarding as it may provide an individual with DPD a sense of worth and likability. Two sets of beliefs are central to the cognitive model of DPD—personal ineffectiveness and a view of the world as dangerous. Given these beliefs, the individual with DPD comes to feel vulnerable and becomes attuned to signs of risk in his or her environment. Based on these beliefs they come to develop an adaptive assumption: "If I have the support and protection of others, I can feel secure." Dependent behavior, as such, stems from the development and activation of dependent beliefs.

Given their dependence on others, individuals with DPD become fearful at anticipated signs of abandonment and engage in behaviors to avert anticipated ruptures. These behaviors can range from submissive to overtly aggressive (Bornstein, 2012a; Murphy, Meyer, & O'Leary, 1994). Should these relationships end, individuals with DPD search for new relationships on which they can depend. Turning to others for protection, however, precludes them from having experiences that might allow them to experience the success of coping with life's challenges. A feed-forward process is put into play in which dependent behavior facilitates the strengthening of dependent beliefs. Clinical signs of such beliefs might be evident in complaints such as Sara's about her boss's lack of direction, or other helpless responses to situations where one would ordinarily expect reasonable competence or mastery. For example, the dependent individual might turn over all aspects of decision making to the therapist, such that he or she has significant trouble deciding when or how often to schedule appointments, or what to contribute to the agenda. This behavior should be judged by how extreme it is in the context of the individual's reasonable capability, in contrast with other normative expectations. DPD stands out as distinctly more helpless or inhibited than usually encountered with individuals who are depressed or anxious. The individual with DPD is fearful of self-assertion to the point of compromising normal development and core self-esteem. Adults may struggle with difficulty in asserting themselves within their family in important areas such as values and/or finances, allowing intrusive or controlling parents to dictate their standard of living, career choice, or religious adherence.

DIFFERENTIAL DIAGNOSIS

DPD is not uncommon. Epidemiological studies indicate that it has a prevalence of between 0.4 and 1.5% in the general population (Grant et al., 2004; Samuels et al., 2002; Torgersen, Kringlen, & Cramer, 2001), and 1.4 and 2.2% in community outpatient samples (Mattia & Zimmerman, 2001; Zimmerman, Rothschild, & Chelminski, 2005). These estimates may be conservative inasmuch as DPD often co-occurs with a symptomatic disorder (Paris, 1998), particularly depression (Bockian, 2006), anxiety (Ng & Bornstein, 2005), and eating disorders (Bornstein, 2001). Although some may expect there to be a strong link between DPD and substance abuse, the findings are inconsistent (Disney, 2013). Bornstein (2011) suggested that dependency did not promote substance abuse, but rather dependency was a consequence of substance abuse. This information suggests that individuals with DPD may not be uniquely vulnerable to substance abuse. Instead, the disorders likely share a common feature, such as affect dysregulation, which then promotes substance abuse and dependency behaviors. Despite these distressing symptoms, a common reason individuals with DPD seek treatment is to address the impact of their dependent behaviors on family members, friends, and coworkers (Bornstein, 2012a; Paris, 1998).

CONCEPTUALIZATION

The possibility exists that, like other forms of psychopathology, DPD may be multiply determined. Genetic, biological, environmental, and developmental factors may all play a role. Preliminary evidence suggests, for example, that infants and toddlers with an "inhibited" temperament type may be at risk for developing a range of conditions, including anxiety disorders, avoidant personality disorder, and DPD (Bornstein, 1992, 2012a; Paris, 1998). Moreover, recent research suggests that DPD may be moderately heritable (Torgersen, 2009; Torgersen et al., 2000). Early experience also may play a role—correlations have been observed between attachment security and risk for DPD (Brennan & Shaver, 1998; West, Rose, & Sheldon-Keller, 1994). Along the same lines, it has been proposed that overprotective, controlling, or authoritarian parents contribute to the development of DPD (Bornstein, 1992, 2012a; Hend, Baker, & Williamson, 1991; McCranie & Bass, 1984). A study by Thompson and Zuroff (1998) examined the reaction of anxious mothers to their daughter's demonstration of competence in performing a study task. Interestingly, when their daughters succeeded, anxious mothers often responded with criticism. When their children performed poorly, however, they received support and guidance from their mothers, suggesting that a reinforcing cycle may exist between parenting practices and the development of behavioral competencies during early childhood. Together, these factors may provide an experience of an inability to tolerate and regulate emotions, as well as a belief that it is necessary to rely on others to survive. As a result, individuals with DPD have limited experience in effectively caring for themselves, reinforcing the reliance on others. It is worth acknowledging that much of this research is correlational or employed retrospective designs.

The cognitive-developmental model suggests that maladaptive cognitions, negative affect, and support-seeking behaviors reciprocally reinforce one another to promote DPD patterns. Based on early developmental experiences, individuals experience negative affect as intolerable and fail to develop effective strategies for modulating their own emotional experience. Infants and toddlers mainly use simple strategies, such as shifting their attention away from an upsetting stimulus or event, to manage their distress. Should these simple strategies fail, they whimper, cry, or become clingy, eliciting the support of their caregivers. Much of the responsibility for affect regulation at these early ages, then, rests with the caregiver. Over time, as language capacity develops, responsibility for managing negative moods gradually shifts to the child and, ultimately, the teen and adult. In individuals with DPD, however, this normative developmental process may go awry if self-soothing thoughts and self-instructions fail to become internalized. The belief that negative moods are intolerable, and that "I can't cope, I *have* to have support to get through this" is reinforced by the experience of relief of negative affect through external support. Second, others are perceived as competent protectors who serve to reduce negative affect. As parents of individuals who develop DPD commonly demonstrate an authoritarian, controlling, or overprotective parenting style, these children typically have limited experience in learning more sophisticated, language-mediated ways to self-soothe. In addition, they are likely rewarded through comfort and praise for seeking support from caretakers.

Finally, individuals with DPD come to view the world as a dangerous place. Viewing others as (at least potentially) benevolent, supportive, and effective, they turn to them for support. Feelings of anxiety increase, as a consequence, when support is unavailable or the individual is asked or expected to function independently. We hypothesize that this would be most common in complex or ambiguous situations, situations in which the availability of support is unclear, or when the individual is confronted by an unfamiliar or difficult task. Should supportive relationships end, individuals with DPD will engage in attempts to reengage the supporter or find alternative means of support. By automatically seeking support as negative affect arises, individuals do not provide themselves with opportunities to challenge their negative perceptions of their ineffectiveness, incompetence, and inability to care for themselves. A cognitive-developmental model of DPD is presented in Figure 8.1.

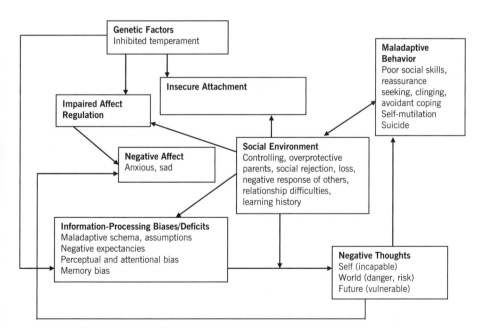

FIGURE 8.1. Cognitive-developmental model of DPD.

The motivation to rely on others for support is thought to be complex. In some instances, individuals with DPD believe they are incompetent, ineffective, and inept in managing their own lives (Bornstein, 2012a). Seeking guidance and support is a means of reducing anxiety related to the perceived immensity of caring for one's self. In other instances, support-seeking behaviors may be motivated by a desire to attain approval from others (Bornstein, 2005b). Social approval is rewarding as it may provide an individual with DPD a sense of worth and desirability, as well as safety in the world. Two sets of beliefs are central to the cognitive model of DPD—personal ineffectiveness and a view of the world as dangerous. Given these beliefs, the individual with DPD becomes attuned to signs of risk and comes to develop an adaptive assumption: "If I have the support and protection of others, I can feel secure." Dependent behavior, as such, stems from the development of dependent beliefs about self, others, and the world.

KEY TREATMENT GOALS

We propose that DPD represents a deviation from normative developmental processes of acquiring affective, social, and behavioral competencies necessary for autonomous functioning. We further propose that biological, cognitive, developmental, and social factors reciprocally interact over the course of development in placing individuals at risk for DPD. With this in mind, there are numerous opportunities for clinical intervention. Interventions might, for example, focus on developing affect regulation, social skills, or behavioral competencies; changing maladaptive beliefs and expectations; or changing social interaction patterns to apply skills more effectively in context. As factors underlying and maintaining DPD vary from individual to individual, and the presence of comorbid conditions may complicate treatment, it is important to develop a clear and parsimonious case conceptualization that can be shared with the individual and which can serve as a guide for treatment. Factors of interest include:

1. *Maladaptive beliefs about the self and world.* As noted, beliefs about personal ineffectiveness and beliefs about the world as a dangerous place are key areas to target for cognitive modification. Maladaptive self-statements (e.g., "I brought this on myself," "These things always happen to me") may not be entirely unfounded, as low self-efficacy tends to drive dependent behaviors and negatively impact social relationships. Testing these beliefs and assumptions is central to the treatment for DPD.

2. *Developmental history.* A collaborative review of an individual's developmental history provides insight as to how maladaptive beliefs were developed and dependent behaviors perpetuated. During discussion, the

clinician can highlight how parenting styles could interfere with the development of secure attachment, limiting independence and fostering specific dependent attitudes and behaviors in significant relationships.

3. *Affect regulation.* Individuals with DPD typically rely on support seeking as an emotion regulation strategy. Thus, alternative, more adaptive strategies for managing negative emotions—strategies that enhance their sense of competency and effectiveness, are an important treatment target.

4. *Dependent behaviors in context.* Passive, submissive behavior and excessive reassurance seeking (Joiner, 2000) are forms of dependent behavior that increase the risk of social rejection and depression. Specific behavioral patterns, and how they can affect relationships with others, are quite important treatment issues for individuals with DPD. The key goals are generally to increase appropriate assertiveness and reduce clinging, reassurance seeking, and oversolicitous actions that annoy others and undermine the individual's self-confidence. Context and interpersonal effectiveness are both important in altering these behaviors, as certain discrete behaviors may constitute important relationship skills when applied in a receptive context, and with more relaxed and assertive communication skills.

Overall, the treatment goal for DPD is to (1) challenge maladaptive beliefs of ineffectiveness and vulnerability by discussion of parenting styles as separate from childhood abilities; (2) understand how maladaptive beliefs and dependent behaviors functioned during childhood, but are maladaptive during adulthood; (3) develop affect regulation strategies that also provide experience of self-efficacy; and (4) develop behavioral strategies to promote independence and appropriate social relationships. Successful treatment of DPD alters the quality of the way that the individual engages with others, driven less by anxiety, fear, and insecure attachment and more by self-direction. Optimally, the individual will give greater attention to previously neglected matters of self—self-direction, self-respect, self-confidence, self-expression, self-exploration, and self-interest—while also using improved skills to meet his or her basic need for attachment security.

COLLABORATIVE STRATEGY

A warm and individual approach is especially important with the individual with DPD, as relatively controlling, emotionally unavailable, demanding, or intrusive caretakers shaped his or her emotional world. This individual is apt to be highly sensitive to perceived demands and the potential for criticism from the therapist, but unlike the individual who is avoidant, will view the therapist as friendly and helpful rather than threatening and critical. In fact, individuals who are dependent may go overboard in flattering and praising the therapists' skill. Because the individual with DPD will endeavor to become the ideal patient, there are several advisements to keep in mind in beginning and maintaining the therapeutic relationship. Warmth and patience are essential, but must be tempered by objectivity and therapeutic focus.

Individuals who are dependent can easily evoke a friendly, flattering, even caretaking stance toward the therapist, and this can cause blurring of interpersonal and therapeutic boundaries. They may not be especially sexually seductive unless there are also some histrionic tendencies, but will idealize and strive to please the therapist. It may be necessary to discourage their attempts to bring gifts or other nurturing efforts (e.g., fluffing your sofa pillows or picking up your trash). In the course of therapeutic interaction and dialogue, it's very important to encourage their autonomy of thought and behavior. This is the individual who needs his or her therapist to pause and ask "What do you think?" before offering suggestions. The individual with DPD may respond very well if given specific instructions, perhaps in a handout form, on the individual's collaborative role in therapy. This helps to set expectations for his or her active participation from the very beginning, and prompts his or her independent efforts in agenda setting, mood reporting, and problem selection. It also demystifies the process of what is to happen in sessions, so he or she is a bit less likely to take on the submissive individual role. Finally, asking for feedback at the end of sessions is an important tool in fostering a sense of shared power and authority.

CLINICAL APPLICATION OF THE INTERVENTION

We propose a multicomponential treatment beginning with a thorough assessment, followed by cognitive and behavioral interventions, as well as the development of affect regulation skills.

Assessment

We begin with a careful assessment, confirming the diagnosis of DPD and clarifying whether the individual manifests symptoms of other conditions. Several semistructured diagnostic interviews have been developed and might be considered, including the Structured Clinical Interview for DSM-IV Axis II Personality Disorders (SCID-II; First, Gibbon, Spitzer, Williams, & Benjamin, 1997) and the Personality Disorder Examination (PDE; Loranger, 1989). In addition to diagnosis, the individual's current mood and use of nonsuicidal self-injurious behaviors should be assessed. This information is helpful not only to assess severity and risk but also proves useful in understanding the emotional state and means of self-regulation. Objective self-report questionnaires can facilitate this process.

The Beck Depression Inventory–II (BDI-II; Beck, Steer, & Brown, 1996), Beck Anxiety Inventory (BAI; Beck & Steer, 1993a), Beck Hopelessness Scale (BHS; Beck, 1988a), the Beck Scale for Suicide Ideation (SSI; Beck, 1991), and the Columbia–Suicide Severity Rating Scale (Posner et al., 2011) are psychometrically strong and clinically useful. As DPD often co-occurs with other conditions, it can be helpful to complete a lifetime diagnostic interview to determine whether the individual has a history of affective or anxiety disorder.

An individual's developmental history, specifically a review of family history, relationships, and development, are primarily accomplished through clinical interview. With regard to childhood factors that may have promoted dependency, one might ask about shyness and inhibition, perception of parents, and response to new or challenging situations. Brief self-report questionnaires, such as the Inventory of Parental Bonding Instrument (PBI; Parker, Tupling, & Brown, 1979) and the Adult Attachment Scale—Revised (AAS-R; Collins & Read, 1990) can be useful in identifying themes and experiences for discussion. The PBI assesses an individual's recollections of parental caring and protection, whereas the AAS-R assesses fears of being abandoned or rejected, comfort with emotional closeness, and perceived dependability of others. Quite often, individuals are able to provide a narrative, to describe the experiences that support their feelings of vulnerability and the value of their dependent behavior. Although the information gleaned from these measures is retrospective, they provide insight into individuals' *current* perceptions of their relationships and their upbringing. As a result, the individual and clinician can discuss factors that promoted a schema of dependency, identify factors that maintained dependency behaviors and beliefs, and highlight examples of how, although adaptive in the individual's developmental environment, these beliefs and behaviors may not be so in his or her current environment. The process of exploring the developmental narrative and current self-report also facilitates a therapeutic relationship that is supportive and motivating, yet not undermining of the individual's ability and independence.

Finally, it can be helpful to assess specific beliefs, attitudes, and perceptions associated with DPD. Objective self-report rating scales, including the Young–Brown Schema Questionnaire (Schmidt, Joiner, Young, & Telch, 1995; Young, 1990), the Personality Disorder Belief Questionnaire (PDBQ; Arntz, Dreessen, Schouten, & Weertman, 2004), and the Personality Belief Questionnaire (PBQ; Beck et al., 2001) can be useful in this regard.

Cognitive Interventions

Individuals with DPD frequently view themselves as incompetent, ineffective, and vulnerable. They view the world as dangerous, and believe they need the support of others. Standard cognitive-behavioral therapy (CBT) techniques, including mood monitoring, rational disputation, and behavioral experiments, can be helpful in testing the validity and utility of maladaptive beliefs associated with DPD. Our clinical experience has been that individuals often recognize that these beliefs are not entirely reasonable, and that their actions "aren't working for me." That said, they experience difficulty developing a viable alternative narrative—another way of looking at their current experiences and of understanding their history. An individual, thoughtful approach is useful in developing this new narrative. To be sure, this can be accomplished through a rational examination of the validity of the individual's beliefs in the here and now with respect to current situations (as is commonly done in CBT for depression or anxiety). We also facilitate this process by examining the validity of the individual's perceptions of his or her experiences as a child (a "developmental analysis" of his or her beliefs) and the ways in which these beliefs are manifested within the therapeutic relationship, forming a tripartite approach (Figure 8.2). Simultaneously using three sets of CBT techniques—rational analysis, developmental analysis, and examination of beliefs within the therapy relationship—offers the best chance of changing long-standing maladaptive beliefs and assumptions. The individual is given a model, a rationale for understanding how these beliefs developed over the course of his or her life and of how his or her behavior maintains them. The maladaptive beliefs are then challenged and areas of competency, effectiveness, and worth are identified.

Behavioral Interventions

A central focus in CBT for DPD is the development of adaptive behavioral skills. Understandably, individuals may be hesitant to demonstrate competence for fear that they may lose social support and acceptance. The development of interpersonal effectiveness skills may help to reduce this apprehension. In addition, many individuals with DPD seek treatment due to distress their dependency causes others. As in CBT for anxiety, individuals

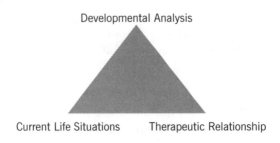

Developmental Analysis

Current Life Situations   Therapeutic Relationship

FIGURE 8.2. Therapeutic triad in CBT for DPD.

are encouraged to approach the things they fear, behave in a more assertive or courageous manner, and note how others respond. As in CBT for anxiety and depression, the development of behavioral skills is done in a systematic, graduated manner. Modeling by the therapist, role play during sessions, *in vivo* practice, and observations of others who are more assertive and autonomous all can be used. Explicit attempts are made to increase awareness of and discourage the maladaptive behaviors, such as excessive reassurance seeking. For example, we worked with a young woman who repeatedly sought reassurance that she was smart. Inasmuch as she had graduated from a prestigious medical school, there was no reason to believe she wasn't "smart." First, we identified this behavior as a form of reassurance seeking and explained that it had the undesirable effects of undermining her self-confidence, and encouraged others to see her as insecure. Over the course of therapy we examined the meaning of this belief for her, evidence of its validity, and the effect of her repeatedly seeking reassurance on her relationships. As important, however, was our collaborative decision to make the therapist's office a "no-reassurance zone." She initially found this exceedingly difficult, and pleaded with the therapist (5–10 times an hour) to reassure her that she was smart. Moreover, she was encouraged not to seek reassurance from others outside of therapy and to observe the effects of this change on her mood and relationships. The opportunity for her to see improvements in her relationships as she behaved in a less dependent manner was an important motivator for further change.

Affect Regulation

Seeking reassurance is but one way of coping with anxiety associated with DPD. Developing a broader range of skills for tolerating negative moods (e.g., mindful acceptance), coping with stressful situations (e.g., social problem solving, assertiveness training), and managing negative moods (e.g., relaxation, rational disputation, schema-focused CBT) all can be helpful. Strategies to challenge negative self-thoughts (i.e., examination of evidence, behavioral experiments, identification of positive or desirable aspects of the self) and interpersonal effectiveness skills may assist the individual to modulate his or her distress. Our goal is to help the individual to develop alternative, adaptive strategies to regulate emotions that do not undermine his or her developing sense of competency and effectiveness (Bornstein, 2005b, 2012a).

As part of our initial assessment, Sara completed a battery of objective self-report rating scales (Table 8.1). The pattern of her responses indicated that she was experiencing moderate to severe feelings of depression, anxiety, and pessimism. She noted that she felt "intensely sad," "worried nonstop," and was highly self-critical. She viewed herself as unattractive

TABLE 8.1. Results of Sara's Self-Report Rating Scales

Beck Depression Inventory = 27	Severe dysphoria
Beck Anxiety Inventory = 18	Moderate anxiety
Beck Hopelessness Scale = 12	Severe pessimism
Beck Scale for Suicidal Ideation = 0	No current suicidal thoughts

and undesirable, and believed she "hasn't measured up" in that she had graduated from college but was employed as a secretary. She stated that she "really needed to find someone [she] could love, someone to marry," but was unsure her search would be successful. These feelings were most severe at night while she was alone in her apartment, and when her boyfriend, Ken, did not immediately respond to her text messages or phone calls. There was no history of suicidal gestures or attempts, suicidal thoughts, or nonsuicidal self-injury.

Several measures were administered to assess maladaptive beliefs commonly associated with vulnerability for psychopathology. Clinically significant elevations were apparent in Sara's responses on the Young–Brown Schema Questionnaire—Revised (Young, 1990). She endorsed a range of items suggestive of sensitivity to emotional separation (e.g., "People haven't been there to meet my emotional needs," "For the most part, I haven't had someone to depend on for advice and emotional support"), fear of abandonment (e.g., "In the end, I'll be alone"), social isolation (e.g., "I don't fit in"), personal defectiveness (e.g., "It's my fault that my parents could not love me enough," "I cannot understand how anyone could love me"), and vulnerability to harm (e.g., "I feel the world is a dangerous place," "I'm a fearful person"). Her responses on the AAS-R (Collins & Read, 1990) were suggestive of feelings of insecurity in current relationships. She noted that she "very much" worries about being abandoned, and fears that her "desire to merge sometimes scares people away." She noted that she is "very comfortable depending on others," that she does not find it difficult to trust others, and that she "often worries that my partner does not really love me."

When asked about her experiences of anxiety and depression on a day-to-day basis, Sara stated, "It gets bad . . . I just think about how I'll be alone forever, and I worry if Ken is giving up on me." Automatic thoughts included "Who would want me?" "I can't handle this," and "This just goes on and on." There was, when Sara spoke, a sense of resignation to her predicament. She felt vulnerable, alone, and had few thoughts as to how her life might change for the better. Her approach to life was passive, and her attempts to develop a broader range of supports were largely unsuccessful. As she stated, "I call [her friends], but they don't call me."

Given Sara's high level of distress, our initial interventions focused on alleviating her feelings of depression and anxiety. Standard CBT techniques including mood monitoring, thought records, rational disputation of maladaptive thoughts, mastery, pleasurable events scheduling, relaxation training, and adaptive self-statements were introduced. Given her dependency and desire for support, Sara was very interested in garnering the therapist's approval. She invariably came to sessions on time, and reliably completed her CBT homework assignments. She took the time, in fact, to rewrite her thought records such that they would be neat and legible. Standard CBT interventions were quickly effective in reducing her feelings of depression and anxiety. Within 8 weeks, her feelings of depression and anxiety had been reduced to more "moderate" levels (BDI = 16, BAI = 10). At this point, however, Sara's progress in treatment stalled. Despite our best efforts, her experience of depression and anxiety remained stable over the next 2 months. Sara had reached an impasse, and we offered her a referral for a medication consultation (which she declined).

Given the lack of continued progress in addressing her feelings of depression, we shifted our focus from behavioral activation and rational disputation to a more explicit focus on her social relationships. She stated that she felt alone, and had never dated anyone for longer than a few months, with her current boyfriend of 3 months (Ken) being the longest relationship thus far. She remarked, "No one stays around that long . . . they just leave." When asked for an example, she described an incident in which she had met a young physician's assistant who was working in a local general medical practice. They'd had a nice first date, and had agreed to get together again. Over the course of the evening, she learned that his birthday was coming later that month. With this in mind, she baked him a cake and personally delivered it to the physician's office the following Monday. As the young physician's assistant was with a patient, she left it with a secretary. As she stated, "All the secretaries in the office were tittering . . . it was so exciting. Who brings a guy a cake?" She was very pleased and quite excited by her thoughtful gift. To her surprise, however, he was unable to schedule a second date. "Just too busy this week. It's crazy here," he would explain. After a week of her calling to offer other times, he remarked that he was considering a new position in another state, and so would likely be leaving town later that year. They never had the second date. Sara did not see how her overeager, even obsequious behavior might have affected their relationship, perhaps by annoying or embarrassing him with nurturing actions before they really knew each other. When asked her thoughts about this, Sara remarked, "What have I got to do? *Nobody* wants me. I'm just a Yugo." "A Yugo?" I asked. She then described an old Yugo automobile her parents had owned during her childhood. She noted, "It was a terrible car but, as you know, it was the most popular car in America for a while." When asked how this applied to her experience with the physician's assistant, she responded, "I'm like the Yugo, everybody drives me, but nobody wants me." She then explained, "What guys want is a Maserati, cute and sexy . . . but that's not me. Nobody will want me." She went on to share a more painful part of her relationship history, that of having short-lived relationships entirely focused on clandestine sexual activity, where there was no dating and no real personal involvement, further reinforcing her sense of undesirability and helplessness. These beliefs, that "Nobody will want me" and that she was, in fundamental ways, flawed and unde-sirable, served as a clinical focus over the next several weeks. Attempts to dispute them rationally were largely unsuccessful.

Given the continuing impasse, a developmental analysis of the belief that she "is just a Yugo" and its function in her life was initiated. Sara noted that she had believed she is undesirable and flawed from an early age, remarking, "Even my mother didn't love me." She explained that her mother gave her cards and gifts for her birthday and holidays, but "never really showed she cared. She never gave me hugs or kisses." When asked to elaborate, she described an incident when she was in the first grade. She had been admitted to the hospital for a tonsillectomy, and recalled her mother "sitting in a reclining chair" across the room. "We were there for at least two days and she never said anything. She just sat there." Sara's narrative was one of emotional deprivation, leading to the belief that she was undesirable and unlovable, even to her mother. She disclosed that her brother (number four of five children) had been very challenging as a child and had been diagnosed with attention-deficit/hyperactivity disorder. Given the large family and the difficult brother, her parents had planned to have no more children. As she noted, "then I came . . . I was the one they didn't want." Seeking an avenue to change this emotionally charged and highly maladaptive set of beliefs, the therapist asked an innocuous question—"She was sitting silently for days? What was she doing?" Sara responded by recalling that she was making her a needlepoint pillow with her name on it, recalling how "She'd sit for hours with her needles and yarn, she was so careful." At this point Sara began to cry and softly muttered "gold bumper." When invited to continue, Sara remarked, "She did love me . . . she just showed it in ways I didn't see as a kid." She reflected that her brother had been so difficult that her mother "just needed a place to rest, a time to relax." As for the bumper, she remarked, "There must have been something about me that Mom thought was good, that was worth-while . . . a Yugo with a gold bumper isn't completely worthless. It's not a great car, but it does have some good parts . . . some things that somebody will like." These insights—that her mother did, in fact, love her; that she did have desirable characteristics; that others might find her worthwhile—represented a turning point in therapy, a nexus of change. That said, it is important not to overstate the importance of cognitive change. We don't wish to underestimate the importance of behavioral change and social context. All three components are important. The insights Sara achieved in CBT—the establishment of a new narrative, a new way of understanding herself and her experiences growing up—permitted her to begin the hard work of changing long-standing behavioral patterns and social relationships. Our goal with Sara was to help her to create a new social environment, a setting in which her new beliefs and expectations could be practiced and nurtured.

PROGRESS, LIFESPAN, AND TERMINATION CONSIDERATIONS

As our case study suggests, progress in CBT with individuals who are highly dependent can be fitful; periods of steady improvement may be followed by periods of stasis. Slow, salutary progress is to be expected as individuals develop affect regulation skills, practice new patterns of behavior, and develop new beliefs. As many individuals with DPD seek rapid improvement, counseling patience and perseverance in therapy at the outset can pay dividends as treatment proceeds.

It is important to consider developmental expectations of dependency. As Freeman and Leaf (1989) rightly note, the normally dependent behavior of an infant or young child would be seen as entirely inappropriate in an adult. Other dependent behaviors, such as seeking support, guidance, and reassurance from others, are context dependent. In addition, elderly individuals naturally become increasingly dependent on others as they lose abilities with age. At the opposite extreme, absolute independence holds its own challenges, as it interferes with learning, collaboration, and reciprocal support among family members and friends. Seeking guidance and support when confronted with a life-threatening illness, a natural disaster, or a financial calamity is entirely sensible. *Not* to dial 911 when one experiences sudden chest pain would be maladaptive. Thus, it is important with individuals of all ages to determine whether the individual has a skill or competency deficit, or is failing to acknowledge competencies he or she does, in fact, possess. Dependency, as such, must be understood in the context of an individual's developmental level, skills, and competencies, and the nature of the challenges presented by his or her environment.

Dependency and autonomy are most usefully thought of as dimensions of cognitive, social, and emotional competencies that can vary over time and across settings. At the same time, cognitive, social, and emotional competencies develop over the course of a lifespan, and the stresses and challenges of life vary from day to day. Behavior that is inappropriately dependent in one setting may be entirely reasonable in another. With this in mind, we suggest that the goals of treatment should be determined collaboratively with individuals, and might address each of the three dimensions that serve as a foundation of DPD:

1. Experience of depression, anxiety, loneliness, and trepidation. Have they developed affect regulation skills to allow them to cope with the vagaries and disappointments of daily life?
2. Persistent negative beliefs about their own abilities and desirability. Do they continue to view their world as inherently dangerous and themselves as vulnerable?
3. Development of adaptive patterns of social behavior. Are their important relationships reasonably reciprocal in terms of support and initiative, or do they assume a role of underassertion, seriously neglecting self-interests in favor of protecting the dependency?

The process of termination should be carefully considered. Individuals with DPD often want to continue therapy, keeping their therapist as a guiding resource. They will, quite naturally, feel ambivalent about completing treatment. With this in mind, it can be helpful to taper sessions over time and encourage individuals to assume increasing responsibility for the focus of the sessions. Booster sessions can be offered and, as important, it can be helpful to explicitly address beliefs they may have about their ability to function independently of the therapist. The perception that they are "being abandoned" or that "No one understands me as well as you" are worthy of examination. Treatment of adults who are highly dependent can, and very often does, change the nature of their relationships with other family members. In fact, one of the primary goals may be to alter the quality of the way individuals relate to significant others. This can present challenges as individuals come to behave in ever more assertive and independent ways. Their behavior is no longer what their spouse, parents, or children had come to expect. Conflicts and tensions at home are not uncommon. In some families, conflicts between adult children and their parents may continue with regard to financial matters, as prolonged dependency on parental income can function as a maintaining factor. Should this occur, couples or family therapy sessions could be scheduled to educate family members about the nature and course of treatment, discuss their concerns, and enlist their support for the therapy process.

COMMON CHALLENGES AND CLINICIAN SELF-CARE

Multiple factors interfere with progress in individuals with DPD, such as narrow view of the self, perceived slow progress, and maintenance of the therapeutic relationship. Individuals with DPD are acutely aware of their distress—they come to therapy feeling depressed, anxious, and lonely. Our experience has been that CBT strategies can be very helpful in guiding individuals to an understanding of how their beliefs and attitudes contribute to their distress. They recognize how viewing themselves as incapable and unlovable contributes to their negative moods and they acknowledge that these beliefs "don't work for me." They often experience difficulty, however, articulating an alternative narrative. The challenge is in identifying a sensible new way of understanding their lives and themselves. In our case, Sara was able to describe, in great detail, a lifetime of experiences demonstrating that she was undesirable ("a Yugo") and incapable. However maladaptive these beliefs were, she *knew* them to be true, to be valid. The clinical challenge was in developing an alternative understanding—that she had desirable characteristics, her mother did love her, and she was more capable than she had believed. It was not sufficient to garner evidence that was inconsistent with the validity of her maladaptive beliefs—one must also help her to develop a new and equally viable understanding of herself and her world.

Progress in treatment for an individual with DPD may be difficult for the individual and the clinician. It is important to remain aware that there are likely to be plateaus and periods when treatment seems stalled. While symptomatic improvement can be expected within 10–20 sessions, it can take 1–2 years to address well-consolidated maladaptive beliefs and behavior patterns. Although standard CBT techniques can be effective for alleviating feelings of depression and anxiety, changing long-standing maladaptive beliefs and interpersonal patterns can take time. As a clinician, being mindful of the pattern can help place what could seem like a lack of progress into perspective, as this may represent a plateau in which a new issue is being faced.

Maintaining appropriate roles within the therapeutic relationship is a common challenge in treating individuals with DPD, as they often press individuals into meeting their needs for friendship, rather than engaging in a process of change. For example, individuals with DPD may attempt to steer the therapeutic conversation to topics of interest or praise of the clinician, rather than discussing issues related to change. Although the former may lead to a smoother session, therapeutic drift and loss of fidelity are important concerns. When this occurs, it is helpful to review treatment process and case conceptualization, examining factors that have maintained behaviors or distress. It is important for the clinician to be mindful of potential reinforcing factors of boundary violations, such as enjoyable discussions and sessions. As these issues occur, the clinician is reminded to examine the function of these behaviors for the individual in maintaining dependency behaviors, and highlight them to the individual as appropriate.

Finally, individuals with DPD come to therapy seeking reassurance, guidance, and support. Their relationships with their therapists are, in many ways, representative of other important relationships in their lives. They invariably will seek reassurance and direction, strive to please you (one individual a number of years ago prepared his thoughts records in calligraphy; they were works of art), and offer gratuitous thanks for your expert assistance. It's not uncommon for individuals to bring gifts after a productive session, lest you think therapy is approaching termination. Their natural tendency will be to encourage you to assume the role of a more directive, supportive sage. However helpful this may be during initial sessions it can, over time, facilitate dependence on the therapist. With this in mind, it can be useful to encourage autonomous thought and action. Ask the individual to identify specific problems and patterns, and to take the lead in challenging maladaptive beliefs. In our case example, it was Sara who had the insight and made the comment "gold bumper," rather than the therapist who suggested it to her.

Working with individuals with DPD can be both difficult and gratifying. Their dependency on the clinician in many ways makes them model individuals—they attend sessions regularly, participate actively, complete their CBT homework tasks, are polite, complimentary, and appreciative. These characteristics, however, are reflective of the underlying dependency issues. Thus, it is the clinician's task to remain objective, neutral, and solution focused. Exercises in which the individual demonstrates a lack of dependency or desire to please the clinician, such as arriving late to session, are encouraged. Not surprisingly, individuals who are dependent find this *very* difficult, offering an opportunity to examine associated thoughts and feelings.

At the same time, it is not uncommon for individuals who are highly dependent to ask for additional sessions and make "emergency" calls to the therapist during evenings and weekends. Balancing the individual's desire as well as the clinician's desire to be available during times of crisis can be quite challenging. To balance these desires, it is recommended that focus remain on encouraging autonomous action and developing the individual's ability to cope independently with stressful events. In session, attempts to cope independently can be discussed as evidence of competence, and challenge the need for dependency in maintaining relationships.

CONCLUSION

The capacity to depend on others—to turn to friends, family members, mentors, colleagues, and experts in time of need—is essential to human survival. For individuals with DPD, dependency presents as an evolutionary factor gone awry, inhibiting individual development and disrupting interpersonal relationships. As Freeman and Leaf (1989) suggest, that dependent personality disorder "represents . . . an abdication of autonomy" (p. 426), the goal in CBT for DPD is to help individuals balance the desire for dependency and the social expectation for autonomy to promote adaptive interdependency.

Cognitive-behavioral approaches for treating personality disorders developed during recent years show promise. A clear and parsimonious formulation based on research on factors associated with vulnerability for DPD offers a useful foundation for clinical practice. As is so often the case in practice, maintaining a collaborative therapeutic rapport facilitates the difficult task of changing long-held maladaptive beliefs and behavior patterns. Technical flexibility—being able to shift nimbly from one evidence-based set of strategies to another while maintaining strategic focus—offers the best opportunity for sustained clinical gains. In working with Sara, the goals were simple: to provide her with skills for managing acute distress, change maladaptive tacit beliefs about herself and the world, develop more adaptive behavior patterns, and help her to develop more and better relationships. A wide range of cognitive and behavioral techniques and strategies were brought into play in the service of achieving these goals. They were, in the end, quite useful in helping her to overcome her feelings of depression and anxiety and become a more autonomous and fulfilled young adult.

The model proposed is based on research from the cognitive-behavioral and developmental psychopathology literatures. While we have endeavored to stay close to the empirical literature, it is worth noting that a great deal remains to be done. Basic longitudinal research on the normative development of dependency and controlled trials of the effectiveness of alternative treatments for the condition need to be completed. The construct of dependent personality disorder, as a categorical diagnostic entity, may need to be revisited, and a dimensional framework for understanding genetic, molecular, neurophysiological, affective, and cognitive substrates of dependent behavior developed. Studies examining not only the efficacy and effectiveness of our interventions but the mechanisms of change will be needed before we can have confidence that we have adequately resolved this important clinical problem. Although our models and interventions are promising, their effectiveness has not yet been demonstrated.

CHAPTER 9

Avoidant Personality Disorder

Christine A. Padesky
Judith S. Beck

Jeb and Marge arrive in a couple counselor's office for a first appointment.

THERAPIST: How can I help you?

MARGE: We've been married 15 years but I feel like I live alone. Jeb doesn't talk to me about anything important.

THERAPIST: How do you see it, Jeb?

JEB: (*to Marge*) I know I don't make you happy. I'm sorry I'm not the kind of guy you want. I've screwed everything up.

MARGE: But you *are* the guy I want. I just want you to express yourself so I don't feel so alone.

(*Jeb is silent and looks down at the floor.*)

THERAPIST: Is it true you don't express yourself, Jeb?

JEB: (*sadly*) I don't know. I guess not.

Jeb and Marge have been married for 15 years and have two young children. They met at work where both are software engineers. Marge fell in love with Jeb partly because he was very kind and even-tempered. She also respected his intelligence and work ethic. Jeb has great difficulty expressing his thoughts and feelings and simply says about Marge, "She is a wonderful woman and perfect for me." Over the years, Marge became increasingly frustrated that Jeb was so quiet in conversations. Although he tended to be reticent while they dated, Marge believed over time he would relax and open up more with her. However, he still seems reluctant to express opinions, even about simple matters such as what he wants for dinner. His tendency to say "I don't know. What would you like?" now grates on her. She has tried to fight with Jeb to get him more engaged but he agrees with her complaints and promises to do better. When he knows she is upset with him, he tends to work late. When she asks him to talk with her about problems, he tries to change the topic of conversation to their children's activities or other noncontroversial subjects. Marge tells the therapist that she suspects the qualities she interpreted early in their relationship as equanimity are really his attempts to avoid conflict. Recognizing that Jeb fits criteria for avoidant personality disorder (APD), the couple therapist refers Jeb to a cognitive-behavioral therapist for individual therapy in the hopes that he will learn to communicate his thoughts and feelings more easily and can bring these skills back to the couple's therapy.

CLINICAL SIGNS AND SYMPTOMS

Most people use avoidance at times in their life, especially to relieve anxiety or when faced with difficult life choices or situations. APD is characterized by pervasive behavioral, emotional, and cognitive avoidance, even when personal goals or wishes are foiled by such avoidance. Cognitive themes that fuel avoidance in APD include self-deprecation, beliefs that unpleasant thoughts or emotions are intolerable, and an assumption that exposure of the "real self" to others or assertive self-expression will be met with rejection.

People with APD express a desire for affection, acceptance, and friendship, yet frequently have few friends and share little intimacy with anyone. In fact, they may experience difficulty even talking about these themes with the therapist. Their frequent loneliness, sadness, and anxiety in interpersonal relationships are maintained by a fear of rejection, which inhibits the initiation or deepening of relationships. As Jeb's history illustrates, people with APD often have difficulty expressing themselves even with a spouse or close friend.

How does a therapist diagnose APD when clients who exemplify APD have difficulty answering therapist questions and revealing their central issues? Therapists can hypothesize that avoidance might be a central feature of a diagnosis when clients, like Jeb, frequently say "I don't know" in response to questions that most clients answer readily. According to the fifth edition of the *Diagnostic and Statistical Manual of Mental Disorders* (DSM-5; American Psychiatric Association, 2013), APD should be diagnosed when patients have displayed pervasive difficulties in a range of situations, at least by early adulthood, related to significant and impairing social inhibition, beliefs that they are inadequate, and an acute and maladaptive sensitivity to others' assessments of them. They must also meet at least four additional criteria, which involve avoidance, restraint, inhibition, or preoccupation with negative evaluation from others. They typically avoid work or social activities that require significant interaction with others, especially when they are uncertain of being accepted or believe they are taking an interpersonal risk, they fear criticism or rejection , they feel inadequate or inferior, or they predict they will feel ashamed or embarrassed. Key features of the "anxious (avoidant) personality disorder" described in ICD-10 reflect these criteria. The diagnosis is made when patients have at least three of the following characteristics:

- Persistent and pervasive feelings of tension and apprehension.
- The belief that one is socially inept, personally unappealing, or inferior to others.
- Excessive preoccupation with being criticized or rejected in social situations.
- Unwillingness to become involved with people unless certain of being liked.
- Restrictions in lifestyle because of need to have physical security.
- Avoidance of social or occupational activities that involve significant interpersonal contact because of fear of criticism, disapproval, or rejection.

ICD-10 also notes that "associated features may include hypersensitivity to rejection and criticism" (World Health Organization, 1992).

A typical person with APD believes "I am socially inept and undesirable," and "Other people are superior to me and will reject or think critically of me if they get to know me." As the therapist elicits thoughts and uncomfortable feelings stemming from these beliefs, patients frequently begin to avoid or "shut down" by changing the topic, standing up and walking around, or reporting that their minds have "gone blank." As therapy proceeds, the therapist may find that this emotional and cognitive avoidance is accompanied by beliefs such as "I can't handle strong feelings," "You [therapist] will think I'm weak," "I'm defective and my emotional reactions prove it," and "If I allow myself to experience negative emotion, it will escalate and go on forever." People with APD have a low tolerance for dysphoria both in and out of the therapy session and use a variety of activities including substance abuse to distract themselves from negative cognitions and emotions.

Sometimes people with APD come to therapy at the insistence of a spouse or family member. When they initiate therapy on their own, they often present with complaints of depression, anxiety disorders, substance abuse, sleep disorders, or stress-related complaints, including psychophysiological disorders. They may be attracted to cognitive therapy because it is generally a time-limited treatment and they (erroneously) believe this form of therapy requires little self-disclosure or revelation of personal history.

DIFFERENTIAL DIAGNOSIS

Features of this disorder overlap with other diagnostic categories, most notably social anxiety disorder; panic disorder with agoraphobia; and dependent, schizoid, and schizotypal personality disorders. To make a differential diagnosis, it is important that the therapist inquire about the beliefs and meanings associated with various symptoms as well as the historical course of avoidant patterns.

Social anxiety disorder shares many of the features of APD. But individuals with APD display much broader patterns of avoidance. As the two disorders are often comorbid, a diagnosis of APD should be considered when patients meet criteria for social anxiety disorder. One distinction between APD and social anxiety disorder may be that people with APD, like Jeb, are often nearly as anxious and reluctant to reveal personal opinions with intimate others such as spouses as they are with other people. People with social anxiety disorder alone usually have a few intimates with whom they feel relaxed and can converse with comfort.

People with panic and agoraphobia often show similar behavioral and social avoidance to those with APD. However, the reasons for this avoidance are quite different. Instead of fears of criticism or rejection, avoidance in panic and agoraphobia is fueled by fears of a panic attack, sensations associated with panic attacks, or distance from a safe place or person who can "rescue" them from personal disaster (physical or mental).

Dependent personality disorder and APD are marked by similar self-views ("I am inadequate") but are differentiated by their views of others. Those with dependent personality disorder see others as strong and able to care for them. Those with APD see others as potentially critical and rejecting. Thus, people with dependent personality disorder seek close relationships and feel comforted by them; people with APD are often fearful of establishing close relationships and feel vulnerable within them.

People with APD are often socially isolated, as are those with schizoid personality disorder and schizotypal personality disorder. The main difference between these personality disorders and APD is that people with APD desire acceptance and close relationships. People diagnosed with schizoid or schizotypal personality disorder prefer social isolation. Those with schizoid personality disorder are indifferent to criticism or rejection from others. Those with schizotypal personality disorder may react to negativity from others but more often such reactions are fueled by paranoia ("What are they up to?") rather than the self-deprecation common to APD.

As mentioned previously, patients with APD often seek treatment for related symptomatic disorders. It is important that proper diagnosis of APD be made early in therapy because these symptomatic disorders can be treated successfully with standard cognitive therapy methods as long as the therapist includes strategies to overcome the characteristic avoidance that otherwise might cause roadblocks to treatment success.

CONCEPTUALIZATION

Patients with APD wish to be closer to other people yet they generally have few social relationships, particularly intimate ones. They fear relationships because they are certain they will be rejected and view such rejection as unbearable. As a result, they develop maladaptive coping strategies of avoidance. Their social avoidance is usually apparent. Less obvious is their cognitive and emotional avoidance, in which they avoid thinking about things that lead to dysphoric feelings. Their low tolerance for dysphoria also leads them to distract themselves from their negative cognitions. This section explains social, cognitive, behavioral,and emotional avoidance from a cognitive perspective.

Social Avoidance

Core Beliefs

Patients who are avoidant have several long-standing dysfunctional beliefs that interfere with social functioning. These beliefs may not be fully articulated but reflect patients' understandings of themselves and others. As children or adolescents, they invariably knew one or more significant person (parents, teachers, neighbors, siblings, peers) who were highly critical and rejecting of them. They developed core beliefs about themselves as a result of interactions with these people, such as "I'm inadequate," "I'm defective," "I'm unlikable," "I'm different," and "I don't fit in." They also developed negative beliefs about other people: "People don't care about me," and "People will criticize and reject me." Core beliefs such as these are reinforced over time by negative meanings the child attaches to subsequent experiences and the discounting of positive information contrary to these core beliefs. As a result, these beliefs become overgeneralized and rigid.

Underlying Assumptions

Not all children with critical or rejecting significant others become avoidant. People with APD make certain assumptions to explain negative interactions: "If this person treats me so badly, then I must be a bad person,"

"Since I don't have friends, I must be different or defective," and "If my parents don't like me, how could anyone?"

Fear of Rejection

As children, and later as adults, people with APD make the error of assuming that others will react to them in the same negative fashion as the critical significant person (or people) did. They continually fear that others will find them lacking and will reject them. They are also afraid they will not be able to bear the dysphoria they believe they will experience if they are rejected. Thus they avoid social situations and relationships, sometimes severely limiting their lives, to avoid the pain they expect to feel when someone inevitably (in their judgment) rejects them.

This prediction of rejection leads to dysphoria, which itself is extremely painful. But the prospect of rejection is even more painful because the person who is avoidant views others' negative reactions as justified. Rejection is interpreted in a very personal manner, as being caused solely by personal deficiencies: "He rejected me because I'm inadequate," "If she thinks I'm unintelligent [unattractive, etc.], it must be true." These attributions are generated by negative self-beliefs and, in turn, reinforce these dysfunctional beliefs, leading to more feelings of inadequacy and hopelessness. Even positive social interactions do not provide a safe haven from expectations of rejection: "If someone likes me that means he doesn't see the real me. As soon as he gets to know me, I'll be rejected. It is better for me to withdraw now before that happens." Thus people with avoidant personality seek to avoid dysphoria by avoiding relationships, both positive and negative ones.

Self-Criticism

Patients who are avoidant experience a string of self-critical automatic thoughts, both in social situations and in contemplation of future encounters. These thoughts produce dysphoria but are rarely evaluated, as patients assume them to be accurate. They arise from the negative beliefs described previously. Typical negative cognitions include "I'm unattractive," "I'm boring," "I'm defective," "I'm a loser," "I'm pathetic," and "I don't fit in."

In addition, both before and during social encounters, people with APD have a stream of automatic thoughts that predict—in a negative direction—what will happen: "I won't have anything to say," "I'll make a fool of myself," "He won't like me," and "She'll criticize me." Patients may or may not be fully aware of these thoughts initially. They may primarily be aware of the dysphoria that these thoughts evoke. Even when recognized, they assume their perceptions are valid and so do not consider testing their accuracy. Instead, people with APD actively avoid situations they believe may engender self-critical cognitions and dysphoria.

Underlying Assumptions about Relationships

Avoidant personality beliefs are also associated with dysfunctional assumptions about relationships. People with APD believe that they are basically unlikable or unacceptable but that if they can hide their true selves, they may be able to deceive others, at least a little or for a while. They believe they should not let anyone get close enough to discover what they "know" to be true about themselves. Typical underlying assumptions are "If I put on a facade, others may (temporarily) accept me," "If others really knew me, they wouldn't like me," "If others get to know me, they'll find out I'm really inferior," and "It's too risky to let people get close because they'll see the real me."

When they do establish relationships, people with APD make assumptions about what they must do to preserve the friendship. They may go overboard to avoid confrontation and may be quite unassertive. Typical assumptions are "If I please her all the time, she might think I'm okay," "If I don't do whatever he wants, he won't like me," and "If I express a different opinion or preference, they'll criticize me." Avoidant patients may feel as if they are constantly on the brink of rejection: "If I make a mistake, he'll change his whole view of me," "If I displease him in any way, he'll end our friendship," and "If I show any imperfection, she'll notice it and reject me."

Misevaluation of Others' Reactions

Patients who are avoidant have difficulty evaluating others' reactions. They may misread neutral or even somewhat positive reactions as negative. Like people with social phobia, some APD patients are likely to focus on their own internal negative thoughts, feelings, and physiological reactions, more than on the facial expressions, tone of voice, and body language of those with whom they are interacting. They often hope to elicit strongly positive reactions from people whose opinions are irrelevant to their lives, such as store clerks or bus drivers. It is very important to them that no one thinks badly of them, because of their assumption: "If anyone judges me negatively, the criticism must be true." It seems quite risky to be in positions in which they can be evaluated, because (their perception of) negative or neutral reactions from others confirm their beliefs that they are unlikable or defective. They lack inner criteria with which to judge themselves in a positive manner; instead, they rely solely on their perception of others' judgments.

Discounting Positive Data

Even when faced with evidence, incontrovertible to others, that they are accepted or liked, people with APD discount it. They believe they have deceived the other person or that the other person's judgment is faulty or based on inadequate information. Typical automatic thoughts include "He thinks I'm smart, but I've just fooled him," "If she really knew me, she wouldn't like me," and "He's bound to find out I'm really not very nice." These types of cognitions help explain Jeb's struggle in couples therapy with his wife. Recall that Marge wanted him to "express himself" and be more emotionally intimate. Despite her sincere statements on many occasions that she loved him, he persisted in his belief that her love was based on her misperception of him, as he had always hidden his true self. He wanted the marriage to continue but was afraid to speak up and express his thoughts, emotions, dreams, and desires. Jeb believed if he did express himself honestly, Marge would see his true self and reject him.

Cognitive, Behavioral, and Emotional Avoidance

In addition to social avoidance, most people with APD also demonstrate cognitive, behavioral, and emotional avoidance. They avoid *thinking* about matters that produce dysphoria and behave in ways that permit them to continue this avoidance. A typical pattern emerges:

1. Patients who are avoidant become aware of a dysphoric feeling. (They may or may not be fully aware of the thoughts that precede or accompany the emotion.)
2. Their tolerance for dysphoria is low so they do something to distract themselves and feel better. They may discontinue a task or fail to initiate a task they had planned to do. They may surf the Internet, turn on the television, pick up something to read, reach for food or a cigarette, get up and walk around, and so forth. In short, they seek a diversion in order to push away uncomfortable thoughts and feelings.
3. This pattern of cognitive and behavioral avoidance is reinforced by a reduction in dysphoria and so it eventually becomes ingrained and automatic.

Patients acknowledge their behavioral avoidance, at least to some extent. They invariably criticize themselves in global, stable terms: "I'm lazy," or "I'm resistant." Such pronouncements reinforce beliefs about being inadequate or defective and lead to hopelessness. Patients do not view avoidance as their way of coping with uncomfortable emotions. They generally are not aware of the extent of their cognitive and emotional avoidance until such a pattern is made clear to them.

Attitudes about Dysphoric Moods

Patients who are avoidant often have dysfunctional attitudes about dysphoric emotions: "It's bad to feel upset," "I shouldn't feel anxious," and

"Other people don't feel scared or embarrassed." Avoidant patients believe that if they allow themselves to feel dysphoric, they will be engulfed by the feeling and be unable to recover: "If I let my feelings get unbottled, I'll be overwhelmed," "If I start feeling a little anxious, it will get worse and worse and I won't be able to tolerate it," and "If I let myself feel bad, I'll spiral downward, get into a deep hole, and I won't be able to function."

Excuses and Rationalizations

Patients who are avoidant have a strong desire to establish closer relationships. They often feel quite empty and lonely and want to improve their lives by making closer friends, performing better in their jobs, and feeling more self-confident. When they think of what they must do to realize their desires, the short-term cost of experiencing negative emotions seems too high. They make a myriad of excuses for not doing what is necessary to reach their goals. "I won't enjoy doing that," "I'll be too tired," "I'll feel worse [more anxious, bored, etc.] if I do it," "I don't feel like doing it now," and "I'll do it later." When "later" comes, they invariably use the same excuses, continuing their behavioral avoidance. In addition, avoidant patients may not believe they are capable of reaching their goals. They make certain assumptions: "There's nothing I can do to change my situation," "What's the use of trying? I won't be able to do it anyway," and "It's better to lose by default than to try and inevitably fail."

Wishful Thinking

Patients who are avoidant may engage in wishful thinking about their future. They hope they will achieve wonderful relationships and jobs. But they generally do not believe they will be able to reach their goals through their own efforts: "One day I'll wake up and everything will be fine," "I can't improve my life by myself," and "If my life gets better, it won't be through my own efforts." For example, whenever Marge stopped pressing for intimacy, even for a day, Jeb hoped that the issue was settled and she now accepted the status quo. He didn't think he had any control over improving their relationship—it would have to be Marge who changed.

Therapy-Interfering Beliefs

Avoidant patients bring the same beliefs and assumptions about themselves and others to the therapy situation. "If I trust my therapist's apparent care and compassion, I'll get hurt," "If I focus on problems in therapy, I'll get too overwhelmed," "If I reveal negative aspects of my history and life, my therapist will judge me negatively," and "If I try the new behaviors my therapist suggests, I'll be rejected" (J. Beck, 2005). These cognitions can interfere with the patient's ability to fully engage in and benefit from treatment if the therapist does not elicit and help the patient evaluate them.

Conceptualization Summary

Patients who are avoidant hold deep-seated negative beliefs about themselves, others, and unpleasant emotional experiences. They see themselves as inadequate and worthless, others as critical and rejecting, and dysphoric emotions as overwhelming and intolerable. These beliefs often stem from childhood interactions with significant people who were critical and rejecting. Socially, they avoid situations in which other people could get close and discover the "real" them. Behaviorally, they avoid tasks that engender thoughts that make them feel uncomfortable. Cognitively, they avoid thinking about matters that produce dysphoria. Their tolerance for discomfort is quite low, and they rely on distraction when they begin to feel anxious, sad, lonely, or bored. They are unhappy with their current state but feel incapable of changing through their own efforts. They may have difficulty fully engaging in treatment when their dysfunctional beliefs are activated and they may employ their characteristic coping strategies in session, as well as between sessions. For a list of the typical core beliefs about the self and others, conditional assumptions, overdeveloped and underdeveloped coping strategies, and therapy-interfering beliefs and behaviors of the patient who is avoidant, see J. Beck, 2005.

KEY TREATMENT GOALS

Based on this cognitive formulation of APD, there are three main treatment goals:

1. *Target cognitive and emotional avoidance.* Until the patient actively participates in therapy, progress will be slow. The therapist helps patients overcome cognitive and emotional avoidance in session and between sessions so patients can become more aware of thoughts, feelings, and the maintenance role avoidance plays in their problems.
2. *Work on building skills.* Patients with APD often need to develop skills of self-reflection as well as interpersonal skills such as self-expression, assertion, and conflict negotiation.
3. *Evaluate the automatic thoughts, underlying assumptions, and core beliefs that maintain avoidant patterns.* Develop alternative cognitions that are more reality based and functional and that support the initiation and maintenance of intimacy and appropriate assertiveness in relationships.

These goals are pursued collaboratively with the patient, using guided discovery whenever possible (J. Beck, 2005; Kuyken, Padesky & Dudley, 2009). Ultimately, the overall goal of treatment for patients with APD is to live more productive and more satisfying lives, which is likely to include the establishment of new relationships and an increase in their comfort within existing relationships. Although perhaps not fully achieved by the end of therapy, treatment success can be assessed by the degree to which APD patients are able to freely make day-to-day and long-term decisions in accordance with their basic values, express themselves with others, and achieve the level of intimacy desired in relationships without undue interference from unhelpful beliefs and formerly ingrained patterns of avoidance.

COLLABORATIVE STRATEGY

Two barriers to collaboration that can be expected with patients with APD are their fear of rejection and distrust of others' expressions of caring. They often have a host of negative cognitions about the therapist, just as they do about other people. Identifying and testing these dysfunctional thoughts during treatment is essential to forming an active collaborative relationship and can serve as a model for doing so in other relationships.

Even when patients who are avoidant are aware of automatic thoughts about the therapist or therapy relationship, they are usually unwilling at first to reveal them. They often infer criticism. When, for example, therapists ask questions about homework assignments, avoidant patients may think "[My therapist] must be thinking I didn't do the homework very well." Patients with APD expect disapproval. If they tear up in session, they may think "My therapist must be disgusted with me when I cry like this." They may also discount the therapist's direct expressions of approval or caring, believing: "You like me only because you're a therapist and you're trained to like everybody," or "You may think that I'm okay now, but if I told you about my relationship with my mother, you'd think I'm terrible."

A therapist can be on alert for signs of these hidden thoughts. When patients display a change of affect in session, the therapist can ask, "You're looking a little upset right now. What just went through your mind?" As many APD patients try to mask their emotions, therapists can anticipate the tendency of these patients to mind-read in the session itself. When discussing a sensitive topic, the therapist might ask, "I wonder, are you predicting what I'm feeling or thinking now?" At the end of sessions it is important for therapists to ask, "When were you the most concerned about what I was thinking or feeling during our session today?" If the patient disavows any concern, the therapist might gently probe: "How about when we discussed your difficulty finishing this week's assignment?" If the patient is reluctant to offer any thoughts in early sessions ("I don't know" or "I wasn't thinking anything"), the therapist can pursue a line of questioning similar to this dialogue between Jeb and his individual therapist in their third session:

THERAPIST: What went through your mind just now, Jeb, when I asked if you ever felt angry with Marge?

JEB: Nothing really.

THERAPIST: The reason I ask is that you looked a little bit nervous.

JEB: No, I'm not really nervous.

THERAPIST: Well, it would be understandable if you were. Some patients worry that I'll criticize them if they say the wrong thing or if they say something I disapprove of.

JEB: Well, you don't seem critical. You seem pretty nice so far.

THERAPIST: (*smiling*) Well, thanks for that. Even so, have you had any thoughts that I might judge you? Or disapprove of something?

JEB: I guess that might have crossed my mind.

THERAPIST: It's so good you told me that [providing positive reinforcement]. Would you be willing to let me know the next time you have a thought like that?

JEB: I guess so.

THERAPIST: That would be really important. Meanwhile, could we practice right now? Can you tell me about one time when you thought I might have criticized or judged you?

Once elicited, there are several ways to evaluate automatic thoughts related to therapy. Initially, therapists ask patients how they could find out whether their predictions were accurate and encourage patients to ask direct questions. Therapists can then forthrightly reveal what they were actually thinking: "Oh, it's so interesting that you thought I was thinking negatively of you for leaving the party. What I was actually thinking was . . " It is helpful for patients to rate how much they believe the therapist's feedback (using a 0–100% scale) and to monitor changes in their degree of belief as their trust in the therapist grows. After several such direct interchanges, patients can be encouraged to evaluate their negative beliefs about the therapist in light of their past experiences: "Do you remember how I reacted when you told me you left a social event early, and when you didn't finish a homework assignment, and when you played a computer game instead of calling your mother? How would you describe my usual response when you tell me about a problem?" Patients can also test their automatic thoughts by engaging in small experiments.

As the following example demonstrates, patients can be asked to describe an experience they are certain the therapist will find unacceptable and to evaluate the validity of this belief in small stages. Jeb was 100% confident that his therapist would judge him negatively if he revealed to her that he had gone upstairs shortly after the start of their daughter's birthday party and that Marge had become angry with him for not helping out. Talking to the parents of his daughter's friends had been a homework assignment and, during the subsequent session, his therapist asked him about it. As he was sure his therapist would be critical of him, Jeb answered generally, stating that it hadn't gone great but now it was over. His therapist sensed Jeb's reluctance to discuss it further and inferred he might be concerned about her reaction. She used this situation as an opportunity for an in-session behavioral experiment about taking small steps toward self-revelation in relationships. First, the therapist set the stage by helping Jeb identify the assumptions and predictions that led to his reluctance to self-disclose:

THERAPIST: Were you able to talk to any of the parents?

JEB: (*quietly*) I don't really want to talk about it.

THERAPIST: Well, that's okay, but can you tell me—what do you predict will happen if you do tell me about it?

JEB: (*after a long pause*) You'll be disappointed. You'll think less of me.

THERAPIST: And if I think of less of you, what do you think will happen?

JEB: I don't know. I guess you might want to give up on me.

THERAPIST: Well, no wonder you don't want to talk about it. (*pause*) Jeb, based on your experience with me so far, how else might I react?

JEB: I guess you could understand the reasons for what I did, but I'm not sure.

THERAPIST: Would it be helpful if you told me and it turned out that I did understand? That I didn't think less of you and could help you with the problem? Would that be a relief?

JEB: Yes. Yes, it would.

THERAPIST: And, if it turned out that I *didn't* understand your reasons, what could you and I do to work that out?

JEB: What do you mean?

THERAPIST: Sometimes in relationships, people don't understand each other's reasons at first. They even might be disappointed or upset with the other person. But that doesn't need to be the end of the story. What could you and I do to work it out if you tell me and I have a negative reaction to what you say?

JEB: I don't know. I guess we could talk about it. But I really think you'd be disappointed.

THERAPIST: Let me write this down. Two things could happen if you tell me: one, I might understand and that would be a good outcome. Or two, I might not understand, be disappointed in you and then give up on you. Is that right?

JEB: Yes.

THERAPIST: I'm going to draw a continuum here on this piece of paper. On one end I'm going to write "I understand." On the other end I'll write "I don't understand, am disappointed, and give up on you." Is it possible that there are other outcomes in between these two end points?

Jeb and his therapist generated a few possibilities for the therapist's reactions in the midrange of the continuum (e.g., therapist would understand but not be able to help; therapist would not understand and yet feel curious and not disappointed; therapist could find out that the homework assignment she had suggested was inappropriate). They also developed a plan for working through any discomfort in their relationship that could result from the revelation. For example, the therapist agreed to be honest with Jeb about her reactions to what he told her and to problem-solve any negative impact on their therapy relationship. Finally, the therapist proposed Jeb tell her about the situation in small steps so he could judge for himself the risks and rewards of self-disclosure:

THERAPIST: You don't have to tell me everything if you don't want to. You could just tell me one small part and then decide if you want to tell me more.

JEB: I guess that would be okay. Well, a bunch of parents came in with their kids and I hung up their coats and they started talking to me.

THERAPIST: How were you feeling?

JEB: Nervous, really nervous.

THERAPIST: And you were thinking . . . ?

JEB: That I didn't know what to say to them.

THERAPIST: Let's stop there. How did it feel to tell me that?

JEB: It was all right. . . . But I haven't told you the worst part yet.

THERAPIST: How do you think I'm reacting so far?

JEB: Okay, I guess.

THERAPIST: You're right. I'm not surprised you were nervous—in fact, I think we had predicted that, right?

JEB: Yeah.

THERAPIST: Can you tell me what happened next?

JEB: I was just feeling so uncomfortable. I should have stayed at the party and helped Marge, but I went upstairs. It's pathetic that I had to hide. I missed most of my daughter's party. I mean, I'm pathetic for being so weak.

THERAPIST: You went upstairs? Did you do anything else you thought was even worse?

JEB: No, not really. I went back downstairs toward the end and helped for a while. But I should have stayed down the whole time.

THERAPIST: And you probably would have, if your nervousness hadn't kicked in so strongly. But I don't see how that makes you pathetic and weak. Doesn't it just say that you tend to avoid when you get nervous? This sounds like another example of the avoidance cycle we've been talking about. I wonder, were you predicting that if you stayed downstairs the parents would judge you?

JEB: Yes.

THERAPIST: Then no wonder you got anxious. But before we continue talking, how do you feel about telling me this?

JEB: It's okay. I don't feel as bad as I thought I would.

THERAPIST: Did I react the way you expected?

JEB: No, you didn't.

THERAPIST: It's going to be so important for you to remember that. Is it okay if we write it down?

Because patients who are avoidant are reluctant to reveal when they predict their therapist will think badly of them, it is important for the therapist occasionally to ask directly whether a patient has been afraid to tell him or her something. Unless patients with APD express these suppressed topics or details, they may continue to believe that their therapist would have rejected them (or at the very least, viewed them negatively) if this information were known. The therapist might say, for example, "You know, sometimes patients are reluctant to tell me certain things because they predict they'll feel too upset or that I'll react negatively to it. You don't have to tell me what it was, but could you tell me whether there has been a time when you were hesitant to say something?"

Avoidant patients often assume that once they establish a relationship, they must continually try to please the other person. They believe that if they assert their own desires, the other person will respond negatively. In therapy, this can lead to the patient's superficial agreement with what the therapist says and an unwillingness to give the therapist negative feedback.

One way to encourage patient assertiveness in therapy is to elicit feedback. Since patients who are avoidant usually provide global, positive statements, it can be helpful to ask them to complete a therapist feedback form at the end of sessions (J. Beck, 2006) because they may be more willing to provide negative feedback in a written form than they are face-to-face. Patients can describe or rate the therapist on a checklist of qualities including process (e.g., "The therapist listened well and seemed to understand me today") and content (e.g., "The therapist explained the homework clearly enough"). If the patient provided any ratings that were not in the highest rating category, the therapist can review the form in the next session, first providing positive reinforcement. ("It's good you indicated that you found me moderately empathic so I can try to improve. Do you remember when you thought I wasn't quite empathic enough?") By taking a nondefensive stance and discussing possible changes in session content and/or process, the therapist can reward patients for assertive criticism, correct misperceptions, problem-solve legitimate dissatisfactions, and demonstrate the change potential of relationships. Then patients can be encouraged to give direct verbal feedback, especially negative feedback, when relevant. At the end of the session, the therapist might say, "At the beginning of this session, we looked at your feedback sheet. Do you remember I was glad you told me that I wasn't being quite empathic enough? How did I come across to you this week? Was there anything I said that bothered you or that you thought I didn't understand? Anything you'd like us to do differently next session?"

Saying aloud thoughts about the therapist and working out problems in the therapeutic relationship can provide powerful learning experiences. When patients discover some of their thoughts about their therapist are inaccurate, it is helpful to hypothesize that the patient's beliefs about other people's reactions might also sometimes be inaccurate. Patients can do experiments to test these beliefs, practice assertiveness, and problem-solve difficulties (J. Beck, 2005). Role-playing and guided-imagery practice are very helpful prior to *in vivo* assertiveness.

CLINICAL APPLICATION OF THE INTERVENTION

Standard cognitive therapy approaches (Beck, Rush, Shaw, & Emery, 1979; J. Beck, 2011; Greenberger & Padesky, 1995; Padesky, 1995; Salkovskis, 1996) can be used with patients with APD to help them manage depression, anxiety disorders, substance abuse, and other symptomatic problems. Guided discovery using standard cognitive-behavioral methods for testing automatic thoughts and underlying assumptions can help them begin to counter self-criticism, negative predictions, maladaptive assumptions, and misevaluations of others' reactions. Mindfulness techniques can help patients who are avoidant gain distance from their thoughts and to experience and tolerate negative emotion nonjudgmentally. Acceptance and commitment methods can be used to help them identify their core values and move toward making difficult behavioral changes in the service of these values. Compassion therapy interventions (Gilbert, 2010) are used to help avoidant patients undermine their highly critical internal voice and increase self-compassion. Special techniques, outlined below, can help patients with APD overcome the cognitive and emotional avoidance that otherwise may hamper therapy interventions.

Overcoming Cognitive and Emotional Avoidance

Although patients with APD experience a range of dysphoric emotions, it is not desirable simply to teach them to reduce depressed and anxious moods. Their avoidance of thinking about things that lead to unpleasant emotions and their negative assumptions about dysphoric moods can hamper standard cognitive therapy treatment. It is important patients allow themselves to experience negative emotions to gain access to key cognitions and learn to evaluate them. Significant and lasting cognitive change occurs only in the presence of negative affect. Therefore, cognitive and emotional avoidance can prove a serious impediment to effective treatment.

It is helpful to diagram the process of avoidance (Figure 9.1) so that patients can see there is an alternative explanation for their avoidance—they are not "weak" or "lazy"; rather, they are fearful of negative emotion and so employ a coping strategy that brings them (short-term) relief. The diagram can help them understand more concretely why they avoid and can lead to a discussion of how to prevent avoidance. Through Socratic questioning, patients can identify the long-term consequences of avoidance (being unable to reach goals that are very important to them) and the benefits of doing the hard work needed to overcome this highly ingrained coping strategy. It is useful for patients to review the diagram daily if they are tempted to avoid (or have engaged in avoidance) to discover how the temptation to avoid plays out in various situations. If applicable, the therapist and patient can explore the origin of the avoidance of dysphoria. Often such avoidance was initiated in childhood, when a patient may indeed have been more vulnerable and less able to cope with unpleasant or painful feelings.

One of the best ways to begin increasing emotional tolerance is to evoke emotion in the session by discussing experiences about which patients report discomfort. If there are signs of cognitive avoidance, the therapist can direct them back to the feelings to begin to identify and test the beliefs leading to the avoidance. A therapy excerpt illustrates this process:

THERAPIST: Can you summarize what we've just talked about?

JEB: I guess you're saying that I need to tolerate feeling bad when Marge is mad so we can talk things out instead of me just shutting down or leaving the room.

THERAPIST: That's it.

JEB: But I usually feel so bad, I can't stand it.

THERAPIST: When Marge got angry Saturday night, what were you feeling?

JEB: Ashamed. I let her down again. I thought she was probably disgusted with me. And I was also really anxious.

THERAPIST: How strong were those feelings, from 0 to 100%?

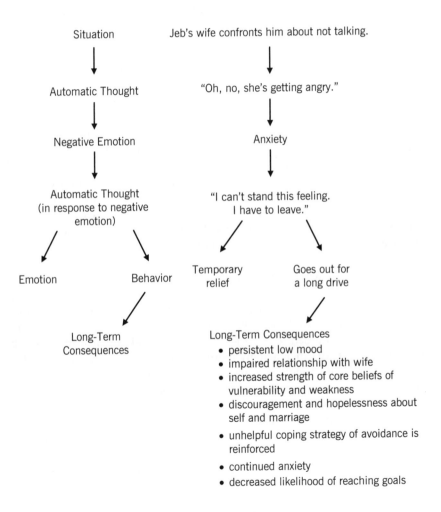

FIGURE 9.1. Diagram of avoidance patterns.

JEB: One hundred percent. I hate feeling so bad. So I apologized and then I left the house and drove around for a while.

THERAPIST: What do you think would have happened if you had stayed in the house with Marge?

JEB: Oh, I would have felt much worse!

THERAPIST: I thought your negative emotions were already at 100%?

JEB: Well, maybe 90%, but I would have felt worse and worse if I had stayed.

THERAPIST: What would it have looked like if you had stayed? [eliciting an image] If you had felt worse and worse?

JEB: I would have started to shake and cry and then I would've collapsed in a heap on the ground.

THERAPIST: How long did you stay in the situation on Saturday night before you left?

JEB: About 3 minutes, probably.

Jeb's therapist gathered more information about his fear of experiencing strong emotions in this situation. Then they discussed situations in which he was not able to leave after 3 minutes (a situation at work and a few instances when he and Marge were driving together in a car). Jeb could not recall any time when he had actually "collapsed in a heap on the ground" even though he often felt very deflated when someone was upset with him. His therapist then proposed that they test his predictions and increase his tolerance for negative emotions through discussion and role plays in session. She proposed doing an experiment for just a few minutes initially and then with gradual increases in the duration and intensity of his distress.

Repeated exposure may be necessary to build tolerance for dysphoria and erode patients' dysfunctional beliefs about experiencing uncomfortable emotions. To desensitize patients, therapist and patient can construct a hierarchy that lists increasingly painful topics to discuss in therapy. The therapist can elicit patients' predictions of what they fear will happen before they discuss each succeeding topic, test the predictions, and accumulate evidence that disconfirms their faulty beliefs (e.g., "It'll be too painful to discuss," "If I start feeling bad, the feeling will never end"). They can also construct "emotional tolerance practice" or "overcoming avoidance experiences" for homework. The assignments may involve initiating and continuing an action for a certain amount of time ("Talk to X for 5 minutes before getting off the phone") or structured reflection ("Think about telling my boss that I want more time off"). Patients are asked to predict what they fear will happen during these experiments and compare actual results with their expectations.

Patients who are avoidant often have difficulty identifying automatic thoughts for homework (or even in the therapy session itself). Usually, asking patients in the session to imagine and minutely describe a situation as if it were happening right then (while focusing on their bodily reactions and trying to reexperience the negative emotion) helps them identify thoughts. Therapists can also suggest a thought that is opposite to the one they infer the patient had. ("So when you walked into the party, were you thinking how glad you were to be there and how easy it would be to talk to people? . . . No? So what were you thinking?") Providing an extreme contrast in this way can spur patients to recognize what they were actually thinking. Role plays also can be used to capture automatic thoughts. After patients relate who said what in an interaction, patients play themselves, and the therapist takes the part of the other person. Patients are instructed to capture their automatic thoughts during these reenactments.

If these methods are unsuccessful, the therapist can compile a checklist of hypothesized thoughts, based on the patient's previously identified thoughts and beliefs and on the case conceptualization. Patients can review the checklist to see if any of these thoughts occurred in the situation under discussion. They can also use the checklist to identify cognitions while still in a distressing situation.

When patients are able to identify their thoughts but fail to do homework assignments, it may be useful to plan and rehearse homework using imagery, as in the following example:

THERAPIST: Okay, Jeb, so you've decided to initiate a discussion with Marge and tell her that you'd rather take a vacation at the lake instead of visiting her family [summarizing]. I'd like you to imagine beginning this discussion with her and tell me if anything gets in the way.

JEB: Okay. *(eyes are closed)* She looks so happy that I've brought this up. But my automatic thought is I can't disappoint her by telling her my idea. She'll be mad.

THERAPIST: What happens next?

JEB: I tell her I want to talk about our children's summer schedule instead.

THERAPIST: Let's go back to the beginning where she looks happy and you think you can't disappoint her. If you do have that thought, what could you say to yourself?

JEB: What you and I talked about. That it's my vacation, too, and her family doesn't always treat me well. That it might be really fun for our family to go to a lake and just relax together.

THERAPIST: That's good. And what could you tell yourself if she does get disappointed and angry?

JEB: I'm not sure. I'm afraid my mind goes blank when she's mad.

THERAPIST: Do you remember what you concluded last week when you told me she got mad at you for driving around instead of coming straight home from work?

JEB: Yeah. That I survived her anger and I actually always do. And that she has a right to her feelings and that she really does love me even when she's angry.

THERAPIST: Great. And how about the idea from last week that you're entitled to have preferences and that she actually wants you to express them, even if she disagrees?

Following further discussion, the therapist asks what he thinks will be important to remember. They write these ideas down on an index card and the therapist encourages Jeb to read the card (and other relevant cards they have composed in previous sessions) daily.

If patients continue to be reluctant about doing homework assignments, the therapist can employ a point–counterpoint technique. Jeb can argue with his "avoidance" voice why he is better off not doing an assignment, while the therapist answers with (and models) an "antiavoidance" voice. Then he and his therapist can switch roles so Jeb has practice using the antiavoidance responses. This technique may uncover additional interfering automatic thoughts, the responses to which Jeb can write down on index cards to read daily—and especially before undertaking an assignment that he knows he is likely to avoid.

These experiences in and between therapy sessions help patients identify dysphoric thoughts and tolerate negative feelings. As such tolerance grows, patients who are avoidant may begin to change the way they relate to family members (e.g., they may become more assertive, participate more actively in conflict). They also may experience more intense sadness, fear, or anger as they bring into awareness memories and reactions they have avoided for so many years. At this point, it is helpful to teach cognitive and behavioral approaches to manage these moods.

The therapist can point out that even though the patient now understands the importance of negative feelings and is willing to tolerate them, it is not necessary or desirable to experience intense feelings all the time. Patients can be instructed to keep diaries of feelings and thoughts when they occur, and then to use automatic thought records to test the "hot thoughts" most closely connected to their feelings (J. Beck, 2011; Greenberger & Padesky, 1995).

It may also be helpful to do couple or family therapy if the patient is in a relationship or living with family members. Therapy sessions can provide a safe forum for patients to test the validity of relevant interpersonal beliefs. One patient, for example, feared that her husband had been angry with her for some time because she did not work outside the house. In one of their couple sessions, the therapist encouraged her to ask her husband about this. Her husband told her it was not true but did reveal other situations that distressed him. These difficulties were then resolved through joint problem solving.

Couple or family therapy may also be indicated when avoidant patterns are supported by the patient's social system. For example, the wife of another patient held her own negative assumptions about emotional expression ("Talking about feelings leads to conflict and irreparable harm"). Family therapy can address dysfunctional assumptions held by family members and can provide a forum for teaching constructive skills for communication and problem solving (e.g., Beck, 1988b; Dattilio & Padesky, 1990).

Skill Building

Sometimes patients with APD have skill deficits because of impoverished social experiences. In these cases, skill-training exercises should be included in the therapy, so the patient has a reasonable chance of success, both in social interactions designed to test beliefs and in naturally occurring social situations. For some, social skills training will begin with nonverbal cues (e.g., eye contact, posture, and smiling). Patients can practice in therapy sessions, at home, and then in low-risk social situations. More advanced social skills training may include instruction regarding conversational methods, assertiveness, sexuality, and conflict management. And patients with meager social experience may need educational information to evaluate experiences more accurately (e.g., "If you wait until the last minute on weekends to make plans, most people will already be busy").

Patients' negative beliefs about themselves may create obstacles to trying out newly developed skills. They may need to be encouraged to act "as if" they possessed a certain quality. For example, one patient had the thought: "I won't be able to make small talk at the party. I'm not confident enough." After a role play demonstrated that she did have conversational skills, the therapist encouraged her to act as if she were confident at the party. She discovered that she could appropriately engage in conversation. During behavioral skills training, it is important to elicit automatic thoughts, especially ones in which patients disqualify their progress or the training itself: "These exercises are teaching me to fool people so they don't see my inadequacy," and "Only a real loser has to learn how to talk at this age." Therapist and patient can work together to test the validity and utility of these beliefs.

Identifying and Testing Maladaptive Beliefs

A major portion of the therapy involves helping patients identify and test the cognitive underpinnings of avoidant patterns. It is important to provide experiences in which patients develop a new perspective about themselves and others on both the intellectual level (e.g., using Socratic questioning) and the emotional level (through experiential techniques). By discussing important early experiences in which the belief originated or became strengthened, patients can gain an understanding of the developmental roots of the negative beliefs, paying particular attention to how these beliefs led to coping strategies that might have been helpful, at least some of the time, at an earlier period in the patient's life (J. Beck, 2005). Next, alternative new beliefs can be identified (Mooney & Padesky, 2000; Padesky, 1994) that the patient wishes were true (e.g., "I'm likable," "Other people will show understanding if I make a mistake"). Old and new beliefs are tested through experiments, guided observation, and role-play reenactments of early schema-related incidents. Patients are directed to begin to notice and remember data about themselves and their social experiences that support the new, more desirable beliefs (Greenberger & Padesky, 1995; Padesky, 1994).

Jeb identified the following core beliefs: "I'm weak and pathetic," "Other people are superior and will judge me negatively," and "It is important to hide who I really am." As he described his childhood, Jeb realized that his core beliefs were very close to his father's description of him. His father was in the military and "had a chip on his shoulder," always looking for a fight. Jeb had severe allergies and asthma as a child, which irritated his father. When Jeb had to stop or forgo an activity due to his medical condition, his father labeled him as "weak." He was quite critical when Jeb failed to make a sports team or spent most of his time on the bench. His father often said, "Get out of here! You're pathetic!" Due to his difficulties participating in sports, Jeb was also teased and disregarded by many boys his age and began to engage in more and more solitary activities. As he grew older, Jeb tried to get closer to his father by faking an interest in military history and football. In fact, Jeb was interested more in science and computers but because he knew this would annoy his father, he hid these interests. Jeb's father was killed in a motorcycle accident when Jeb was 17. While this freed Jeb to pursue his true academic interests, his father's judgments followed him into adulthood.

Jeb's therapist suggested they use psychodrama to reenact some of these scenarios from Jeb's childhood. She asked Jeb to identify a specific scene that he thought helped plant these core beliefs in his mind. Jeb described the situation in enough detail for the therapist to know how to role-play his father. As the role play began, Jeb eyes filled with tears as he quickly became a frightened 8-year-old boy. As the role play progressed, the therapist asked "8-year-old Jeb" what he was thinking and feeling. After the role play, his therapist noted how closely the young Jeb's thoughts and emotions mirrored how he described feeling when Marge became angry with him.

Next, therapist and patient switched roles and the therapist asked him to notice what he thought and how he felt as he role-played his father. For the first time, Jeb began to understand how unhappy and angry his father was with his own life. He remembered his mother once saying to him when he was a young teen, "Ignore your father. He doesn't want to be here and he's taking it out on you." At the time, Jeb thought she meant he didn't want to be stateside because he always bragged about how much he liked serving overseas. After the role play, he wondered if his mother meant that his father didn't want to be in their family. He telephoned his mother the next week and learned that his father was not very mature when they married. His father was not happy when Jeb was born because he preferred drinking with his buddies to staying home with a wife and child. Jeb realized that his father's explosive anger and demeaning comments reflected his father's unhappiness more than anything Jeb was doing as a child that was "weak" or "pathetic."

Another psychodrama allowed Jeb to try out this new perspective. Drawing on his own experiences as a father, Jeb considered how most fathers would handle an 8-year-old son with severe allergies and asthma. Jeb concluded that most fathers would be far more sympathetic and caring than his own father had been. Then they discussed a hypothetical father who spoke cruelly to his son when the child's activities were limited by medical problems. His therapist asked Jeb what he would want to say to that father. After writing down the main ideas, Jeb agreed to play himself as an 8-year-old possessing the wisdom of his adult self. His therapist took on the role of Jeb's father in the scene they had role-played the week before:

FATHER: I can't believe you sat on the bench for almost the whole basketball game. You're so pathetic!

JEB: Why are you saying such mean things to me? I can't help that my asthma made me miss so many practices.

FATHER: You annoy me! I don't want you around.

JEB: You always seem so unhappy and angry. Why are you angry?

FATHER: I'm angry that I have to be here watching such a weak kid. You're pathetic!

JEB: I'm sorry I have asthma. But I wouldn't seem pathetic to you if you took some interest in me. I'm really a good kid.

FATHER: But I didn't want to have a kid. I want to be traveling the world, fighting for our country.

JEB: I know you like to fight. But I wish you wouldn't fight me. I didn't attack our country.

FATHER: No, but you sure messed up my life. I now have two people to be responsible for. I had more fun with your mother before you came along.

JEB: I'm sorry you don't want a family. But it really isn't fair to take it out on me. I'm only 8 years old. I didn't ask to be born.

FATHER: (*softening*) Yeah. I know. I'm just angry that I can't really do what I want.

Once Jeb understood how his father's criticism of him was related to his father's anger and frustrations, Jeb was better able to reconsider his core beliefs. His therapist asked him how he would like to view himself and others. Although skeptical that these were true, Jeb identified two core beliefs that he preferred: "I'm a good man" and "Others can accept me as I am." At this stage of therapy, his therapist began to introduce prediction logs, positive-experience logs, and imagery rehearsal of new behaviors. In prediction logs, Jeb recorded his expectations for different social experiences (e.g., "I'll try to talk to three people at the party tomorrow night but no one will want to talk to me") and actual outcomes ("Two people were friendly and one was okay"). Keeping track of what actually happened in situations over time helped Jeb see that his negative core belief did not predict his current experiences well at all.

In addition, Jeb kept a list of social interactions that supported his new beliefs. This positive-experience log required Jeb to shift his attention from rejection experiences to ones involving acceptance or social enjoyment. When he became self-critical and his negative core belief was activated, he reviewed this log to help reactivate his more positive core beliefs.

Finally, as Jeb began changing his beliefs and recognizing his good qualities, he became willing to enter more social situations (e.g., actively joining conversations when he and Marge were with friends, inviting coworkers to lunch, and arranging a party for Marge's birthday). He prepared for these new experiences through imagery rehearsal with his therapist. Jeb concretely imagined these situations and reported to the therapist any difficulties or embarrassment he experienced. They then discussed possible solutions to these social dilemmas, and Jeb rehearsed his desired behaviors and conversations in imagery before *in vivo* practice.

PROGRESS, LIFESPAN, AND TERMINATION CONSIDERATIONS

The final phase of therapy involves developing a plan to maintain progress, as patients with APD can easily become avoidant again. Progress maintenance involves work in both the behavioral and cognitive realms. Ongoing behavioral goals often include activities such as the following: establishing new friendships; deepening existing relationships; taking on more responsibility at work (or changing jobs); expressing preferences and opinions; acting in an appropriately assertive way with others; tackling previously avoided tasks at work, school, or home; and trying new experiences, such as taking a class, pursuing a new hobby, or volunteering.

These goals may feel risky to the patient. If thinking about them engenders distress, the anxiety can be framed in a positive way. Anxiety can be viewed as a sign the patient is making progress by entering new territory (Mooney & Padesky, 2000). Emergence of anxiety signals the reactivation of dysfunctional attitudes that could derail the patient from achieving personally important goals. Thus, anxiety is used as a spur to look for interfering automatic thoughts and underlying assumptions. The patient can review what helped in therapy to devise a system to recognize and respond to these negative cognitions and attitudes after therapy is terminated.

It is important for patients to attenuate their residual dysfunctional attitudes, and to strengthen their new, more functional beliefs. A core belief worksheet (J. Beck, 2006) helps patients identify and reframe data that initially seemed to support the old belief and to identify positive data supportive of the new belief. Patients can also keep diaries, on a daily or weekly basis, that record relevant positive experiences.

Two entries from Jeb's diary read:

> 3/5   Marge seemed irritated when I told her I thought Jimmy [his son] and I should go to the game instead of staying home and doing yard work. At first I felt bad and thought, "I've upset her. I'm a pathetic excuse for a husband." Then I realized that was my old way of thinking. The new idea, which I do believe, is that it is okay for Marge to have her feelings and she doesn't always have to be happy with me. I'm a good man and it is okay for a father to want to take his son to a ballgame. Jimmy was excited and we had a good time. When we got home, Marge had settled down. She said she realized that it was important that I express my preferences.

> 3/8   Thinking about asking boss for time off. Feeling very anxious. AT [automatic thought]: "He'll get mad at me." Old belief: "It's terrible for people to get mad." New beliefs: "He may not get mad but it's okay if he does," "He won't be mad forever," "This is good practice for me to be assertive," "I'll never get what I want if I let my old beliefs get in the way," "The worst that will happen is he'll say 'no.'"

A belief that is particularly troublesome for the patient who is avoidant is "If people really knew me, they'd reject me." This belief can be reactivated when patients develop new relationships and when they reveal more of themselves to others. If relevant, it is often helpful for patients to review their initial fears of revealing themselves to their therapist and how they think about this now. They can experiment by disclosing a relatively "benign" piece of information about themselves that they have been reluctant to reveal and then examining what transpires. They can continue to do so in a hierarchical fashion, gradually disclosing more about themselves to others.

In addition to daily belief logs and thought records, daily or weekly review of specially prepared index cards is also useful. Patients record a troublesome belief on one side of a card, with evidence against it beneath. On the other side is the more functional belief with supportive evidence. Patients can rate the credibility of each belief, at both an intellectual and emotional level, on a regular basis. Significantly increased confidence in a dysfunctional belief or significantly decreased confidence in a new belief indicates that patients need to do more work in that area.

Toward the end of treatment, the therapist should assess the benefits of spacing sessions. Some patients with APD need encouragement to reduce the frequency of therapy appointments. Other patients may desire and feel prepared to terminate, but may fear hurting the therapist's feelings by making such a suggestion.

Finally, it is helpful for therapists and patients who are avoidant to jointly develop a plan for patients to continue therapy on their own when formal therapy is terminated. Patients might, for example, set aside at least a few minutes each week to do activities aimed at continuing the progress made in therapy. During this time they can review self-assigned homework progress, examine any situations they avoided, investigate obstacles, look ahead to the coming week predicting which situations may be troublesome, and devise a way to deal with likely avoidance. They can review relevant notes or thought records from therapy. And, finally, they can self-assign homework and schedule their next self-therapy session (J. Beck, 2011).

An important goal of progress maintenance is to predict likely difficulties in the months following termination. Patients can be encouraged and guided to devise a plan to handle these troublesome situations. They may find it useful, for example, to compose instructions for themselves if they find they are experiencing the following difficulties:

> "What can I do if I find myself starting to avoid again?"
> "What can I do if I start believing my old beliefs more than my new beliefs?"
> "What can I do if I have a setback?"

Review of these paragraphs at relevant times can help maintain progress. Padesky and Mooney (2012) describe a four-step strengths-based cognitive-behavioral therapy model to build resilience. Therapists can use this model to help patients with APD (1) identify their positive interests and strengths; (2) construct a personal model of resilience; (3) consider how to apply this model to relevant challenges; and (4) practice staying resilient in the face of difficulties, rather than avoiding them.

COMMON CHALLENGES AND CLINICIAN SELF-CARE

Some therapists may experience considerable frustration with patients with APD because progress is usually quite slow. In fact, it can be a challenge to keep patients who are avoidant in treatment as they may begin to avoid therapy, too, by canceling appointments. It is helpful for therapists to realize that patients' avoidance of behavioral assignments, or of therapy itself, provides an opportunity to uncover the automatic thoughts and attitudes associated with this avoidance.

If such avoidance is present, the therapist (and patients, too) may begin to feel hopeless about treatment. It is important to anticipate and undermine hopelessness by focusing on the patient's progress to date, even if it is relatively small. A functional way to deal with avoidance of homework assignments is to focus on the thoughts that interfere with undertaking or completing a task and help patients test and effectively respond to those thoughts in the future.

Typical therapist cognitions about the avoidant patient may include the following: "The patient isn't trying," "She won't let me help her," "If I try really hard, she'll drop out of therapy anyway," "Our lack of progress reflects poorly on me," and "Another therapist would do better." These types of thoughts may lead the therapist to feel helpless, unable to assist the patient in effecting significant change. When these cognitions arise, the therapist can test them by reviewing what has transpired in therapy. It is important to keep realistic expectations for progress and recognize the achievement of small goals. On the other hand, consultation or supervision may be indicated if progress is, indeed, quite minimal.

CONCLUSION

Treatment of patients with APD involves the establishment of a trusting therapy alliance fostered by the identification and modification of patients' dysfunctional thoughts and beliefs regarding this relationship, especially expectations of criticism or rejection. The therapy relationship serves as a laboratory for testing beliefs prior to the APD patient's testing beliefs about other relationships. It also provides a safe environment to try new behaviors (e.g., assertiveness). Mood-management techniques are employed to teach patients to manage their depression, anxiety, or other disorders.

The goal is not to eliminate dysphoria altogether but to increase patients' tolerance for and acceptance of negative emotion. A schematic diagram to illustrate the process of avoidance and a strong rationale for increasing tolerance and acceptance of emotions helps patients become more motivated to experience negative feelings in the session—a strategy that may be implemented in hierarchical fashion. Tolerance of negative affect within sessions may have to precede "emotion tolerance" or "antiavoid-ance" practice outside of therapy. An important key to increasing tolerance is the continual testing of beliefs concerning what patients fear will happen if they experience dysphoria. Couple or family therapy may be indicated, as well as social skills training. Finally, treatment also encompasses the iden-tification and modification of maladaptive automatic thoughts, underlying assumptions, and core beliefs. Beliefs that are more realistic and positive in nature may have to be constructed and validated through a variety of tech-niques, such as positive-experience diaries as described previously.

CHAPTER 10

Obsessive–Compulsive Personality Disorder

Karen M. Simon

"If a thing is worth doing, it's worth doing well."

Mr. S was a 45-year-old white, married engineer with a school-age son. He came for cognitive therapy after a recent exacerbation of a chronic and severe muscular pain in his back, neck, and shoulders. Mr. S had suffered from this condition since his late 20s. Because he originally considered his pain to be a physical problem, Mr. S sought treatment from physical therapists, chiropractors, and massage therapists and he took various muscle relaxants and anti-inflammatory medications. These treatments helped somewhat, but Mr. S had a severe episode of pain in his late 30s that resulted in his missing 3 weeks of work. At that time he was working on an important and complicated project. He then began seriously considering that his neck and back pain might be related to the degree of psychological stress that he was experiencing.

Mr. S had been born in a midsized city in the United States and was raised in a conservative, religious, middle-class family. He was the younger of two children, with a sister 7 years older. Mr. S described his father as being a nice, somewhat anxious man with whom Mr. S had a good but not a close relationship. He was much closer to his mother and stated that he was always concerned about her opinion of him. His mother was very involved with Mr. S when he was a child. He liked the attention but also experienced her as being a critical, judgmental woman who had many rules about the way that people are supposed to behave. Mr. S remembered one particular incident, when he was in first grade, in which a friend had gotten a citizenship award and he had not. Although she did not explicitly state it, he got the impression that his mother was dissatisfied with him and was thinking, "Your friend earned an award, so why can't you?"

Mr. S reported feeling reasonably happy during his childhood. By sixth grade, however, he started becoming concerned about his grades and popularity. In school, he coped with this by either working very hard to do well (while always worrying that he was not doing well enough) or else by procrastinating and trying not to think about what he was supposed to be doing. Socially, he became introverted, avoidant, and emotionally constricted. By being less involved and expressive, the less chance it seemed to him that he had of being criticized or rejected. These patterns of behavior gradually increased throughout his adolescence.

During his second year of college, Mr. S experienced a great deal of anxiety over his inability to perform academically up to his expectations. It became harder for him to complete written assignments because he was concerned that they would not be good enough. In addition, Mr. S felt very lonely and isolated due to his being away from home and his inability to develop friendships or romantic relationships. He became increasingly pessimistic about himself and his future. This culminated in a major depressive episode, during which he lost interest in most activities and spent the majority of his time sleeping. This episode lasted a couple of months and led to Mr. S dropping out of school and joining the army. The increased structure and companionship in the army were helpful, and he functioned well for the 3 years he was in the service. He then returned to school and obtained his engineering degree.

Mr. S had worked as an engineer since his late 20s and had been moderately successful in his career. At the time he sought treatment, he was performing some administrative and supervisory duties, which were less comfortable for him than the more structured, technical, detail-oriented engineering work on which he spent most of his time.

Mr. S was never comfortable or very successful with dating. In his early 30s, he was reintroduced to a woman he had met briefly several years before. She remembered him—which surprised and flattered him—and they started dating. They married 1 year later, and 2 years after that had a child. Mr. S described the marriage as being good but not as close as he would like. He felt emotionally and sexually restrained with his wife, and he realized this was part of his problem. Mr. S did not have any close friends but was marginally involved with various church and civic groups.

CLINICAL SIGNS AND SYMPTOMS

The obsessive–compulsive personality style is common in contemporary Western culture, particularly among males (American Psychiatric

Association, 2000). This may be partially due to the high value that society places on certain characteristics of this style. These qualities include attention to detail, self-discipline, emotional control, perseverance, reliability, and politeness. However, some individuals possess these qualities in such an extreme form that they lead to either functional impairment or subjective distress. Thus, the individual who develops obsessive–compulsive personality disorder (OCPD) becomes rigid, perfectionistic, dogmatic, ruminative, moralistic, inflexible, indecisive, and emotionally and cognitively blocked.

DSM-5 (American Psychiatric Association, 2013) defines the essential features of OCPD as significant impairment in personality and interpersonal functioning co-occurring with pathological personality traits. To meet criteria for impaired personality functioning, the individual must show impairments in his or her identity, self-direction, or both.

Individuals who meet criteria for OCPD tend to derive their identity from their work or productivity and tend to experience a constricted range and intensity of emotions. They also tend to have a rigid perfectionism that interferes with completing tasks and achieving goals. In DSM-5, impairments in interpersonal functioning are defined as difficulty with empathy and intimacy. Pathological personality traits in the individual with OCPD are identified as compulsivity and negative affectivity.

The *International Classification of Diseases—Version 2010* (ICD-10; World Health Organization, 2010) equivalent of OCPD is anankastic personality disorder. Individuals with this personality disorder are characterized by ICD-10 as experiencing "feelings of doubt, perfectionism, excessive conscientiousness, checking and preoccupation with details, stubbornness, caution, and rigidity" (*http://apps.who.int/classifications/icd10/browse/2010/ en#/F60.5*). ICD-10 specifies that the individual with anankastic personality disorder may experience "insistent and unwelcome thoughts or impulses that do not attain the severity of an obsessive–compulsive disorder."

The most common presenting problem of persons with OCPD is some form of anxiety. Compulsives' perfectionism, rigidity, and rule-governed behavior predispose them to the chronic anxiety that is characteristic of generalized anxiety disorder. Many compulsives ruminate about whether they are performing well enough or doing the wrong thing. This often leads to the indecisiveness and procrastination that are frequent presenting complaints. Chronic anxiety may intensify to the point of panic disorder if these individuals find themselves in a severe conflict between their compulsiveness and external pressures. For example, if an individual who is compulsive is approaching the deadline for a project but is progressing very slowly due to perfectionism, his or her anxiety may escalate. The compulsive then may catastrophize about his or her physical symptoms, such as rapid heartbeat and shortness of breath. This may lead to the vicious cycle often seen in patients with panic disorder, in which worry leads to increased physical symptoms, which lead to further increased worry, and so on.

Individuals with OCPD also suffer from specific obsessions and compulsions more than average. Rasmussen and Tsuang (1986) found that 55% of a sample of 44 individuals with obsessive or compulsive symptoms also had OCPD. Furthermore, a longitudinal study of 668 patients found that approximately 21% of their subjects with OCPD (as per DSM-IV) also met criteria for obsessive–compulsive disorder (McGlashan et al., 2000).

Another common presenting problem in OCPD is depression. This may take the form of dysthymic disorder or major depressive disorder. Compulsives often lead rather flat, boring, unsatisfying lives and suffer from chronic mild depression. Some will become aware of this over time, although they may not understand why it is occurring and will come to therapy complaining of anhedonia, boredom, lack of energy, and not enjoying life as much as others appear to. Sometimes they will be pushed into therapy by spouses who view them as depressed and depressing. Due to their rigidity, perfectionism, and strong need to be in control of themselves, their emotions, and their environment, compulsives are very vulnerable to becoming overwhelmed, hopeless, emotionally isolated, and depressed. This may happen when they experience their lives as having gotten out of control and their usual coping mechanisms as being ineffective.

Compulsives often experience a variety of psychosomatic disorders. They are predisposed to developing such problems because of the physical effects of their chronically heightened arousal and anxiety. They frequently suffer from tension headaches, backaches, constipation, and ulcers. They may also have Type A personalities and thus are at increased risk for cardiovascular problems, particularly if they are frequently angry and hostile. Because compulsives frequently view these disorders as having physical causes, it is common for them to be referred to psychotherapy by physicians. Helping them to understand and work on the psychological aspects of these problems can be quite difficult.

Sexual disorders may also be a presenting problem. The compulsive's discomfort with emotion, lack of spontaneity, overcontrol, and rigidity is not conducive to a free and comfortable expression of his or her sexuality. Common sexual dysfunctions experienced by the compulsive are inhibited sexual desire, inability to have an orgasm, premature ejaculation, and dyspareunia.

Finally, compulsives may come to therapy due to problems other people are having in coping with them. Spouses may initiate couple therapy because of their discomfort with the compulsive's lack of emotional availability or workaholic behavior resulting in little time spent with the family. Families with a parent who is compulsive may come for therapy due to the rigid, strict style of parenting, which can lead to chronic fighting between the parent and children. Employers may send employees who are compulsive to therapy because of their continual procrastination or their inability to function effectively in interpersonal relationships on the job.

RESEARCH AND EMPIRICAL DATA

There has been little definitive research on OCPD. To date, most of the knowledge about this disorder has been derived from clinical work. However, there is considerable evidence that OCPD does exist as a separate entity. Several factor-analytic studies have found that the various traits hypothesized to comprise OCPD do tend to occur together (Hill, 1976; Lazare, Klerman, & Armor, 1966; Torgerson, 1980). Adams (1973), in working with children who are obsessive, found that the children's parents had a number of obsessive traits, including being strict and controlling, overconforming, unempathic, and disapproving of spontaneous expression of affect. It has not yet been determined what percentage of children with obsessive–compulsive personality traits develops into adults with OCPD.

There has been some research into the genetic and physiological bases of OCPD. A study by Clifford, Murray, and Fulker (1984) found a significantly higher correlation of compulsive traits, as measured by the trait scale of the Layton Obsessive Inventory, in a sample of monozygotic twins than in a sample of dizygotic twins. In another study, Smokler and Shevrin (1979) examined compulsive and histrionic personality styles in relation to brain hemisphericity as reflected by lateral eye movements. The authors found that the subjects who were compulsive looked predominantly to the right when responding to experimental tasks, which they interpreted as showing a higher degree of left-hemisphere activation, while the subjects who were histrionic looked predominantly to the left. Because the left hemisphere has been associated with language, analytic thinking, and reason, it was expected to be predominant in subjects who were compulsive. The right hemisphere has been associated with imagery and synthetic thinking.

Beck and his colleagues (2001) investigated whether dysfunctional beliefs discriminated among personality disorders, including OCPD. In their study, a large number of psychiatric outpatients (mean age 34.73 years) completed the Personality Belief Questionnaire (PBQ; Beck & Beck, 1991) at intake and were evaluated for personality disorders using a standardized clinical interview. The subjects also completed the Structured Clinical Interview for DSM-IV (SCID-II; First, Spitzer, Gibbon, & Williams, 1995). Their findings showed that patients with OCPD preferentially endorsed PBQ beliefs theoretically linked to their specific disorders. Beck and colleagues (2001) interpreted their results as supporting the cognitive theory of personality disorders.

Although many clinicians report success in treating OCPD with cognitive therapy (e.g., Beck, Freeman, & Associates, 1990; Freeman, Pretzer, Fleming, & Simon, 1990; Pretzer & Hampl, 1994), the definitive outcome research has not yet been conducted. However, there have been a few studies that tend to support the use of cognitive interventions with compulsive traits and OCPD.

Hardy and his colleagues (1995) examined the impact of DSM-III Cluster C personality disorders on outcomes of contrasting brief psychotherapies for depression. Twenty-seven of their 114 depressed patients obtained a DSM-III diagnosis of Cluster C personality disorder, that is, obsessive–compulsive, avoidant, or dependent personality disorder, whereas the remaining 87 did not. All patients completed either 8 or 16 sessions of cognitive-behavioral or psychodynamic–interpersonal psychotherapy. On most measures, patients with personality disorders began with more severe symptoms than patients without personality disorders. Among those who received psychodynamic–interpersonal therapy, patients with personality disorders maintained this difference posttreatment and at 1-year follow-up. Among those who received cognitive-behavioral therapy, posttreatment differences between those with and without personality disorders were not significant. The length of treatment did not influence these results. It should be noted, however, that Barber and Muenz (1996) found that individuals with compulsive personality did better with interpersonal–psychodynamic therapy than with cognitive therapy.

In a study comparing cognitive therapy to medication, Black, Monahan, Wesner, Gabel, and Bowers (1996) examined abnormal personality traits in patients with panic disorder. Cognitive therapy was associated with a significant reduction in abnormal personality traits, as measured by the Personality Diagnostic Questionnaire—Revised (Hyler & Reider, 1987). This was true for compulsive, as well as for schizotypal, narcissistic, and borderline personalities.

McKay, Neziroglu, Todaro, and Yaryura-Tobias (1996) examined changes in personality disorders following behavior therapy for obsessive–compulsive disorder. Twenty-one adults who were diagnosed with obsessive–compulsive disorder participated. At pretest, the mean number of personality disorders was approximately four, whereas the posttest number was approximately three. Their analyses suggest that this change, although apparently small, was clinically relevant because change in number of personality disorders was significantly related to treatment outcome. Although treatment was successful in reducing obsessive–compulsive disorder symptoms, obsessive–compulsive personality was more resistant to change.

DIFFERENTIAL DIAGNOSIS

Assessment and diagnosis of OCPD are not usually difficult if the clinician is aware of, and watchful for, its various manifestations and clinical signs. At the first telephone contact with the compulsive, the therapist may detect signs of rigidity or indecisiveness in arranging the first appointment. Indecisiveness in the compulsive will be based on the fear of making a mistake rather than the fear of displeasing or inconveniencing the therapist, as might be seen in a patient with dependent personality disorder.

Upon first meeting, the clinician may notice that the patient who is compulsive is rather stilted and formal and not particularly warm or expressive. In trying to express themselves correctly, compulsives often ruminate a great deal about a topic, making sure that they tell the therapist all the details and consider all the options. Conversely, they may speak in a slow, hesitating manner, which is also due to their anxiety about not expressing themselves exactly correctly. The content of the compulsive's speech will consist much more of facts and ideas rather than of feelings and preferences. In obtaining historical and current life information, possible indicators of OCPD include the following:

1. The patient was raised in the rigid, controlling type of family discussed earlier.
2. The patient lacks close, self-disclosing interpersonal relationships.
3. The patient is in a technical, detail-oriented profession such as accounting, law, or engineering.
4. The patient either lacks many leisure activities or has leisure activities that are purposeful and goal directed and not merely pursued for enjoyment.

Formal psychological testing may be helpful at times in diagnosing OCPD. The Millon Clinical Multiaxial Inventory–III (Millon, Millon, Davis, & Grossman, 2009) was specifically designed to diagnose personality disorders and is often useful in understanding the various manifestations of OCPD. Typical responses on projective tests are a large number of small-detail responses on the Rorschach, and long, detailed, moralistic stories on the Thematic Apperception Test. The therapist will need to consider whether the time and money spent on projective tests are worthwhile because an accurate diagnosis and understanding of the patient can probably be obtained without them.

The simplest and most economical way to diagnose OCPD is usually just to ask patients directly, in a straightforward, noncritical manner, whether the various DSM-5 criteria apply to them. Most compulsives will quite readily admit to such criteria as not feeling comfortable expressing affection, being perfectionistic, and having difficulty making decisions. However, they might not understand the connection between such characteristics and their presenting problems for therapy.

OCPD has a number of elements in common with other symptomatic and personality disorders that may need to be ruled out for accurate diagnosis (American Psychiatric Association, 2013). The difference between OCPD and obsessive–compulsive disorder is relatively easy to determine. Only obsessive–compulsive disorder has true ego-dystonic obsessions and compulsions, whereas OCPD does not. However, if diagnostic criteria are met for both disorders, both diagnoses should be made.

OCPD and narcissistic personality disorder tend to share perfectionism and the belief that other people cannot do things as well as they can. An important difference is that individuals with OCPD are self-critical, whereas those with narcissistic personality disorder are not. Individuals with both narcissistic personality disorder and antisocial personality disorder lack generosity but will indulge themselves. However, individuals with OCPD are stingy with themselves as well as with others. OCPD shares with schizoid personality disorder an apparent formality and social detachment. In schizoid personality disorder, this results from a fundamental lack of capacity for intimacy, whereas in OCPD, this results from discomfort with emotions and excessive devotion to work.

On occasion, OCPD may also need to be differentiated from personality change due to a general medical condition, such as the effect of a disease process upon the central nervous system. OCPD symptoms may also need to be differentiated from symptoms that may have developed in association with chronic drug use (e.g., cocaine-related disorder not otherwise specified).

CONCEPTUALIZATION

The conceptualization of OCPD used in this chapter integrates the views given above and follows Freeman, Pretzer, Fleming, and Simon (2004) and Pretzer and Hampl (1994). The driving schemas are considered to be: "I must avoid mistakes at all costs," "There is one right path/answer/behavior in each situation," and "Mistakes are intolerable." Most of the problematic aspects of OCPD are seen here as resulting from the strategies these individuals use to avoid mistakes: "I must be careful and thorough," "I must pay attention to details," "I must notice mistakes immediately so they can be corrected," and "To make a mistake is to deserve criticism." The goal of individuals who are compulsive is to eliminate mistakes, not merely to minimize them. This results in a desire for total control over themselves and their environment.

An important characteristic distortion of these individuals is dichotomous thinking. This is shown in the belief: "Any departure from what is right is automatically wrong." Beyond the many intrapersonal problems described previously, such beliefs lead to interpersonal problems because relationships often involve strong emotions and do not have unambiguously correct answers. Relationships are also problematic because they threaten to distract these individuals from work and thus promote mistakes. The compulsives' solution is to avoid both the emotions and the ambiguous situations.

Another prominent cognitive distortion in OCPD is magical thinking: "One can prevent disasters/mistakes by worrying about them." If the perfect course of action is unclear, it is better to do nothing. Therefore, patients who are compulsive tend to avoid mistakes of commission but not omission. They tend to catastrophize about changing their approach to life, believing that nothing except their compulsivity stands between them and sloth, financial ruin, or promiscuity.

Using the example of Mr. S, we will demonstrate how the cognitive therapist can begin to form a conceptualization. A reading of his description at the beginning of this chapter reveals a number of themes, suggesting possible schemas. Mr. S repeatedly expresses a sense of his own inadequacy. This is shown in his description of the interaction with his mother when he was in first grade. His sense of himself as inadequate in comparison to others is suggested by his lifelong pattern of avoidance and isolation. He states that the less involved and expressive he is, the less chance he has of being criticized or rejected. This leads to another theme in Mr. S's history. He seems to have a strong expectation of criticism by others, from his mother and his childhood peers to his current supervisor. Mr. S's strong sense of inadequacy and expectation of criticism seem to stem from his perfectionism. He worries about making mistakes even when his performance is fine, and he can never believe that he is doing well enough. This can be seen as early as grade school and continuing into his current job. Because Mr. S. shows a number of characteristics of OCPD, the therapist will keep the possibility of this disorder in mind as treatment continues. Additional information will influence the therapist's emerging cognitive conceptualization of Mr. S.

KEY TREATMENT GOALS

The cognitive treatment of OCPD addresses several general goals:

1. Educate the patient who is compulsive about the role of perfectionism in producing and maintaining his or her presenting symptoms.
2. Assist the patient who is compulsive in testing the difference between rigidly following long-held rules and routines and flexibly evaluating what works for him or her and what does not.
3. Help the patient who is compulsive evaluate the automatic thoughts, underlying assumptions, and core beliefs that maintain perfectionism and rigidity.
4. Link these general goals to the productivity/work life and personal relationships of the patient who is compulsive, with meaningful personal outcomes targeted as the specific goals of treatment.

Treatment success is evident in reduced tension or pain and distress, along with greater flexibility in applying standards and improved productivity, time management, and personal relationships.

In addition to teaching patients the cognitive theory of emotion, it is important at the beginning of cognitive therapy to establish therapeutic goals. These will relate to the presenting problems and may, for the compulsive, include such things as "getting assignments or work done on time," "reducing the frequency of tension headaches," or "being able to have orgasms during intercourse." It is important to be specific in listing goals; general goals such as "not being depressed" are harder to work with. If the patient is mainly concerned with depression, it is necessary to break this down into its various aspects, such as being able to get up earlier in the morning or being able to accomplish specific occupational or social tasks, to effectively treat the depression.

Relevant and workable goals are then ranked in the order they are to be worked on, as it is difficult and often nonproductive to try to work on several at once. Two criteria to use in ranking the goals are the importance of each problem to the patient and how easily solvable it is. It is often helpful to have rapid success early in therapy to heighten the patient's motivation and belief in the therapeutic process. After goals have been established, it is important to identify the automatic thoughts and schemas that are associated with them.

Early in the course of cognitive therapy, it is vital to introduce patients to the idea that feelings and behaviors are related to their perceptions of, thoughts about, and meanings given to life events. Watching for an affective shift in the session and then asking the patient what he or she had been thinking just before can demonstrate the cognitive model. Another way to demonstrate this would be to describe a situation such as waiting for a friend who is late and listing the various emotions that the person waiting may be experiencing, such as anger, anxiety, or depression, and relating these feelings to thoughts that were probably producing them: "How dare he make me wait for him," "Maybe he was in an accident," or "This just proves that nobody likes me."

Generally, the problem being worked on is monitored each week between sessions, usually on a dysfunctional thought record (DTR; Beck, Rush, Shaw, & Emery, 1979). The DTR allows patients to list what the situation is, how they are feeling, and what their thoughts are when the problem occurs. Thus, a compulsive working on procrastination might become aware that when he or she is avoiding a task at work, he or she is feeling anxious, and thinking, "I don't want to do this assignment because I won't be able to do it perfectly." After a number of similar examples of automatic thoughts have been gathered, it becomes apparent to the compulsive that much of the anxiety and procrastination is due to perfectionism. It is then crucial to determine the assumptions or schemas underlying the various automatic thoughts. In the example of perfectionism, the underlying assumption may be "I must avoid mistakes to be worthwhile." It is often helpful at this point to assist the patient in understanding how he or she learned the schema. Usually it developed out of interactions with parents or other significant figures, although sometimes the schemas are based more on cultural norms or developed in more idiosyncratic ways. Therapy then consists of helping the patient who is compulsive to identify and understand the negative consequences of these assumptions or schemas and then to develop ways of refuting them so that they no longer control the patients' feelings and behavior and lead to the problems that brought him or her to therapy. New, more helpful assumptions are developed in collaboration with the patient as possible alternative schemas to be tried out in his or her daily activities. Usually, one will emerge as the front-runner to take the place of each of the old, maladaptive schemas.

Mr. S's goal in therapy was to eliminate, or at least greatly diminish, the pain he experienced in his back and neck. Unlike many patients who are psychosomatic, he had already come to accept that psychological factors played a major part in his pain. The therapist discussed the cognitive model with Mr. S, and he was quite receptive to it. The homework assignment for the first few weeks was to monitor his pain on the weekly activity schedule. This consisted of ranking the severity of his pain from 1 to 10 on an hour-by-hour basis while also noting what he was doing. At first, Mr. S noticed that the pain was most severe in the evening, when he was home with his family. This was difficult for him to understand, as usually he enjoyed his evenings at home and found them relaxing. Through data gathering, Mr. S realized that he distracted himself from the pain as it was building during the day. At times, distraction is a useful technique for compulsives, particularly with their nonproductive, ruminative thinking. In Mr. S's case, however, distraction interfered with the assessment of the problem. As he became more aware of his pain, he noticed that it would start as a type of tingling, sunburn-like feeling and then progress from mild to a more severe pain. Under prolonged stress, the muscles in his back and neck would spasm, and he would have to spend a couple of days at home in bed.

COLLABORATIVE STRATEGY

Compulsives may enter therapy for a variety of reasons, but they rarely ask for help with their personality disorder. Although they are sometimes aware that certain aspects of their personality, such as being perfectionistic, contribute to their psychological problems, they generally do not seek help for inflexible thinking or overcontrolled emotions and behavior.

The general goal of psychotherapy with patients with OCPD is to help them alter or reinterpret the problematic underlying assumptions so that behaviors and emotions will change. Cognitive therapists are generally willing to accept patient's complaints at face value. Thus, when a patient complains at intake of anxiety, headaches, or impotence, this is frequently the problem that is addressed. Sometimes the compulsive's complaints are more externalized—for example, "My supervisors are very critical of my work for no good reason." This type of problem presentation can be more difficult to work with. The therapist can still directly address the presenting complaint, however, by clearly establishing that because the supervisor's behavior cannot be directly changed through the therapy, the goal will need to be to change the patient's behavior in ways that may lead to the supervisor's acting differently toward him or her.

As in all therapies, it is important at the start to establish a rapport with the patient. This can be difficult with patients who are compulsive because of their rigidity, discomfort with emotion, and tendency to downplay the importance of interpersonal relationships. Cognitive therapy with the compulsive tends be even more business-like and problem focused than usual, with less emphasis on emotional support and relationship issues. Usually, rapport is based on the patient's respect for the therapist's competence and a belief that the therapist respects and can be helpful to the patient. Trying to develop a closer emotional relationship than the compulsive is comfortable with early in therapy can be detrimental and may lead to an early termination.

Compulsives can elicit a variety of emotional reactions from therapists. Some therapists find these patients to be somewhat dry and boring because of their general lack of emotionality and their tendency to focus more on the factual aspects of events rather than the events' affective tones. They can also be experienced as exasperating because of their slowness and focus on details, particularly to therapists who value efficiency and goal directedness. Therapists who tend to like the idealization and dependency that many patients develop in therapy often find patients who are compulsive less rewarding, as they tend not to form this kind of therapeutic relationship. Some compulsives act out their needs for control in the therapy in either a direct or a passive–aggressive manner. For example, when given a homework assignment, they might directly tell the therapist that the assignment is irrelevant or stupid, or else agree to do it but then "forget" or not make the time to get the assignment done. These patients can elicit anger and frustration from therapists and bring up conflicts related to the therapists' own need to be in control.

Another problematic situation may occur when the therapist's schemas are also compulsive. As noted early in this chapter, subclinical compulsive characteristics can be conducive to success in Western culture. The cognitive therapist may have achieved his or her academic and professional success through conscientiousness, attention to detail, self-discipline, perseverance, reliability, and so on. If the therapist is also perfectionistic, rigid, overly controlled, and lacking in insight, he or she may also be blind to the patient's pathology. Such therapists may buy into their patients' perspective uncritically and therefore miss opportunities to help them.

Therapists' reactions to patients who are compulsive can provide valuable information about the patients and the sources of their difficulties. However, therapists should avoid trying to make changes in the patient based on their own values rather than the patient's needs and presenting problems. For example, Mr. S may have been less emotionally expressive than his therapist would prefer, but this was not a source of significant impairment or subjective distress for him and therefore not a focus of treatment.

Strauss and colleagues (2006) studied the role of the therapeutic relationship between patients with OCPD or avoidant personality disorder and their cognitive-behavioral therapists. After studying 30 patients who completed 52 sessions of weekly therapy, they found two factors that predicted greater reduction in symptoms. The first factor was the patients' initial rating of the therapeutic alliance. The second factor was related to the occurrence of a problem in the alliance during treatment, which the patient and therapist then went on to resolve. The collaboration that occurs in therapy and the experience of overcoming the obstacles to collaboration in treatment turn out to be meaningful in terms of the patients' improved functioning in general.

CLINICAL APPLICATION OF THE INTERVENTION

Within the broad structure of cognitive therapy, a number of specific techniques are helpful with patients with OCPD. It is important to structure the therapy sessions by setting an agenda, prioritizing the problems, and using problem-solving techniques. This is useful in working with a number of characteristics, including indecisiveness, rumination, and procrastination. Structure asks that the patient choose and work on a specific problem until it improves to an acceptable level. If the compulsive has difficulty working with the structure, the therapist can have the patient look at his or her automatic thoughts about it and relate this difficulty to the general problems of indecisiveness and procrastination. The weekly activity schedule (Beck et al., 1979), a form on which patients can schedule activities on an hourly basis, can also help them add structure to their lives and become more productive while exerting less effort.

The therapist must be prepared for the patient who is compulsive to use these or other specific techniques in a perfectionistic manner. For example, it is not unusual for patients with OCPD to bring a thick stack of flawlessly printed DTRs to session as their homework for the week. Although this conscientiousness might at first appear to be helpful for their progress in therapy, it is usually better seen as a sample of their problematic behavior. Patients who are compulsive often display their typical vacillation and rumination in their use of the DTR. They may bounce back and forth between the automatic thoughts and rational response columns, never reaching a balanced conclusion. This may be seen as a sample of the thinking process in which they engage privately. It therefore provides an opportunity to address the process as well as the content of their cognitions.

Because of compulsives' frequent problems with anxiety and psychosomatic symptoms, relaxation techniques, meditation, and mindfulness are often helpful. Compulsives frequently have difficulty using these techniques at first, sometimes due to their belief that they are wasting time by taking half an hour to relax or meditate. A cognitive therapy technique that is useful in addressing these issues is to list advantages and disadvantages of a specific behavior or belief. A disadvantage to relaxation techniques for the compulsive may be that they take time; an advantage might be that the patient can actually get more done because he or she is more refreshed and less anxious.

It is often useful to conduct behavioral experiments with patients with OCPD. For example, instead of directly trying to dispute a certain belief held by a compulsive, the therapist can take a neutral, experimental attitude toward it. Thus, if an individual who is compulsive claims not to have time to relax during the day, the therapist may suggest an experiment to test this claim. The patient may compare productivity on days he or she uses relaxation techniques in contrast with the days he or she does not. Compulsives tend to value pleasure much less than productivity. It is often therapeutic to help them become aware of this and evaluate with them the assumptions behind their value system concerning the place of pleasure in their lives.

Several cognitive and behavioral techniques can be useful in helping patients who are compulsive cope with chronic worrying and ruminating. Once patients agree that this is dysfunctional, they can be taught a mindful approach of noticing, labeling, and redirecting their thoughts. If they continue to believe that worrying is helpful or productive, they may agree to limit it to a certain time period during the day. This at least helps them to minimize their worrying for the rest of the day. Graded task assignments, in which a goal or task is broken down into specific definable steps, are often helpful. These steps serve to counter patients' dichotomous thinking and perfectionism by demonstrating that most things are accomplished by degrees of progress, rather than by being done perfectly or in their entirety right from the beginning.

After Mr. S learned to monitor his pain more consistently, he discovered that three types of situations were associated with his muscular tension. These included (1) having tasks or assignments to do, (2) having procrastinated and thereby having many things not completed, and (3) being expected to participate in social situations with new people. Mr. S and his therapist decided to work initially on the first situation, as it occurred much more often than the third, and tended to lead to the second. For example, he once noticed that he was experiencing a moderate degree of back pain while standing and rinsing off the dishes before putting them in the dishwasher. He was thinking that the dishes needed to be perfectly clean before putting them in the dishwasher. This thought was making the task stressful and take much longer than it should. Collecting a number of similar examples helped Mr. S see that his perfectionism resulted in numerous tasks each day becoming sources of stress that produced pain. He then began to look for the general assumptions or schemas underlying his automatic thoughts. Mr. S. developed the diagram shown in Figure 10.1 as a model of his behavior.

The therapist and Mr. S then further discussed the meaning of this pattern of thinking and behavior:

THERAPIST: So you find that you experience a lot of stress when having to do a task because you believe that no matter how well you do it, it won't be acceptable?

PATIENT: Yes, and I think that's why I tend not to make decisions or to procrastinate so I don't have to deal with these feelings.

THERAPIST: So you avoid and procrastinate in order to reduce your stress?

PATIENT: Yes, I think so.

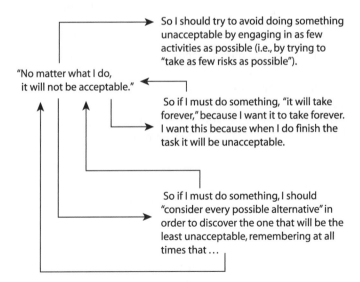

FIGURE 10.1. Mr. S's model of his behavior.

THERAPIST: Does that actually work for you as a way of reducing stress?

PATIENT: No, putting things off usually just make it worse. I like to think I'm a pretty responsible person, and it really bothers me not to be getting things done. I've had some of my worst back pain after I've been procrastinating all week.

THERAPIST: You wrote on the diagram that you believe what you do won't be acceptable. What if you did something that wasn't acceptable to certain other people? What about that would upset you?

PATIENT: What do you mean?

THERAPIST: Do you think it's possible for someone to do something that someone else would consider unacceptable, yet not get upset about it?

PATIENT: Yes, I've known some people like that. I guess for me, though, I feel like I am personally unacceptable or deficient if I don't function up to a certain level, which often seems impossible for me to do.

Thus, Mr. S's core schema or belief was that if he did not always function perfectly, then he was personally unacceptable. Given there was little chance that he could perform well enough to be acceptable, his primary symptoms were a form of anxiety (i.e., the physical stress in his back). At times, though, Mr. S would give up and conclude that no matter what he did would be unacceptable. At these times, he would become hopeless and depressed, like he did during college.

After uncovering Mr. S's core belief, the focus in therapy was to change it, as the belief seemed to be the primary source both for Mr. S's current symptoms and heavily contributed toward his OCPD. As the therapist and Mr. S discussed his belief over the next few sessions, he came to understand better how he had internalized the very high standards he believed his mother had for him. In addition, he became very self-critical, as he had experienced his mother to be when he did not meet her expectations. He also expected others to be very critical of him.

The therapist and Mr. S started examining the validity of his beliefs by first looking at whether they appeared to be accurate interpretations of the past. For one homework assignment, Mr. S listed all the times he could remember in the past that others had been very critical of him, and also listed possible alternatives as to why they might have acted that way. Mr. S also had the thought that probably others had been disapproving of him on many occasions but just had not said so. The therapist and Mr. S then discussed what he could do about this belief:

THERAPIST: So it still seems to you that most others are disapproving of you, even though you can think of very few times when you have had clear evidence that this was true?

PATIENT: Yes, I still often think that others aren't pleased with what I am doing, and then I am very uncomfortable around them.

THERAPIST: How do you think you could find out if these thoughts are accurate or not?

PATIENT: I don't know.

THERAPIST: Well, in general, if you wanted to know what someone is thinking, what would you do?

PATIENT: I guess I would ask them.

THERAPIST: Would that be possible for you? Do you think you could ask for feedback the next time you believe someone is disapproving of you?

PATIENT: I'm not sure. They might not like my asking them or they might not tell me the truth.

THERAPIST: That is a possibility and maybe we can think of a way to determine that later on. In the meantime, what if we start with someone you believe to be pretty honest and nonjudgmental? Who do you think would fit that description?

PATIENT: My boss is a decent guy and I'd really like not to have to worry that he is judging me all the time.

THERAPIST: Can you think of a relatively safe way you could ask your boss how he is feeling about you or your work?

PATIENT: I suppose I could say something like this: "Jack, you seem to be concerned about something. Is anything bothering you about the way my project is going?"

THERAPIST: That sounds pretty good. Would you be willing to accept that as your homework for next week? Would you be willing to ask your boss his thoughts once this week when you think he is disapproving of you and record both what you expect him to say and what he actually says?

PATIENT: Okay, I'll try that.

This was an example of setting up a behavioral experiment to test a specific dysfunctional belief. Over the next couple of weeks, Mr. S did, on several occasions, ask others what they were thinking when he thought that they were evaluating him critically. He found that on all but one occasion, he had misinterpreted what others were thinking about him. On that occasion, one of his bosses at work was mildly annoyed with him, but this was due to Mr. S being late in getting him some work. The patient realized from this that his procrastination caused more problems and dissatisfactions for him than his level of performance.

Mr. S, like many compulsives, had the belief that it was often functional to put things off because this enabled him to perform better. The therapist had him evaluate this belief in a homework assignment by rating his level of performance from 1 to 10 on a variety of tasks. He then compared the average level of performance on those tasks he had done immediately. He found that his average level of performance was slightly higher on tasks that he did without procrastinating. Mr. S attributed this to the increased stress he would feel about tasks he avoided.

Another technique that proved helpful to Mr. S was having him compare the values and standards he had for himself with those he had for others. He came to realize that he was much more critical and demanding of himself than he was of others, and he agreed that it did not make much sense to have two different sets of values. The therapist then built on this understanding by having him note when he was being self-critical and ask himself what he would be thinking if he observed someone else performing at the same level. Mr. S found that this technique helped him to be more understanding and less critical of himself. This technique does not work with many compulsives, however, because patients who are compulsive are frequently as critical and demanding of others as they are of themselves.

The therapist and Mr. S also identified the primary cognitive distortions and maladaptive modes of thought that Mr. S frequently used. These included:

1. Dichotomous thinking ("If I don't do this task perfectly, I have done it terribly").
2. Magnification ("It is horrible if I don't do this well").
3. Overgeneralization ("If I do something poorly, it means I am an unacceptable person").
4. "Should" statements ("I should do this perfectly").
5. Mind reading ("Others are judging me, even though they haven't said so").

Mr. S monitored the use of these thought patterns on DTRs, and identified how they increased his stress level and often lowered his level of performance.

As Mr. S learned to recognize and understand the distortions in his thought processes, he became increasingly effective at responding rationally to his automatic thoughts. This helped Mr. S change the habitual cognitive and behavioral patterns that led to his muscular pain. A couple of sessions were spent in working on his social anxiety, which was also related to his perfectionism and fears of being unacceptable. As a result of the progress he had already made in these areas, Mr. S found that he was experiencing less social anxiety. He also found he was able to continue making progress by using the same techniques he had learned to help with his anxiety about doing tasks.

After 15 sessions over a 6-month period, Mr. S was experiencing little back pain, and when he did, he was generally able to recognize the source of his stress and his dysfunctional automatic thoughts, and then modify them. At a 6-month follow-up session, Mr. S reported having remained relatively pain free. He had one difficult weekend before he had to make a speech, but he had been able to cope with this and prepare the speech, and the presentation went well.

PROGRESS, LIFESPAN, AND TERMINATION CONSIDERATIONS

For most patients it is easy to slip back into familiar but dysfunctional cognitive and behavior patterns. This is particularly true with patients who have personality disorders, as their problems are deeply ingrained. Cognitive therapy has advantages over some other forms of therapy in coping with this. Patients become very conscious of the nature of their problems, and they learn effective ways of coping. They learn how to use tools such as the DTR, which they can use outside the therapy context to work on problem areas.

It is crucial when nearing the end of therapy to warn patients about the possibility of relapse, and to have them watch for minor recurrences of the problems that brought them to therapy. These are indications that the patients need to do some more work—either by themselves with the tools they learned in therapy, or with their therapist. It is important that patients realize it is common to need occasional booster sessions so they will not be ashamed to get help if a problem recurs. Most cognitive therapists build this into the therapy by gradually stepping down the frequency of sessions and scheduling periodic booster sessions after the main part of the therapy has been completed.

As the patient makes progress—feeling better and increasing in confidence—it is important to document what strategies or techniques helped with what problems or symptoms. Ideally, this would be an ongoing homework assignment that is reviewed periodically in therapy sessions. Thus, at termination each patient has a personalized "treatment manual" to guide their efforts in maintaining their gains and coping with slips and relapses.

Well before termination, it is important to normalize the episodic use of booster sessions and returns to treatment in the coming years. Just as it is not considered a failure to need a dentist in the future after repairing one's teeth in the present, circumstances are likely to arise in patients' lives that may benefit from a return consultation with their cognitive therapist. When patients' symptoms increase and their efforts to intervene do not work sufficiently well, it is counterproductive to catastrophize and blame themselves.

Although any significant life transition may lead to increased symptoms and distress, this is most likely to occur when individuals who are compulsive enter retirement. Unless they have prepared for this transition in therapy, it is unlikely that they have made more than financial preparations. The transition from the structured and productive life of the working individual to the unstructured, seemingly "unproductive" life of the retiree can be extremely stressful to individuals with OCPD. Maintaining their sense of identity as useful, valuable individuals in retirement tends not to happen easily without preparation. They are vulnerable to anxiety and depression as well as to marital discord when they attempt to change household routines that have been the domain of the spouse for many years.

COMMON CHALLENGES AND CLINICIAN SELF-CARE

Once the therapist has the knowledge and tools described in this chapter, the primary challenge to effectively treat patients with OCPD may be the therapist's own automatic thoughts and schema. The therapist will be alerted to the possibility of his or her own problematic distorted thoughts by the experience of strong emotions before, during, or after sessions with the compulsive patient. If the therapist dreads certain appointments or experiences strong feelings of frustration or irritation during therapy sessions, it would be appropriate for him or her to complete DTRs. If the therapist is not able to successfully challenge his or her automatic thoughts, consultation or supervision is the ethical next step.

CONCLUSION

Based on considerable clinical experience and some research support, cognitive therapy appears to be an effective and efficient treatment for OCPD. Compulsives often respond particularly well to certain aspects of cognitive therapy. These include its problem-focused nature, use of homework assignments, and emphasis on the importance of thought processes. Individuals with OCPD seem to prefer therapeutic approaches that are more structured and problem focused to approaches that focus primarily on the therapeutic process and the transference relationship as the means of change (Juni & Semel, 1982).

CHAPTER 11

Depressive Personality Disorder

David A. Clark
Catherine A. Hilchey

Clayton, a middle-aged information technology (IT) technician, described himself as the "proverbial pessimist." He always looked on the negative side of life, readily predicting doom and gloom not only in his personal life but in the world at large. He adopted a rather nihilistic, fatalistic view of life, belittling his own significance in comparison to the enormity of the world around him. Clayton expressed a considerable degree of self-criticalness, even self-loathing that had stalked him since early adolescence. Although possessing a dry and cynical humor, he was also harsh and judgmental toward others, often appearing irritable, hostile, and impatient in his interpersonal relations. People found him quite abrasive, so Clayton was not well liked by coworkers or neighbors. This contributed to his preference for an introverted, solitarily life style. Although meticulous and conscientious in his work, he never achieved his potential because of an incapacitating doubt about his self-worth and competence.

When asked to describe his emotional state, Clayton used words like "gloomy," "joyless," and "empty," rather than "sad" or "depressed." For sure, he went through periods of feeling depressed and had tried various antidepressants with limited success, but the more usual mood state was that of gloom, with feelings of inadequacy. He had come to the conclusion that he was incapable of joy and felt chronically disinterested in his work, family, and daily living. He confessed that he was an excessive worrier who could brood for days over his personal failings and shortcomings. When he finally decided to seek cognitive therapy for his enduring state of negativity, Clayton was in the midst of a divorce. However, he accepted this fate with a kind of resignation, believing that he had been a terrible husband and deserved the rejection. He felt guilty for the dark cloud he continually brought to his family and was convinced his wife and children would be much better off without him. Clayton was also struggling with an increase in suicidal ideation, which he had expressed to his estranged wife. She was the one who finally convinced Clayton that he couldn't let things go any longer—he needed to talk to a therapist!

Clayton's clinical presentation is characteristic of depressive personality disorder (DepPD). In DSM-IV-TR (American Psychiatric Association, 2000), DepPD was considered a "provisional" diagnostic personality type, lacking sufficient empirical validation to include in the official nomenclature of personality disorders. Located in the section titled "Conditions Requiring Further Research," DSM-IV-TR defined DepPD as a pervasive pattern of depressive thinking and behaviors that begins in adolescence or early adulthood and occurs in many different life domains. Although recognition of a depressive temperament or personality type can be traced back to the earliest days of 20th-century psychiatry (Kraepelin, 1921), DepPD has struggled to emerge from the "diagnostic hinterland."

The *International Classification of Diseases* (ICD-10; World Health Organization, 1992) and DSM-5 (American Psychiatric Association, 2013) both recognize persistent depression in the form of chronic depression, dysthymia, or other persistent mood disorders. However, neither diagnostic system recognizes DepPD as a distinct diagnostic personality type on par with other personality disorders like paranoid, borderline, avoidant, and so on. The DSM-5 Personality and Personality Disorder Work Group concluded that DepPD did not meet the threshold for inclusion as a diagnostic personality type, probably due to concerns that it overlaps with dysthymic disorder. Instead they concluded that DepPD is better represented as a constellation of pathological personality traits (Huprich, 2012). Thus, DepPD was removed from the DSM-IV-TR's "Conditions for Further Study" and incorporated into the proposed research model for personality disorders called the "alternative DSM-5 model for personality disorders. Elements of DepPD can be found within the specific personality facet called *depressivity*, which falls under the negative affectivity and detachment personality domains (American Psychiatric Association, 2013). Depressivity is defined as "feelings of being down, miserable, and/or hopeless; difficulty recovering from such moods; pessimism about the future; pervasive shame and/or guilt; feelings of inferior self-worth; thoughts of suicide and suicidal behavior" (American Psychiatric Association, 2013, p. 779). Depressivity appears to capture most of the negative internal representation and affect disturbance seen in DepPD but it fails to include the disturbance in interpersonal relatedness that is an important aspect of the personality disorder

(Huprich, 2012). One of the negative effects of "downgrading" DepPD to the level of personality trait within a proposed research model of personality disorders will be to discourage research on the construct and bias practitioners against recognizing personality manifestations of depression in their patients.

Despite its diagnostic uncertainty, there has been a small but consistent research literature on DepPD. This chapter draws on that research, first highlighting the clinical signs and symptoms that define DepPD. We will adopt the DSM-IV-TR criteria for DepPD since these are the most common criteria used in the extant research and they fit best with the personality disorder conceptualization adopted in this text. In addition, issues of differential diagnosis will be considered, especially how DepPD is distinct from major depression and dysthymia.

CLINICAL SIGNS AND SYMPTOMS

Individuals with DepPD feel chronically down, dejected, or gloomy most of the time, regardless of their circumstances. They often exclaim that they have never been able to feel joy, happiness, or positive emotion for an appreciable period of time. Their self-evaluation is overwhelmingly negative and highly self-critical, which results in feelings of inadequacy, worthlessness, and low self-esteem. They often brood over past failures and mistakes, and hold to a negative, pessimistic expectancy about the future. Individuals with DepPD are as critical and judgmental of others as they are of themselves. As a result they are often not well liked by others and so may lead a fairly solitary, introverted lifestyle. Often people with DepPD will comment "I've never been happy, even as a child," and they may confess that they don't really know what it is like to experience happiness. They often feel guilt or remorse over past failings and a sense that they have missed out on life. They may overcompensate by throwing themselves into their work to make up for the deficiencies in their life. Individuals with DepPD are often harsh and judgmental toward others, emphasizing the failings and shortcomings of others (American Psychiatric Association, 2000). Their interpersonal style can be more introverted and unassertive, whereas in others it is actually overassertive, even abrasive or aggressive (Bagby, Watson, & Ryder, 2012). In sum, the person with DepPD is a chronically miserable, negative, highly pessimistic individual who feels empty and cheerless most of the time and has difficulty in forming healthy interpersonal relationships.

According to DSM-IV-TR (American Psychiatric Association, 2000), DepPD is characterized by a generalized pattern of depressive thinking and behavior that is present by early adulthood. This pervasive negativity is evident as a predominant mood state of feeling down and unhappy, self-referent beliefs indicative of low self-esteem, heightened self-criticalness, rumination or worry, a negative judgmental interpersonal attitude, pessimism, and/or guilt or remorse. These criteria are broadly similar to the research criteria proposed by Akiskal (1983). DSM-IV-TR (American Psychiatric Association, 2000) makes it clear that DepPD should not be diagnosed if it occurs exclusively in the presence of major depressive episodes or the symptoms meet criteria for dysthymic disorder. When using DSM-5 (American Psychiatric Association, 2013) to diagnosis DepPD, the other specified personality disorder category can be used followed by a statement that the reason is presence of depressive personality traits. Given the absence of DepPD in DSM-5 we suggest the clinician also refer to the DSM-IV-TR criteria for DepPD (American Psychiatric Association, 2000, p. 789) when offering a "formal" diagnosis of the personality disorder.

PREVALENCE

DepPD has a prevalence rate of 2% in the general population (Ørstavik, Kendler, Czajkowski, Tambs, & Reichborn-Kjennerud, 2007), with a much higher rate reported in outpatient mental health settings (Bagby et al., 2012). It is much more common in women than men but has been reported across many cultural groups (Huprich, 2012; Ørstavik et al., 2007). It has a high comorbidity rate with dysthymia and major depression, as well as other personality disorders, such as avoidant, borderline, self-defeating, and obsessive–compulsive (Huprich, 2009). Approximately 40–60% of individuals with DepPD have current major depression and comorbidity rates with dysthymia span a wide range, from 18 to 95% (Huprich, 2009). In a large outpatient study by McDermut, Zimmerman, and Chelminski (2003), 57.6% of individuals with DepPD were concurrent for major depression, whereas only 18.2% were comorbid for dysthymia. However, in other studies comorbidity rates for dysthymia ran between 49 and 80% (Ryder & Bagby, 1999; Ryder, Schuller, & Bagby, 2006). Major depression differs from DepPD by its acute onset, briefer duration, and greater presence of neurovegetative symptoms (Bagby et al., 2012). Of course major depressive episodes that take a more chronic course are harder to differentiate from DepPD.

DIFFERENTIAL DIAGNOSIS

The greatest diagnostic challenge for the clinician is differentiating DepPD from dysthymia. There has been considerable discussion in the research literature on the key characteristics that distinguish these two disorders.

Low self-esteem and feelings of hopelessness are prominent symptoms for both conditions (Ryder et al., 2006). A more recent review paper by Bagby and colleagues (2012) concluded that DepPD is characterized less by mood disturbance and neurovegetative symptoms than dysthymia, and more by persistent and pervasive psychological symptoms of negativity, pessimism, and self-criticalness. Klein (1999) also noted that depressed mood is more prominent in dysthymia, and that individuals with DepPD often do not experience depressed mood most of the day more days than not for at least 2 years. Instead chronic anhedonia may be more evident in DepPD (Bagby et al., 2012). We would also add that disturbance in interpersonal relations, especially ambivalence, may be more characteristic of DepPD (Huprich, 2009). In sum, the cognitive therapist should be able to distinguish DepPD from dysthymia but it will require a fine-grained clinical assessment and advanced knowledge of depressive phenomenology to make the differential diagnosis. Table 11.1 presents the critical clinical features of DepPD that are useful for making a differential diagnosis.

Despite these diagnostic complexities, there are groups of individuals who fit the DepPD criteria who cannot be accommodated in other depressive diagnoses (Huprich, 2012). It turns out that depressive personality pathology is well recognized by practicing clinicians. In a random national sample of experienced psychiatrists and psychologists, Westen (1997) found that 77% reported treating DepPD, which was the second most common personality disorder. This was more recently replicated in another national sample of psychiatrists and clinical psychologists in which depressive personality pathology again emerged as a highly recognized diagnostic prototype that clustered with anxious–avoidant, dependent–victimized, and schizoid–schizotypal to form a hierarchical superordinate domain labeled the internalizing spectrum (Westen, Shedler, Bradley, & DeFife, 2012). Thus it would appear that most clinicians recognize the need for a depressive personality distinction when delineating personality pathology.

TABLE 11.1. Differential Diagnostic Features of DepPD

- Affect is predominantly gloom, unhappiness, and cheerlessness rather than sadness.
- Core self-schemas of worthlessness, inadequacy, insignificance, and incompetence.
- Cognitive profile characterized by pervasive negativity, pessimism and criticalness toward self and others.
- Strong feelings of guilt, remorse, and regret.
- Chronic anhedonia; an inability to feel accomplishment or pleasure.
- Elevated level of trait hostility or irritability.
- Proneness to pathological worry or brooding.
- Negative, critical, sometimes abrasive interpersonal style.

CONCEPTUALIZATION

There are no published works on cognitive theory or therapy for DepPD. The closest might be a chapter in the previous edition of this volume (Beck, Freeman, & Davis, 2004) that described a cognitive case conceptualization and treatment of passive–aggressive personality disorder (negativistic personality disorder). However, there are important differences between the DSM-IV-TR (American Psychiatric Association, 2000) diagnosis of passive–aggressive personality disorder and DepPD that makes the passive–aggressive personality disorder conceptualization of little relevance for DepPD. Passive–aggressive personality disorder is characterized by critical-ness, passive resistance, and anger toward others, whereas DepPD involves internally directed anger, profound sense of unworthiness, absence of positive affect, and pessimism about the future. Figure 11.1, then, depicts a proposed cognitive case formulation for DepPD that is based on the cognitive theory of personality disorders presented in Beck and colleagues (2004). We discuss the various elements of the cognitive formulation by referring back to the case presented at the beginning of this chapter.

Like other personality disorders, it is important to recognize the influence of early childhood experiences in the development of personality pathology. In DepPD, lack of family or social support, parental criticism, and parental loss/separation are often reported (Huprich, 2012). Clayton experienced a number of difficult childhood experiences from which he developed a belief in his own inadequacy and unworthiness. His parents divorced while he was in elementary school and for the next several years he was shunted between parents. Both parents remarried to partners with children and so Clayton felt he had no family unit. His father was highly critical of his efforts, often making disparaging comments that he was "just like his mother." He felt ignored by his peers and went through a couple of years of bullying while in middle school.

Although DepPD is a pattern of persistent and pervasive negativity, nevertheless negative life events, especially those involving loss and failure, will play a critical role in exacerbating depressive symptoms and may be responsible for treatment seeking. Clinically, it is important to identify proximal life stressors that may have led to referral. A detailed analysis of the client's evaluation and responses to stressors can provide an important understanding of the function of depressive personality pathology in the individual's daily life. Clayton had a number of negative life events that seemed to converge at a single point in time that resulted in his willingness to seek treatment. His wife asked that he leave the house and she was filing for divorce. At the same time he learned from his family physician that he was at elevated risk for heart disease and had to stop smoking and lose weight. These stressors combined with years of feeling unfulfilled and disillusioned with a "dead-end" job. It is interesting that Clayton took a very

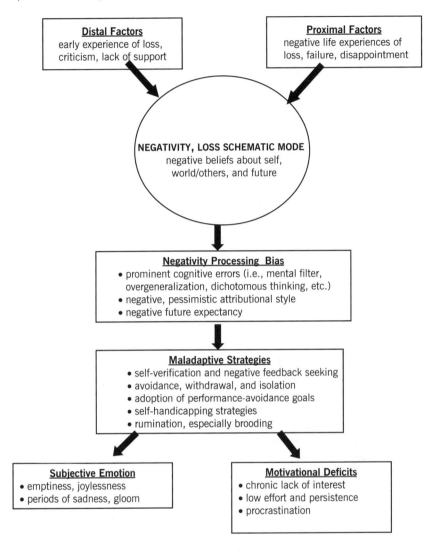

FIGURE 11.1. Cognitive conceptualization of DepPD.

passive, accepting response to these adverse events. He expressed a pro-found sense of resignation, stating that he always expected his life would go from bad to worse, and there was little or nothing he could do or wanted to do about it.

A key part of the cognitive case formulation is the identification of the client's core beliefs about the self, personal world, others, and future that define the personality pathology. Beck and colleagues (2004) noted that the maladaptive schemas in personality disorders are much more persistent, pervasive, impermeable, compulsive, and less easy to control than the schemas in individuals without personality disorders. Like major depression, DepPD is characterized by prepotent, hypervalent schemas that together constitute a negativity or loss mode (Beck et al., 2004; Clark & Beck, 1999). The self-schemas in the loss mode are oriented toward negative beliefs of worthlessness, failure, and incompetence. The world is viewed as harsh, cynical, and unpleasant, while the future is considered empty, hopeless, and futile. Other people are seen as uncaring, incompetent, and punishing. The core beliefs in DepPD are very similar to the belief structure identified with major depression, except that in personality pathology we see a chronic, almost continuous activation of the loss mode. Clayton believed he was an utter failure, that he had really messed up his life. He could easily recount all his past experiences of failure and believed that he was incapable of happiness. He believed his job did not deserve more than mediocre effort, and there was little he could do to alter a life destined for loneliness and misery. He was highly self-critical but also believed people were inherently stupid and incompetent. He ascribed to a nihilistic philosophy of life, believing that human life had no meaning other than the unfortunate depletion of valued earth resources.

The chronic activation of negative schemas about the self, world, and future is associated with an entrenched biased cognitive processing. Cognitive errors such as negative mental filter, overgeneralization, dichotomous thinking, and selective abstraction predominate (i.e., Beck, 1987), so that negative interpretations and evaluations seem the only plausible view to the person with DepPD. In major depression or dysthymia, the cognitive errors are primarily seen in self-referent information processing. In DepPD, the negativity processing bias is much broader and more pervasive so that it extends to the processing of a wider range of information, such as perceptions and interpretations of other people. Thus criticalness toward self and others emanates from a negative inferential style in which the person with DepPD believes negative events are caused by enduring, generalized deficiencies in one's self, family, friends, and acquaintances (see Abramson, Metalsky, & Alloy, 1989). In addition, cognitive bias is apparent in how the future is viewed, with negativism and pessimism dominating the person's expectations for themselves and significant others.

This negativistic processing bias was readily apparent in Clayton's daily life. Clayton mentioned that because of downsizing, he was being given more responsibilities at work. He was sure he would be one of the IT technicians let go, but when he was retained he viewed this cynically as a ploy by the company to retain "cheaper labor." Soon Clayton was assigned tasks that challenged his skills and knowledge. He was convinced his incompetence would become apparent to all, and that he would make costly mistakes that would eventually lead to his dismissal. Clayton found work increasingly stressful as he became preoccupied and worried about "screwing up." He tried to compensate by working longer hours but with each new assignment, he was convinced this would be the task that would lead to his eventual downfall. Clayton could not see his work situation any differently than a test of his competence, which he was sure to fail. He also spent a considerable amount of time thinking about his "pathetic future," imagining himself alone, unemployed, adrift in this world with no friends or family. Clayton rejected a more positive possibility of his current circumstances as utter foolishness, mere brainwashing by "positive thinking" gurus who made their fortunes deluding people to the reality of life.

In DepPD, the chronic activation of the negativistic, loss mode is characterized by the prominence of certain behavioral strategies that serve a self-protective function. The strategies develop to deal with the overwhelming negativity, criticism, and failure individuals with DepPD expect to encounter in their personal world. Although intended to counter low self-esteem and an entrenched negative self-schema, the strategies end up reinforcing the person's negative world view and ensuring continued activation of the loss mode.

Several behavioral and interpersonal strategies are emblematic to DepPD. The first strategy is negative *self-verification* and *feedback seeking*. According to self-verification theory, people are motivated to seek opportunities that verify and confirm their self-conceptions (Swann & Read, 1981). Since individuals who are depressed have a negative self-view, they will seek out, attend to, and embrace more rejecting social interactions because these experiences engender a feeling of security and control (Sawnn, Wenzlaff, Krull, & Pelham, 1992). Although negative feedback is unpleasant, even for individuals with DepPD, nevertheless they are drawn to and prefer negative feedback because it is consistent with their negative self-view (Timmons & Joiner, 2008). Not only is there research evidence to support self-verification and negative feedback seeking in depression (see Timmons & Joiner, 2008) but this formulation is entirely consistent with cognitive theory. In DepPD, a negative self-schematic organization is so entrenched that we would expect negative feedback seeking to become especially characteristic of the person's social interactional style. And yet negative feedback seeking is ultimately maladaptive because it reinforces the negative, pessimistic beliefs about self and others for people with DepPD.

There were several examples of negative self-verification and feedback seeking, especially in Clayton's interpersonal style with others. He would often brood over past social interactions, dwelling on comments that suggested negative evaluation or rejection by others. He would make critical, cynical comments that would make him less endearing to others. He would come across as self-centered and arrogant around others, often disclosing his criticism of others. He quickly picked up on any negative remark and would become irritable and defensive whenever he detected the possibility of criticism. In sum, Clayton was hypervigiliant for any signs of negativity that might be directed his way, and he stewed over negative thoughts about himself, other people, and his experiences in the world.

A second prominent behavioral strategy in DepPD is avoidance, withdrawal, and social isolation. Avoidance is a common coping strategy in depression (Ottenbreit & Dobson, 2008) and is a prime target for change in behavioral activation therapy (Martell, Addis, & Jacobson, 2001). Avoidance is also a prominent feature of DepPD. Because of their pessimistic disposition, the person with DepPD expects to fail and so will choose to avoid challenging situations. The absence of positive affect deprives the individual with DepPD of an important source of motivation to meet challenges and difficulties. As a result, the default option is avoidance, isolating one's self from others. Over the years Clayton had settled for a less challenging job but with the company reorganization, he was being forced to take on more responsibilities that he found highly threatening. He could not avoid these new job demands and so experienced a significant increase in anxiety over his performance.

Third, individuals with DepPD tend to adopt performance-avoidance goals in an effort to avoid proof of their worthlessness (Rothbaum, Morling, & Rusk, 2009). Like all individuals, people with DepPD adopt a goal-setting orientation to establish self-worth. However, the existence of negative self-beliefs in DepPD means that goal setting becomes defensive, or focused on seeking to avoid the negative judgments about competence and worthiness (Rothbaum et al., 2009). So the person with DepPD aims to avoid proof of worthlessness rather than adopting goals based on attaining positive judgment, or learning just for the sake of learning. Self-verification and negative feedback seeking are strategies that serve the goal of avoiding proof of worthlessness (Rothbaum et al., 2009). Clayton had clearly adopted performance-avoidance goals in his life. He frequently compared himself with others, trying to avoid looking less competent or worthy by criticizing and denigrating the skills and accomplishments of friends and colleagues. In fact, the heightened negative judgmental attitude toward others stems from the adoption of performance-avoidant goals.

Fourth, the person with DepPD utilizes self-handicapping strategies, such as withdrawal, procrastination, and rumination, to enhance self-worth (Rothbaum et al., 2009). For example, Clayton would procrastinate on an unfamiliar work project in order to avoid feeling incompetent. He would spend his time working on more familiar, mundane tasks that were less important to his employer. Although completing less important tasks gave him a sense of control, it sabotaged opportunities to gain a greater sense of accomplishment by solving a less familiar but more important work project. Rumination, or brooding, can also be seen as a self-handicapping strategy as the individual spends hours fretting about a hypothetical scenario that in most likelihood will never happen.

KEY TREATMENT GOALS

As indicated in Figure 11.1, the ultimate goal of cognitive therapy for DepPD is to reverse the motivational deficits and joylessness that characterize DepPD. Treatment success will be determined by improved energy, interest, and effort in daily activities, as well as increased periods of positive affect. There are several components of the case formulation that are addressed in order to achieve improved affect and motivation.

1. *Loosen the negative self-schema organization.* In cognitive therapy of depression, correction of negative self-beliefs is a key treatment goal. In DepPD, the negative self-belief has been so chronically activated, that negative beliefs have become almost self-evident truths. Thus an initial goal in cognitive therapy of DepPD is to reduce strength of belief or conviction in one's inherent worthlessness and to instigate a cognitive shift from the inevitability of negativity to the possibility of positivity.

2. *Build a coherent, more balanced, positive self and world view.* It is unlikely that individuals with DepPD have had much experience with a more realistic view of the self, world, or future that is balanced between positive and negative possibilities. Therefore, a second treatment goal is to create a cognitive shift toward a more realistic self- and other-evaluation. This is expected to be a slower and more time-consuming process in DepPD than in major depression where the therapist is building on past experiences of realistic thinking.

3. *Correct pessimistic explanatory style and negative future expectancy.* Self-blame for past failures and disappointments must be addressed in cognitive therapy for DepPD. The goal is to shift from a stable, global, and internalized attribution for negative experiences to a more specific, less enduring, and possibly externalized attribution for the causes of disappointments and failures. At the same time, pessimistic predictions about future highly significant personal events must be addressed so that a more balanced future outlook is adopted.

4. *Heighten present-moment awareness.* Individuals with DepPD spend much of their time caught in rumination about past failures and pessimism about future possibilities. Their ability to "live in the moment" is limited at best and emotional experience is filtered by an overwhelming sense of negativity. Thus an important goal of therapy is to reorient the patient to the present moment and to teach a deeper appreciation of the immediate sensory aspects of emotional experience. For example, people with DepPD often claim they have never been happy. If so, do they know what it's like to feel happiness or joy? The ability to attend to present experience and momentary positive affect is an important goal of treatment.

5. Encourage learning-based goal setting. As noted previously, individuals with DepPD often evaluate their self-worth by comparing their performance with others. It's important to encourage a healthier goal reorientation so the patient learns to engage in activities for the intrinsic joy of learning rather than competing against others. For Clayton this meant seeing new job tasks as an opportunity to learn new skills rather than as an opportunity to judge how he was performing relative to his coworkers.

6. Reduce negative feedback seeking. Because of their entrenched negative self-beliefs, individuals with DepPD exhibit biased attention and recall of negative interpersonal and performance-related feedback. Educating the patient on the effects of negative self-verification includes addressing the functional value of self-verification. Learning to identify and correct negative feedback seeking is an important goal of treatment.

7. Correct behavioral self-handicapping. Teaching patients how to recognize self-handicapping behaviors in their daily interactions will require repeated fine-grained analysis of their responses across a range of daily activities. Eventually the therapist will see the habitual ways that an individual with DepPD reacts in a self-handicapping manner, seeking to avoid defeat and failure but ends up creating a more negative outcome that reinforces a sense of worthlessness. Correcting self-handicapping habits such as procrastination, passivity, or impulsivity will be difficult since these are likely semiautonomous behavioral response patterns.

8. Reduce rumination and brooding. A final treatment goal targets excessive rumination over past failures, mistakes, and disappointments. This begins by introducing the patient to the futility of rumination and worry, addressing both positive and negative beliefs about rumination, and teaching how to "let go" of ruminative issues and concerns.

COLLABORATIVE STRATEGY

In cognitive therapy of DepPD, establishing a productive therapeutic relationship is particularly challenging because of the excessive negativity and pessimism of the patient with DepPD. Because negativity is a pervasive perspective, the therapist and therapy process will come under the patient's harsh criticism and pessimism. There are several aspects to this negativity that must be addressed within the course of treatment.

The patient might express considerable misgivings and low expectation for the success of treatment. Treatment outcome expectations, or "beliefs about the consequences of participating in treatment" (Constantino, Arnkoff, Glass, Ametrano, & Smith, 2011, p. 184) may include positive or negative beliefs about the benefits of treatment, treatment credibility, or the therapist's competence. As well, negative expectancy for treatment success could be attributed to the self (e.g., "My situation is hopeless, there is nothing you can do to help me," "I'm beyond hope"), a more generalized negative belief in psychological treatment ("I don't believe that just talking is going to solve anything"), or it could be based on past experiences. However, given the presence of dispositional pessimism, the patient with DepPD could enter treatment with a negative expectancy based on no prior treatment experience. Whatever the basis of the skepticism, low expectancy can have an adverse effect on treatment outcome. A recent meta-analysis found that positive expectancy had a small but significant impact on better treatment outcome (Constantino et al., 2011).

Given a propensity for criticalness, it is likely that the negativity about treatment by the patient with DepPD will become obvious early in the therapy process. It is important that the cognitive therapist address negative treatment expectancy and any negative beliefs about the therapist early in treatment. In fact, it might be necessary to target negative treatment beliefs first before trying to address other aspects of the negative self-schema. Ultimately, it is important to establish a collaborative therapeutic relationship despite the patient's skepticism and misgivings about treatment. This could be achieved by doing a cost–benefit analysis associated with giving therapy a try versus giving up immediately. Another strategy might be to explore with the patient past experiences where more positive outcomes were achieved than expected because of the patient's collaborative efforts. It would also be important to help the patient correct dichotomous thinking so that treatment outcome is not viewed as either a "cure" or a "complete failure," but rather to see it in terms of "degrees of improvement." A collaborative relationship could be established if the patient with DepPD adopts the view "Why not put some effort into therapy, give it a chance, and see how much I can improve?"

Homework compliance may be especially problematic in patients with DepPD because of the negativity and chronic anhedonia that characterizes this condition. The importance of engaging the client in homework is no less important because patients with DepPD are unable or unwilling to commit to active therapy assignments. Homework compliance is known to improve treatment outcome in depression and anxiety (Kazantzis, Whittington, & Dattilio, 2010). It is critical that the cognitive therapist address negative beliefs about homework, encouraging a "try-it-and-see" approach, and that homework development, implementation, and evaluation are conducted in a highly collaborative manner.

Finally, individuals with DepPD have a tendency to personalize and misinterpret comments in a negative, even self-disparaging, manner. This negative interpersonal style will be apparent in the therapeutic relationship. It is likely that the patient with DepPD will misinterpret a therapist's comment, causing rupture in the therapeutic process that could lead to premature termination of treatment. One way to deal with this potential problem is to frequently request patient feedback whenever the therapist offers an analysis, interpretation, or directive to the patient. Another way is to maintain a calm, interested, and hopeful stance in response to the patient's negative style, disconfirming negative interpretations and providing genuine, caring alternatives.

CLINICAL APPLICATION OF THE INTERVENTION

Assessment

Assessment is a critical part of case conceptualization and treatment. As noted previously, detecting depressive personality traits can be particularly difficult when the individual has major depression or a dysthymic disorder. Thus the cognitive therapist should conduct a thorough clinical and personality assessment of DepPD before developing a case formulation.

Several structured interviews and self-report questionnaires have been developed to assess DepPD or depressive personality traits (see Bagby et al., 2012, for a comprehensive review). The Structured Clinical Interview for DSM-IV Axis II Personality Disorders (SCID-II; First, Gibbon, Spitzer, Williams, & Benjamin, 1997) can be used to assess for DepPD, although reliability and validity data are limited (Huprich, 2005). Alternatively, the Diagnostic Interview for Depressive Personality (DIDP) is available, which is a 63-item semistructured interview developed specifically to assess DepPD (Gunderson, Phillips, Triebwasser, & Hirschfeld, 1994). The measure has good criterion-related validity and a cutoff score of 42 accurately detects DepPD.

In terms of self-report questionnaires, the 41-item Depressive Personality Disorder Inventory (DepPDI) has demonstrated adequate construct validity for assessing depressive personality traits (Huprich, Margrett, Bathelemy, & Fine, 1996). More recently caution has been raised about the DepPDI's validation since it has shown low convergence with two other DepPD measures (Huprich, 2004) and its discriminant validity with the Beck Depression Inventory–II (BDI-II; Beck, Steer, & Brown, 1996) is problematic (Chamberlain & Huprich, 2011). It is likely that any self-report questionnaire of depressive personality traits will be influenced by mood state. Thus one must be cautious when interpreting elevated scores on the DepPDI when clients are clinically depressed. Chamberlain and Huprich (2011) found that seven DepPDI items loaded with the BDI-II items, indicating they are tapping into depressive state. With this caveat in mind, individuals who score above the recommended cutoff of 170 should be more closely assessed for DepPD.

Unfortunately, the few standardized measures of personality disorder thoughts and beliefs are of limited utility to the assessment of DepPD. The Personality Belief Questionnaire (PBQ; Beck & J. Beck, 1991) does not have items on depressive personality beliefs (Beck et al., 2004). The Young Schema Questionnaire–3 (YSQ-3; Young, 2006) has three new subscales that may be of particular relevance to DepPD—Approval Seeking, Punitiveness, and Pessimism/Negativity—and as well as the original YSQ, has Failure and Negativity subscales that may be relevant for depressive personality.

To our knowledge no empirical studies have validated the YSQ with depression personality pathology. The YSQ Shame, Defectiveness, Insufficient Self-Control, Failure to Achieve, and Social Isolation subscales have predictive validity for depression (Oei & Baranoff, 2007). Nevertheless, caution must be exercised when interpreting elevated scores on the YSQ Failure and Pessimism/Negativity subscales because these scores could reflect a heightened depressive state rather than presence of depressive personality traits. The more recent YSQ-3 might be the most helpful version of the YSQ when assessing the cognitive basis of DepPD.

Interventions

As with treatment of major depression, cognitive restructuring, behavioral activation exercises, and empirical hypothesis testing will be key treatment components of cognitive therapy for DepPD. However, there are three modifications to cognitive therapy that are important in the treatment of DepPD.

In the initial stage of treatment, a greater emphasis is placed on goal setting and goal orientation. In DepPD, there is a dearth of positive goal-directed activity because of chronic anhedonia, or if goals do exist, they are oriented toward avoidance of failure and worthlessness. Developing a hierarchy of goals that promote engagement in life activities and direct treatment is critical to success. The therapist will also need to spend more time discussing how patients with DepPD evaluate their goal-directed activity. Clayton at first expressed little or no interest in maintaining contact with his family. The therapist needed to spend considerable time working with him in discerning what type of estranged father and husband he could be in light of his impending divorce, and then what he would have to do to fulfill his new parental role.

Second, a more concentrated form of cognitive restructuring is needed in light of the chronic activation of the negativity schema organization. This means that many interpersonal and achievement-related experiences in the person's daily life need to be assessed for misinterpretations of blame, self-criticalness, and guilt. Not only will the therapist need to work on building alternative, more adaptive interpretations, but greater attention must be directed toward building "cognitive self-care"—that is, individuals with DepPD automatically engage in self-criticism for perceived negative experiences. To counter this tendency, the patient must be taught how to respond to disappointment with greater self-compassion, kindness, and understanding (see Gilbert, 2009). Self-compassion is antithetic to DepPD so progress in this area will be slow and difficult.

Affect awareness is a final intervention strategy that should be emphasized with DepPD. Individuals caught in depressive personality pathology have become so attuned to negative affect that they may have difficulty evaluating their momentary emotional state, or recognizing shades of positive affect. Attending to positive affect, recognizing it, gauging its intensity, and learning how it can be enhanced must be built into the later sessions of treatment. To ensure lasting change, cognitive therapy must not be content with simply turning down the volume of negativistic self-schemas but it must also strengthen the dominance of more positive, healthy beliefs about the self, world, and future. An important part of this cognitive shift is learning to feel joy, happiness, and contentment when they occur. This will require that the patient learn how to actively construct positive affective states by combining intention, selective attention, expressive actions, and mindful awareness.

PROGRESS, LIFESPAN, AND TERMINATION CONSIDERATIONS

Course

DepPD remains moderately stable over time, showing at least as much temporal stability over a 10-year period as other personality disorders (Laptook, Klein, & Dougherty, 2006). As well, prospective research indicates that individuals with DepPD are at significantly higher risk of developing dysthymia, in particular (Kwon et al., 2000). In his review, Huprich (2012) concluded that DepPD is associated with a long-term pattern of impaired functioning and poorer response to medication treatment (see Phillips et al., 1998). Approximately half of individuals with DepPD have a lifetime history of major depression (Ørstavik et al., 2007), and individuals with DepPD and dysthymia evidence less improvement in depressive symptoms over a 10-year period (Laptook et al., 2006). Individuals with DepPD have significantly higher suicidality ratings and more suicide attempts than psychiatric outpatients without DepPD (McDermut et al., 2003). Clearly, then, DepPD follows a fairly stable course, having a significant decrement in daily functioning and response to treatment.

Termination Issues

Toward the latter part of treatment, the focus should shift from identifying, evaluating, and correcting negative self-schema to building and maintaining beliefs and behaviors that promote positive affect. This will take considerable time and effort because the person with DepPD has minimal personal experience with feeling happy or content. The cognitive therapist will have to provide opportunities for the patient to learn what it is like to feel momentary happiness, and other positive affective states such as curiosity, excitement, hope, interest, pleasure, contentment, pride, satisfaction, mastery, and so on. Thus therapy should focus on how to notice positive affect and what it feels like to experience these states. Erroneous beliefs about feeling joy or happiness must also be addressed. For example, Clayton believed that feeling happy was an intense emotional experience that left you feeling euphoric and disconnected from reality. He thought that "happy people" were in this sort of state for much of the day. Of course this was totally unrealistic and so Clayton had to discover the nature of "realistic happiness," what it means to feel contented and satisfied with your life. It is important that the patient has a repertoire of strategies and activities that can be used to promote more positive affect and enhance interest in daily activities. Before treatment termination, the cognitive therapist should be convinced of the patient's improved emotion regulation ability, which would include the capacity to repair sad mood and maintain a more positive affective state.

Individuals with DepPD have a propensity for depressive rumination. Consequently, the patient's ability to truncate brooding over past failures and disappointments will be a good barometer of treatment progress. As cognitive therapy progresses, a greater focus on the present becomes the best antidote to brooding and rumination. If the patient with DepPD is able to stay anchored in present experiences, this will provide a bulwark against the tendency to ruminate and worry. Patients who continue to slip into brooding over past negative experiences are not ready for treatment discontinuation since frequent rumination is one of the hallmarks of loss mode activation.

Social relationships are a major focus in cognitive therapy for DepPD. As noted previously, the interpersonal relationships in DepPD may be superficial, deficient, or uneven and conflicted because of the patient's maladaptive interpersonal style. Issues of excessive criticalness of others, social withdrawal, and irritability need therapeutic attention. This will require the correction of maladaptive beliefs about others, exposure to interpersonal situations and, for some individuals, actual interpersonal skills training. Significant improvement in the patient's social relations indicates treatment progress, whereas continued avoidance and isolation from others would contraindicate treatment termination.

Finally, individuals with DepPD will continue to struggle with depressive negativity long after therapy has terminated. Thus a critical part of relapse prevention involves the ability to effectively implement cognitive strategies to identify, evaluate, and correct pessimistic, negative judgments about self and others. Negative evaluations will continue to occur in daily functioning but it is the patient's ability to counter the evaluations with more balanced, realistic alternatives that determines readiness to terminate treatment. Thus booster sessions will be an important part of the relapse prevention plan because individuals with DepPD rarely leave therapy completely recovered. A negativistic orientation will always seem more natural and so booster sessions can help shore up more positive cognitive and emotive strategies that have been learned in the course of therapy. Of course individuals with DepPD who are captive to their negativistic perspective, who find their negative self-beliefs highly plausible, if not self-evident truths, will not be ready for treatment termination.

Clayton's treatment occurred over a 5-year period with the first block of 23 sessions over a 1-year period, followed by a second block of 15 sessions 5 years later. Throughout treatment for chronic major depression he consistently scored in the 20–30 range on the BDI-II, but at termination of the second block of sessions his scores dropped to the 10- to 12-point range. At end of treatment, Clayton reported that he was doing much better, and that he was experiencing more happiness and less depression than at any point in his life. There were a number of intervention strategies that seemed helpful in Clayton's recovery. We worked on learning to enjoy daily activities, being less rigid and perfectionistic at work, reducing anxiety and worry, dealing with intimacy rejection, correcting negative beliefs about self and others, and modifying unrealistic expectations. In addition, Clayton took a stress leave from work and so some sessions focused on a return-to-work plan. Throughout treatment Clayton was taking venlafaxine and a mood stabilizer, and struggled with chronic insomnia. The sudden improvement at the end of treatment coincided with the flourishing of a new romantic relationship. There has been no subsequent contact with Clayton in the intervening 4 years since his last session.

COMMON CHALLENGES AND CLINICIAN SELF-CARE

As discussed previously, individuals with DepPD are at higher risk for major depression, dysthymia, and other personality disorders (Bagby et al., 2012). There is a high probability that treatment-seeking individuals with DepPD are drawn to therapy because they currently experience a major depressive episode or a worsening of their chronic depression. If so, it will be necessary to treat the major depression with standard cognitive therapy for depression (Beck, Rush, Shaw, & Emery, 1979; J. Beck, 1995), but at the same time, take into account the personality issues that characterize DepPD. The treatment goals, intervention strategy, and collaborative style must be modified for the depressed individual with DepPD.

Like other depressive disorders, cognitive therapists must regularly monitor for suicide risk. Pessimism, hopelessness, and emptiness are endemic to DepPD, and yet these are the key cognitive factors that cause heightened suicidality in DepPD. It is important to establish a therapeutic environment in which the patient is able to disclose thoughts of self-harm, regularly assess the patient for suicide risk, and develop a safety plan in case there is an escalation in suicide potential.

Although treatment goals are crucial to all forms of cognitive therapy, this is especially true for treating DepPD. Fear of failure and avoidance goals are prominent in DepPD, so it is important to set realistic, specific approach goals that emphasize learning rather than performance goals that aim to avoid a sense of worthlessness. The goals need to be set collaboratively to increase the patient's commitment to the therapeutic process. Because of pervasive negativity, a considerable degree of therapist direction will be needed with goal setting, but this must not be done at the expense of collaboration.

Evidence gathering may prove less beneficial when doing cognitive restructuring with patients with DepPD than an approach that emphasizes the consequences of negative thoughts and beliefs. Evidence gathering is a key strategy in cognitive restructuring for depression, but the negative constructions in major depression are state dependent. In DepPD, the negative perspective is trait based and so the patient has less access to alternative thinking. What may prove more beneficial is to take a pragmatic approach by asking "What are the personal consequences of continuing to put the most negative construction on your experiences?" Clayton, for example, believed that his work had no value, anyone could do his job, and he was completely expendable. Rather than engage Clayton in an exercise that would determine whether his work had value, the therapist approached the problem by gathering evidence on the consequences of believing your work has no value. They agreed there was no way to prove "worth or value of work" but they could evaluate the effects of a "work value" assumption versus a "work valueless" assumption. After accepting the personal benefits of adopting a "work value assumption" Clayton and his therapist developed an experiential, behavioral plan that reinforced a "work value" belief.

Cognitive therapists treating DepPD may find the work disheartening because the negativity, pessimism, and criticalness are so rigid and pervasive. Treatment progress may be slow and critical remarks may be expressed toward the therapist and the treatment process. It will be important to see this as part of the personality pathology and not to internalize or personalize the remarks. Obviously, it is important to take seriously anything expressed by the patient, but negative evaluation must be seen as part of the negative belief system that should be targeted for change. Rather than become disheartened by the criticism, the therapist should take this as an opportunity to work on cognitive change.

TREATMENT EFFICACY AND OUTCOME

Given its basis in personality pathology, one might expect that treatment of depression in DepPD would be less effective than in individuals without DepPD. Although the treatment outcome literature is scant, the findings are more mixed than might be expected. Klein and Shih (1998) reported that DepPD was associated with a poorer course of depression, with at least half the sample receiving psychotherapy and/or medication. However, Maddux and colleagues (2009) found that presence of comorbid depressive personality did not influence the outcome of medication or 16–20 sessions of psychotherapy for chronic depression.

Two studies have investigated the effectiveness of cognitive-behavioral therapy (CBT) for individuals with DepPD. In the first study (Saulsman, Coall, & Nathan, 2006), 119 patients with major depression were classified as high- or low-depressive personality based on Millon Clinical Multiaxial Inventory–III (Millon, 1994) scores. All participants received 20 hours of group CBT for depression and anxiety. Rate of improvement was comparable between the two groups, although the depressive symptoms of the high-depressive personality group were significantly elevated at pre- and posttreatment as well as 1-month follow-up. More recently, Ryder, Quilty, Vachon, and Bagby (2010) examined the influence of DepPD traits on treatment of 120 patients who had major depression, and were randomly assigned to 16–20 weeks of individual CBT, interpersonal therapy (IPT), or antidepressant medication. Regression analyses revealed that higher DepPD traits were associated with a poorer outcome for IPT but not for CBT or medication. Although these findings are only suggestive, they do indicate that depressive episodes can be successfully treated in individuals' comorbid for DepPD. However, it would appear that the posttreatment symptom level remains elevated, indicating that therapists should not expect as much symptom remission when treating individuals with major depression and DepPD. Unfortunately, there is no empirical research on the effects of treatment on DepPD traits nor do we know whether the more specialized form of CBT described in this chapter would be more effective in the treatment of DepPD. Nevertheless, the treatment studies that have assessed depressive personality traits indicate that cognitive-behavioral interventions can significantly reduce depressive symptomatology even in the presence of negative personality pathology.

CONCLUSION

Given the high comorbidity between DepPD on the one hand, and major depression and dysthymia on the other, CBT practitioners who treat a lot of depression will often encounter individuals with DepPD. Although the official DSM-5 nomenclature does not recognize DepPD, most clinicians report that depressive personality pathology is common in clinical settings. The most distinctive feature of DepPD is the presence of a persistent and pervasive negativity toward the self, the world, the future, and others that is manifest as loss of pleasurable engagement or anhedonia, brooding, poor interpersonal relations, guilt, and elevated irritability. Unlike major depression or dysthymia, depressed mood and neurovegetative symptoms may not be as prominent as cheerlessness or inability to experience positive affect.

The cognitive model recognizes that the loss mode is more chronically activated in DepPD and the negativity processing bias is more generalized across a broad spectrum of life experiences. Because of their chronically activated negative schemas, individuals with DepPD often adopt compensatory strategies that seek to avoid thoughts of worthlessness. Thus they may adopt performance-avoidance goals, generally engage in procrastination and behavioral avoidance, and rely on negative feedback seeking as a form of negative self-verification.

Cognitive-behavioral treatment of DepPD must focus on establishing adaptive goals, and help clients shift from chronic negative schema activation to greater elaboration of more balanced positive beliefs about self, world, future, and others. As well, the CBT practitioner will need to "train" the individual with DepPD in better awareness of positive affect and the adoption of a present, momentary time frame rather than a preoccupation with the past or future. Although treatment of DepPD is slower, more difficult, and more therapeutically challenging, there is evidence that CBT can be effective for depressed individuals with DepPD.

CHAPTER 12

Paranoid, Schizotypal, and Schizoid Personality Disorders

Julia C. Renton
Pawel D. Mankiewicz

Relatively few recognized cases of individuals with paranoid, schizotypal, and schizoid personalities are seen within clinical services. The reason for this appears to be twofold. First, these are not clients for whom seeking psychological therapy would be concordant with their belief sets. Second, when they do present to mental health services, these clients are likely to be allocated to inappropriate clinical pathways. Individuals with these arrays of difficulties might be referred to services for people with psychosis and may be either incorrectly diagnosed or discharged with no further treatment once they are perceived as not meeting diagnostic criteria for schizophrenia. Although these disorders have generally been regarded as "untreatable" (Davison, 2002), evidence has begun to demonstrate that symptoms of severe personality disorders are treatable, particularly with cognitive therapy for emotional distress and unhelpful beliefs associated with these personality disorders (Bateman & Tyrer, 2004). Indeed, a study conducted by Joyce and colleagues (2007) demonstrated that paranoid, schizotypal, and schizoid personality disorders had no adverse effect on treatment response for patients with depression randomized to cognitive therapy interventions (while, for comparison, the effectiveness of interpersonal therapy appeared significantly decreased).

Furthermore, these clients present considerable difficulties in developing engagement within psychological therapy. Adshead and Sarkar

(2012) reflected on how interpersonal (dysfunctional attachment patterns) and social (maladaptive social behaviors) components of such personality disorders manifest in relationships with mental health professionals. As explained by the authors, these individuals generally do not take on the conventional "sick role" in which they are compliant, obedient, and grateful as patients or therapy clients. As a result, conventional and collaborative therapeutic relationships are less likely to develop. Therefore, Evershed (2011) insisted that the cardinal principle of cognitive therapy with such personalities must be the formation of a therapeutic alliance with the client. This process needs to commence at the very beginning of the therapy through a development of mutual understanding of the individual's difficulties (formulation), which should lead to establishing an initial sense of trust and collaboration.

KEY TREATMENT GOALS

Basic treatment goals for any of these three disorders may include the following:

1. Elicit trust within therapy by exploring ambivalence, respecting the individual's autonomy and emotional boundaries, and remaining nondefensive.
2. Explore the impact and accuracy of unhelpful beliefs about others in key interpersonal and social contexts, and work collaboratively to develop alternative, more functional beliefs.
3. Experiment with more adaptive social behaviors and skills to support more functional beliefs and to reduce predominance of suspicion and mistrust.

The description of each disorder is separated within the chapter to illustrate the key differences and nuanced methods in applying cognitive therapy.

PARANOID PERSONALITY DISORDER

Prama is a 27-year-old accountant living in London with her parents. Her parents came to England from India as newlyweds and built a successful business selling packaging items. Prama has one older brother who is also an accountant. Her parents have a fairly isolated family life. They have a couple of distant cousins living in the United Kingdom, who they see only rarely. Her parents do not entertain and have no friends of their own. When Prama and her brother were younger, they were encouraged to concentrate fully on their academic studies. Friendships with other pupils were not encouraged, with Prama's parents telling her, "These girls are your competition," "Beat them or they will beat you," and "They don't care about the Asian girl, they want to see you lose." She recounted that her parents were suspicious in all business interactions with their clients and believed that vigilance was needed as everyone would try and deceive them. Interestingly, Prama recounted that her name meant *knowledge of truth*, which seemed to have a great significance to her parents. She reported being a loner at school, believing that others would have little interest in spending time with her. Despite having no outside interests, Prama describes her parents as uninterested in her or her brother, constantly sending them to their rooms to study while reminding them that they had nothing to offer without academic success. She describes her childhood as boring, bleak, and negative, with pervasive themes of suspicion and threat.

Prama did well at school and went to study economics at university. There she remained isolated and perceived the attempts of others to engage with her as trying to steal her work or spy on her. After university, she returned back to the family home and managed to find work with a large accounting firm. However, her repeated failings to work alongside her colleagues and cooperate in projects led the firm to give her a series of performance warnings and objectives. Her appraisals had repeatedly mentioned her negative attitude toward colleagues. Alongside her performance management, a referral to the occupational health department was made, due to the observed increase in her distress and avoidant behavior. This included her hiding in the rest room for hours to avoid meetings and then staying at work late in the evenings. On meeting with the occupational health department, the doctor wrote to her general practitioner (GP) and asked if he would consider referring her to the Community Mental Health Team (CMHT), believing her to have a psychotic disorder.

On referral to the CMHT, it became apparent that this was not an episode of psychosis or an "at-risk mental state" (ARMS). Rather, the diagnosis of paranoid personality disorder (PPD) was hypothesized and Prama was referred to the outpatient cognitive-behavioral therapy (CBT) service. Prama did not see herself as needing psychological therapy but described feeling "tired of looking over my shoulder and feeling anxious." She also reported being fearful that she would lose her job due to her perceived inability to change and work closely alongside her peers.

CLINICAL SIGNS AND SYMPTOMS

The essential diagnostic feature of PPD is a persistent interpretation of the intent of others as malicious, coupled with an array of distrust and suspiciousness (American Psychiatric Association, 2013). Individuals with this disorder assume that other people will exploit, harm, or deceive them even if no evidence exists to support this expectation. They are preoccupied with doubts about the trustworthiness of friends (if they have any) or colleagues even without justification, and scrutinize the actions of others for evidence of malevolent intentions, often reading hidden meaning. Individuals with PPD rarely confide in or become close to others, fearing that anything they share may be used against them. Such individuals often bear grudges over long periods of time and are unwilling to forgive any slights or wrongs that they perceive have been done to them. They are often very difficult to get along with and have problems with close relationships. These individuals are rarely in intimate relationships, but if they are, there is often a recurrent suspicion regarding fidelity of the spouse/partner.

For comparison, ICD-10 *Classification of Mental and Behavioral Disorders* (World Health Organization, 1992) diagnostic guidelines for PPD are largely similar to those of DSM-5. Distrust and suspiciousness constitute the main diagnostic themes, although these characteristics are not as explicitly central to the diagnosis of PPD as in DSM-5. Additionally, ICD-10 discusses the preoccupation with unsubstantiated "conspiratorial" explanations to events, a combative and tenacious sense of personal rights, and a tendency to experience excessive self-importance, which manifests in a persistent self-referential attitude. While such individuals often hold their ideas with a high degree of conviction, the degree of vigilance they require to maintain their perceived safety often leads them to feel anxious and emotionally exhausted.

Research and Empirical Data

Despite growing recognition of paranoid personalities in clinical and non-clinical populations, there seems to be a paucity of empirical literature on PPD. Bebbington and colleagues (2013) demonstrated that prevalence of different types of paranoid ideation ranged from 2 to nearly 30% in the general population, which followed an almost perfect exponential distribution ($r = .99$) and was corroborated by a number of factors, including interpersonal sensitivity, mistrust, persecutory cognitions, and even ideas of reference. Furthermore, a clinical study conducted by Mankiewicz, Gresswell, and Turner (2013) has shown a considerable and statistically significant correlation between paranoid ideation and psychological distress, which consequently decreased individuals' satisfaction with life. In addition, Carroll (2009) described a symptomatic overlap between PPD and some anxiety disorders, such as social phobia, and argued that persons with PPD may initially present to mental health services with anxiety complaints. Likewise, the literature reviewed by Bernstein and Useda (2007) suggested that similar to social phobia, individuals with PPD are preset with cognitive biases, leading to misinterpretation of social clues.

Such symptoms must inevitably be addressed in psychological therapy to empower an individual to elaborate the deeply held paranoid beliefs. Indeed, cognitive therapy has long been shown to be a suitable treatment for paranoia. For instance, Renton (2002) demonstrated how attentional, interpretational, and memory biases in paranoia could be addressed through cognitive interventions, while Morrison, Renton, French, and Bentall (2008) developed a self-help resource guide based on cognitive therapy principles for those with paranoid beliefs.

Differential Diagnosis

PPD and Delusional Disorder

The main difference between PPD and delusional disorder appears to be the absence of systematized delusions in those with PPD. The thinking within PPD is not strictly delusional, but shows a cognitive style in which threat perception is high and generalized. There are some strong beliefs about the malevolent intent of others within PPD but this is vague and centered around untrustworthiness rather than persecution. The beliefs within PPD often appear less systematized and crystallized but at times might be more pervasive than within delusional disorder. People with delusional disorder may have relationships that predate the onset of their delusional thinking and may be able to maintain these relationships and those that are outside of their delusional system. This is often less possible for those with PPD, as their rigidly held outlook translates into a generalized negative pattern of relationships and a recurrent search to confirm negative suspicions of those around them. By definition, people with PPD do not display tenacious psychotic symptoms, whereas delusional disorder is characterized by persistent nonbizarre delusions in the absence of other psychotic symptoms (such as the tenacious belief that an ex-boyfriend is following, spying, and spreading malicious gossip about an individual in the absence of any other symptomatology or evidence to suggest this is factual). Also, individuals with paranoid personalities seem more likely to consider the possibility that their beliefs might be unsubstantiated, while belief conviction among those with delusional disorder appears almost uncorrectable, especially within initial stages of psychological treatment.

PPD and Schizotypal Personality Disorder

In schizotypal personality disorder, the lack of close relationships is more related to the acute discomfort with, and reduced capacity for, those relationships. Within PPD this avoidance generally relates to themes of suspicion. Although there is also a degree of suspiciousness within schizotypal personality disorder, those with such diagnosis often endorse a wide range of unusual beliefs, magical thinking, and odd presentations that affect many aspects of their functioning.

PPD and Narcissistic Personality Disorder

Narcissistic personality disorder is characterized by an overinflated sense of entitlement and grandiosity (Carroll, 2009), however, it is hypothesized that the core beliefs within narcissistic personality disorder are those of inferiority and unimportance (Behary & Davis, Chapter 14, this volume). These beliefs are only activated under certain circumstances and are mainly observed when the individuals perceived their self-esteem to be under threat. It might be that while persons who are paranoid feel a sense of personal attack and are generally suspicious of the motives of others, those with narcissistic personalities fear a sense of attack to their self-concept rather than their own safety. Persons who are narcissistic manifest persistent self-referential attitudes, but tend to misinterpret the perceived attention of others as flattery and admiration.

PPD and Avoidant Personality Disorder

Although both paranoid and avoidant personality disorders demonstrate severe levels of avoidance of others and social situations (despite a negative impact on personal goals), the difference is demonstrated by the absence of perceived malevolence regarding the actions of others in avoidant personality disorder. It is possible that those with avoidant personalities believe that others will be critical or rejecting, however, this is linked to their perceptions of themselves as inadequate rather than the malevolence of others.

Collaborative Strategy

The engagement of those with PPD is particularly difficult as suspiciousness and mistrust are pervasive throughout all relationships. As for most clients with PPD, therapy poses a great threat. Therapists themselves are likely to be viewed with suspicion and those beliefs about the potential malevolence of others are likely to inhibit engagement with the therapeutic process. Socratic questioning and the assessment of both sides of the patient's ambivalence about therapy are important tools in early collaborative engagement.

When Prama first entered therapy, she was angry as to her referral by her GP and suggested that she was baffled as to why everyone was "picking on me." The therapist asked Prama if she would be willing to work together to consider whether this was true and whether therapy could have any utility for her. Further discussion focused around the advantages and disadvantages of doing nothing versus the advantages and disadvantages of spending some time in therapy looking at the current situation and whether there was any possible ways of making any changes. The outcome of those discussions appears in Figure 12.1.

With PPD, it is important to give time to the engagement process, even though it may feel unlikely that there will ever be a collaborative relationship. Initially, Prama struggled to fill in Figure 12.1, but the therapist encouraged her to reflect on the process and implement this work at home over the week ahead. Upon her return, it appeared that Prama had given a surprising amount of thought to the task and was better able to understand the potential advantages of engaging with the process of therapy. Perhaps the introduction of the concept of pros and cons, coupled with time at home away from the potentially threatening situation of therapy, allowed her to better analyze the difficulties of no action and the potential gains associated with change while remaining in control of this appraisal. Also, there were a couple of surprising additions to the grid. Prama commented that a disadvantage of taking no action was that she would never have children. She told the therapist that she had never mentioned this desire to anyone, and had not even acknowledged it to herself, but that the reflective

Advantages of not engaging with therapy	Disadvantages of not engaging with therapy
I've managed okay up till now.	I'll lose my job.
I'll be safe.	I won't get a good reference.
People can't take advantage of me.	I'll always feel like this.
I won't put myself at more risk.	I might end up with nothing.
	I'll never have kids.
Disadvantages of engaging with therapy	**Advantages of engaging with therapy**
I won't be able to cope with the anxiety.	I'll have a chance of keeping my job.
If I engage with therapy, it's like admitting I'm wrong.	I'd like to get promoted.
People at work might find out and think I'm weak.	I might feel less anxious at the end of it.
I might fail at it.	I would like to feel how others seem to feel in their lives.
It'll make me vulnerable.	I'd like to have a friend.
(Concerns about the therapist?)	I'd like to see if I could be happy.

FIGURE 12.1. Prama's advantages versus disadvantages of engaging and not engaging with cognitive therapy.

process had made her realize that she was troubled by the prospect of never developing any connection with anyone.

As part of this process and the negotiation around the commencement of treatment, the statement "Concerns about the therapist" was added to the grid at the third session and Prama was engaged in a discussion about how the therapeutic relationship might be seen as a potentially threatening one. Subsequently, the therapist endeavored to normalize the anxiety about Prama's engaging herself in the therapy process and anxiety about the prospect of personal change.

Clinical Application of the Intervention

The development of Prama's goals for therapy was more problematic. Due to the rigidity of her belief set, she resisted the therapist's attempts to generate a goal list. Prama focused instead on the need to take definitive action against certain individuals within the workplace. Therefore, they agreed to allow vague goals about understanding the situation rather than "SMART" (short-term, measurable, achievable, realistic, and time-limited) goals prior to the commencement of intervention. This allowed for a flexible either/ or approach to goal setting that satisfied both the client and therapist. For instance, where Prama had identified "Others out to discredit me" as the problem, the corresponding goal was "To examine colleagues' behavior in detail and *either* take action to stop/report this *or* find an alternative way to understand and respond." Prama decided that although all the goals were related, she wanted to begin with her concerns that others were out to discredit her as she felt that this directly underpinned the resistance to coworking that was threatening her job.

Problem Maintenance Formulation

Therapy continued with formulating a series of recent events in the workplace and using this to develop a shared understanding of how such interpretations might become less accurate over time (see Figure 12.2). Prama was able to understand the information-processing changes that occurred with anxiety and to see that this may render her thinking less accurate over time. She outlined a situation where she had been asked by her boss to coauthor a report at work and present it at a meeting by the end of the day and described that she immediately thought "They'll steal my work and pass it off as their own."

Prama and her therapist formulated how this led her to become anxious and fearful, at which time she was only able to incorporate information in keeping with her threat appraisals. In addition, Prama removed herself from the situation (hiding in the rest room), thus not allowing herself to discover that her peer may have wanted to fairly contribute to and share

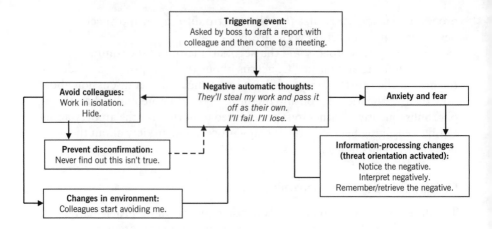

FIGURE 12.2. Prama's problem maintenance formulation diagram.

responsibility for this project. Finally, as a result of this and other unusual responses to work requests, her peers had begun to regard *her* with some degree of suspicion and had begun avoiding her, reinforcing her thoughts about their malicious intent.

Socratic Questioning and Cognitive Interventions

The use of Socratic questioning is even more vital during the engagement and therapeutic process with this client group and needs to be based on the principles of *guided discovery* rather than *changing minds* (Padesky, 1993b), in which the therapist helps the client review the evidence around his or her belief sets as opposed to pointing out any inaccuracies in thinking. This is particularly pertinent for those with PPD as they are likely to have come across people who dismiss their beliefs and have had few experiences with other people where their perspective has been validated.

Following the development of a shared formulation, therapy continued with the use of cognitive techniques within a Socratic framework to help Prama evaluate the accuracy of her thoughts regarding her colleagues and her boss (see Figure 12.3). Prama preferred to begin the task of evaluating the accuracy of her thoughts within the sessions but was happier completing this work alone in between sessions.

Behavioral Experiment

Following up her thought record, Prama and her therapist designed a behavioral experiment to further test the belief that others would steal her work

Event: Asked by boss to draft a report with colleague and then come to a meeting.	
Thought to be tested: They will steal my work and pass it off as their own. **How much do you believe the thought:** 90% **How anxious are you:** 70%	
Evidence supporting the thought:	**Evidence NOT supporting the thought:**
He never normally talks to me. He usually looks embarrassed and walks away when I enter the room. He is older than me and hasn't been promoted to a senior position.	I have shared some data with him before and he's credited me with them in the team report. He's asked us to do a joint report and so will know that some of the work is mine. He's often agreed with comments I had made in team meetings. He is pretty shy and he has said he would hate to be a manager. He is highly respected by his peers.
Following this thought record:	**How much do you believe the thought now:** 30% **How anxious are you now:** 50%

FIGURE 12.3. Prama's negative automatic thought and mood change record.

on future projects. Prama arranged to meet with her colleague and complete their next report the following day. Using a behavioral experiment sheet, Prama outlined the thought to be tested, likely problems and strategies to deal with these, the expected and actual outcomes, and how much the outcomes matched her original thought. Prama was able to consider that her colleague might just want to complete the report as requested and that their two sets of skills and data complemented each other. As a result of both the thought record and the behavioral experiment, Prama was able to develop an alternative thought as to the intentions of her colleague within this situation. Her conviction in the tested belief reduced to 30%.

Developmental Formulation

Prama and the therapist continued to develop a set of conceptualizations looking at specific events in her daily life, use the techniques to evaluate the accuracy of her interpretations, and come up with alternatives. During this process, while continuing to shift her perspective on current difficulties, it became apparent that she still continued to make suspicious and paranoid interpretations of many situations both inside and outside of work. Therefore, the therapist decided to shift the focus from looking at maintenance formulations within the work domain to a more generic, developmental, and historical perspective on her difficulties to encourage the generalization of the learning process onto a range of domains in her life.

It is important to note that this shift of focus was made possible by Prama's ability to challenge her cognitions within the workplace and mediate her behavioral responses. This meant that she was managing to work safely with colleagues without experiencing disabling levels of anxiety and her employers were no longer concerned about her performance at work. Although she was still making paranoid appraisals of a range of situations both inside and outside of work, the imminent threats had been dealt with and she was able to shift the focus of therapeutic work.

Prama found her historical cognitive conceptualization (see Figure 12.4) useful and admitted that particularly the idea of her familial background of "suspicion of others" having been accepted by her as a fact, resonated well. She was able to consider that these beliefs had been central to her interaction with others but also recognized her belief that she was of no value, interest, or utility was true and that despite the initial intention of others, their appraisal of her would lead them to take advantage of her.

Prejudice Metaphor

Prama's therapist next addressed her core beliefs as a key factor in the maintenance of her difficulties. The therapist and Prama decided that they needed to work on her core negative beliefs about herself and her core beliefs about others at the same time. Prama was socialized to Padesky's prejudice metaphor (Padesky, 1993 a) as a way of explaining the mechanisms by which information-processing biases could maintain her negative self-beliefs, despite the available evidence to the contrary. This model illustrates how individuals process information differently depending on whether it is consistent with their own belief set. It helps the client to understand the means by which information-processing biases allow the ignoring, distorting, and making an exception of information contradictory to their own beliefs. Conversely, information that is consistent with their belief set is readily accepted. This strategy helped Prama to understand how her own beliefs persisted much like the prejudicial beliefs of others.

Positive Data Log

Once Prama understood the process of belief maintenance, she was able to think about how she would change the way that she managed information and therefore change her own strongly held threat-oriented beliefs about

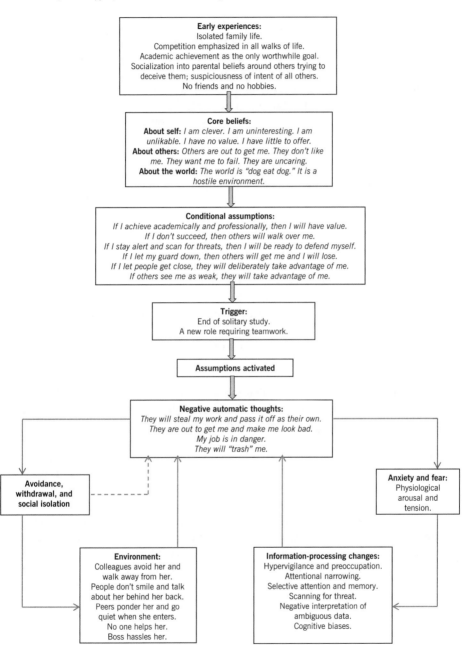

FIGURE 12.4. Prama's developmental cognitive formulation diagram.

others and the unhelpful beliefs she held about herself. In addition, a series of tasks were devised to place Prama in situations where she might gather this information, as her avoidance had previously been pervasive.

Some alternatives to core beliefs were generated by Prama, who used this to help her review her daily activities and generate evidence to log, in line with the new beliefs. Among other beliefs, Prama decided to collate evidence in line with "I can be liked by some people" as an alternative to her original core belief of "I am unlikeable," and "Some aspects of my life are important," as an alternative to "I have little value." She also began to generate a range of activities (mainly within work) that allowed her to engage in situations in which she was more likely to generate evidence.

Progress, Lifespan, and Termination Considerations

Prama continued to attend therapy and work productively with her therapist. She gradually improved the manner in which she interacted with colleagues and mentioned that she had at times accepted a cup of coffee during a work project. This was hugely significant for her as she felt that it highlighted her "letting her guard down." She also recounted that she had answered some basic questions about her home life. The therapist reviewed how far she had come, both within work and within the therapeutic relationship. At this stage of therapy (24 sessions), the therapist commented on statements that had been brought when she was considering the advantages and disadvantages of therapy. The therapist reminded Prama that she had cited never having children and no friend as problematic and asked whether the goal list should be amended to represent this.

On consideration, Prama stated that she did not feel able to consider this at the current time and wanted to consolidate her progress in the workplace. The therapist acknowledged that while her historical core beliefs were still active (although weakened), an alternative set of beliefs had also been created. The therapist and Prama reflected on how this had manifested in changes in the therapeutic relationship and pondered her ability to sustain a positive and helpful relationship without being taken advantage of. Prama recognized this enormous change and expressed pleasure at what she saw as a "relationship with no losers." However, despite this she insisted that she wanted to continue to consolidate her learning at work. She said that she might consider a return to therapy in the future to further challenge her old beliefs within an interpersonal context. During the last few sessions, the therapist worked with Prama to develop a detailed blueprint explaining the role that her history, beliefs, and thinking had on all aspects of her life, and to encourage her to utilize the relevant strategies. Prama was encouraged to use her blueprint on a regular basis to reinforce and generalize the therapy's learning effects.

SCHIZOTYPAL PERSONALITY DISORDER

The main feature seen in individuals with schizotypal personality disorder (StPD) is their acute discomfort with, and reduced capacity for, close relationships, alongside cognitive or perceptual distortions and eccentricities of behavior. They often have subclinical psychotic symptoms or experiences, such as suspiciousness, believing people are talking about them or intend them some harm. They also lack friendships, feel anxious in social situations, and may behave in ways that others perceive as odd.

Clara was referred to the early intervention service (at the age of 32) following concern from the hostel in which she had been living on and off for many years. She had been nearing the top of the housing list after many years of waiting, but had been informed that if she were to make herself voluntarily homeless again that she would be returned to the bottom of the queue. The staff at the hostel had urged Clara to register with a GP for a medical evaluation, due to concerns about Clara's behavior of talking to herself, lack of interaction with others, and other behavior suggestive of paranoia. During her appointment with the GP, she told him that she had heard voices for many years and was convinced that others were planning to harm her, so the GP referred her to mental health services.

Clara was the youngest of five children born to her Dutch mother and English father. They lived a very unconventional lifestyle and her parents subscribed to few social norms. Clara spent a limited time in education during her life and when she did, was rarely in the same school for more than a couple of terms. Clara's descriptions were vague but it seemed that her father probably had mental health difficulties, although never treated. Her parents were not Romany Gypsies but described being inspired by the Romany lifestyle and culture. They deliberately moved frequently between housing, believing that they were giving their children "more experiences," which they believed to be advantageous to them. Despite some hostility from the neighbors, Clara's parents remained adamant that others were envious of their lifestyle and that they should neither be upset at this antagonism nor show any response to it.

Clara's parents tried to inspire all their children to believe that they were "not like other children," that they were "special and unique, and that they should "celebrate their differences." However, they also believed that they should leave them to their own devices to best develop their own personalities. In reality, this meant that Clara spent much of her time alone while her parents smoked marijuana and played guitar. When she was born, two of her older siblings were in secondary school and the other two had already left home. Her eldest sister had no contact with the family since she had left home at age 17. Her parents did have occasional friends who drifted in and out of their lives, and Clara has hinted at the possibility that one of these men may have sexually abused her over the years. She was not prepared to discuss this in any detail.

As a result of this family structure, Clara spent much of her childhood playing alone, and failed to make any friends either locally or at school. When another move sent her to a new school, she was often bullied, called names, and ostracized. At secondary school, Clara tried to dress in a way that she thought would make her an "interesting eccentric" rather than "plain, weird, and bullied," and began experimenting with a range of homemade tattoos, unusual styles, and piercings, which her parents encouraged. At age 14, she confided in her mother that she was hearing the voice of her older sister whom she had never met. Her mother told her that this meant that she had "the gift" and should take time to develop this special power. When she was 17, her parents returned to Holland (where they had met). Clara decided to remain in the United Kingdom and went to live in a hostel. She has been voluntarily homeless on and off over the last 15 years, leaving the hostel at times when she becomes convinced that other residents are talking about her. She believes that her sister is alive and looking out for her and that the voice that she hears is her sister communicating with her via telepathy. She has no other friends and has never been employed, living instead off benefits. Clara does not drink or take any illicit substances, believing that this might interfere with her "communication" with her sister.

Clinical Signs and Symptoms

The predominant diagnostic theme for StPD in DSM-5 (American Psychiatric Association, 2013) appears to be persistent gaps in social and interpersonal functioning alongside subjective experience of considerable distress with, and limited ability to engage in, close interpersonal relationships. A person with StPD demonstrates unusual, eccentric behavior, present in a wide range of interpersonal circumstances. Cognitive deficits may include ideas of reference, strange beliefs or magical thinking, odd perceptual experiences, and suspiciousness or paranoid thoughts, with little or no insight regarding the distorted aspects of these cognitions. In addition, such individuals present with improper or limited affect and excessive social anxiety, and rarely have any close friends.

It is important to note that the World Health Organization's ICD-10 does not recognize a diagnosis of StPD, but rather schizotypal disorder. In ICD-10, schizotypal disorder is classified as a clinical disorder associated with schizophrenia rather than a personality disorder. Thus, DSM-5 designation of schizotypal as a personality disorder might be seen as controversial with those favoring ICD-10 in their clinical practice. ICD-10 (World Health Organization, 1992) still highlights eccentric behavior and appearance and a tendency to social withdrawal, but also focuses on obsessive ruminations without inner resistance, often with dysmorphophobic, sexual, or aggressive contents; vague, circumstantial, metaphorical, over-elaborate, or stereotyped speech; and occasional transient quasi-psychotic episodes with intense illusions, auditory or other hallucinations, and delusion-like ideas.

Research and Empirical Data

Empirical literature on StPD appears scarce. Some evidence suggests that the development of schizotypal personalities is associated with childhood neglect (Johnson, Smailes, Cohen, Brown, & Bernstein, 2000) and hypersensitivity to criticism, passivity, and lack of engagement in childhood along with anxious–avoidant attachment styles (Olin, Raine, Cannon, & Parnas, 1997). These attachment styles seem to predict both positive schizotypy (hallucinatory experiences and unusual beliefs) and negative schizotypy (withdrawal and anhedonia). In a more recent longitudinal study conducted by Lahti and colleagues (2009), it was demonstrated that lower placental weight, lower birth weight, smaller head circumference, higher gestational age, lower childhood family socioeconomic status, undesirability of pregnancy, higher birth order, and maternal smoking during pregnancy were among the early life origins of schizotypal personalities in adulthood.

Furthermore, despite the differences in conceptual understanding of schizotypy across DSM-5 and ICD-10, what remains a constant is that psychological research favors a focus on individual symptoms, as in psychosis. In particular, cognitive-behavioral studies tend to investigate the effectiveness of therapeutic interventions addressing the comorbid emotional distress. Yet, as demonstrated by Mankiewicz (2013), there have been three novel developments in cognitive therapy for such symptoms. First, there is a growing tendency to employ cognitive therapy as a person-based rather than symptom-oriented treatment, in which individually tailored interventions are implemented as a conceptual rather than manualized process (e.g., Chadwick, 2006). Second, it is becoming more necessary to deliver cognitive treatment for complex psychological difficulties as an integrative and multifaceted model that consists of a range of cognitively based interventions, such as mindfulness or metacognitive therapy (e.g., Tai & Turkington, 2009). Finally, due to the availability of research evidence that identifies early life origins of, in this instance, schizotypal features, it seems now possible to deliver cognitive therapy as a preventative intervention that aims to decrease psychological distress of children, enhance coping skills and self-esteem of young individuals, and improve networks for those exposed to severe stressors (e.g., Davies & Burdett, 2004).

Differential Diagnosis

StPD and Schizophrenia, Delusional Disorder, and Mood Disorders with Psychotic Features

The difference here appears to be related to gradations of symptomatology. Although a range of the symptoms will be similar, the degree of conviction or certainty with which the person holds those beliefs is what differentiates between the diagnosis of a psychotic disorder or a personality disorder. As mentioned above, models of psychotic phenomena that emphasize these on a continuum of normal experience will view this diagnosis as reflecting only a degree of experience rather than reflecting any explicit categorization.

StPD and "At-Risk Mental State"

It could be construed that due to the subdiagnostic nature of the symptomatology, both StPD and ARMS are similar. However, while these may be difficult to differentiate in early adolescence, the early development and longitudinal stability of symptomatology over time will point to the diagnosis of StPD.

StPD and Schizoid Personality Disorder

Although both of these involve a marked lack of social interaction, those with schizotypal personalities usually present with odd beliefs and perceptual experiences, magical thinking, and an unusual style of appearance and behavior, whereas those with schizoid personality disorder appear as aloof, detached, and unremarkable.

Collaborative Strategy

Traditionally, those with StPD rarely come into therapy without an external prompt. They are typically difficult to engage due to the interpersonal aspects of therapy that elicit all their socially anxious and paranoid beliefs. Therapists themselves are likely to be the object of suspiciousness and seen as a source of threat. Additionally, many of those with StPD have a range of beliefs about how the world works that differ from those held in traditional mental health services or cognitive therapy (e.g., telepathy, clairvoyance) and these beliefs are central in their sense of self. These intensify their suspiciousness about, and avoidance of, any traditional services. As mentioned previously, the use of Socratic questioning is most important in the engagement and therapeutic process with those for whom a suspicious and threat-alert component is central to their difficulties and interpersonal interactions.

When Clara was referred, an ARMS was considered and rejected due to the longitudinal stability of her symptoms. She was referred to the CMHT to help her access individual permanent housing. On first presentation, Clara looked very unusual. She had very long hair with matted dreadlocks throughout; piercings around mouth, nose, and eyebrows; and visible tattoos on her neck. She wore boots with steel toe caps and military-style clothing. Her care coordinator helped Clara understand that her ability to remain a tenant at the hostel was at risk unless she engaged in therapy. Clara agreed to work with a therapist only because she was highly motivated to retain and improve her housing situation.

Clinical Application of the Intervention

Clara wanted a place to live above all else, so she proceeded with therapy despite her fear and mistrust of such interaction. She realized that therapy was her only means of breaking the cycle of hostels and homelessness. Within therapy, her initial goals reflected this rationale for agreeing to work with services including having a permanent place to herself, to feel safer both "at home" and out, not feeling like she had to be on guard all the time, and to talk to someone other than her sister.

Problem Maintenance Formulation

Due to Clara's readiness to engage and her motivation in addressing her recurrent problems, therapy began by conceptualizing the maintenance of her fear and homelessness cycle (see Figure 12.5).

The role of the conceptualization was important for Clara in that she was able to see an acceptable alternative to either being persecuted or "crazy." Clara identified with the processing that occurred once anyone in the hostel approached her and was able to see how, at times, her interpretation of events went "a little beyond the facts." She particularly identified with aspects of her emotional reasoning, realizing that she viewed her physical sensations of anxiety as a sign that "bad things were afoot."

The therapist and Clara also discussed the issue of her safety behaviors and the way in which these maintained her threat beliefs. The therapist used a number of analogies (e.g., garlic and vampires) to illustrate how safety behaviors prevent disconfirmation of beliefs. Clara appeared to understand the process but needed a period of Socratic cognitive interventions to allow her to question these beliefs prior to experiments to test her beliefs.

Cognitive Interventions

Once Clara and her therapist developed a shared understanding of what was happening when her coresidents approached her, they decided to work

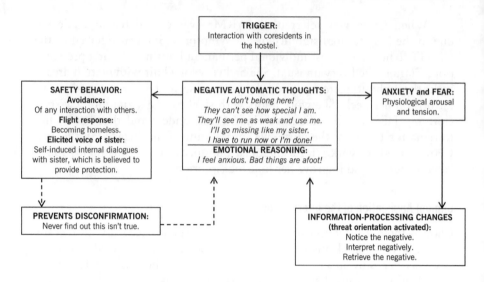

FIGURE 12.5. Clara's problem maintenance formulation diagram.

together to examine the accuracy of these beliefs using a variety of cognitive techniques. The therapist introduced Clara to thought records to help her analyze the evidence for and against her anxiety-provoking thoughts and reduce her conviction in her threat-oriented interpretations.

Pie charts were also used to help Clara find a range of alternative explanations for events she had witnessed. For example, Clara's automatic interpretation of seeing her coresidents gathering and talking in the lounge was "They are plotting against me, I'll go missing like my sister." Initially she had a high conviction in her interpretation (75%), which led to increased anxiety levels (80%). Hence, Clara was encouraged to brainstorm all possible factors that might have contributed to the event in question and rate how much (out of 100%) could be explained by that factor. With the therapist's help, Clara identified the following explanations:

"They might all be watching a TV program"—40%.
"There is often a 'house meeting,' which I always avoid, it might be that"—20%.
"They might just be socializing with each other"—20%.
"It's raining and cold outside so they may be avoiding that"—5%.
"The bedrooms are closed for cleaning"—10%.
"They are plotting against me"—5%.

The factors and corresponding percentages were then transferred onto a pie chart to help her visualize the range of possibilities.

Behavioral Experiments

Clara continued to use a range of cognitive techniques to evaluate situations in which she had felt suspicious and paranoid. After a few weeks, her belief that people in the hostel were plotting against her reduced to 40% and it was at this stage that Clara and her therapist then decided that it would be useful (and possible) to devise a series of experiments to further test this belief to find out whether it was true. First, Clara went into the lounge to test out her belief that the residents will see her fear and set on her. She was able to identify factors that might prevent her from completing the experiment and found solutions to overcome them. She then joined the weekly hostel meeting and was surprised to find that people were kind and welcoming. She was then able to further reduce her conviction levels for her initial beliefs to 20%.

Developmental Conceptualization

A cognitive conceptualization at the historical level allowed Clara to understand how past events affected her beliefs and assumptions (see Figure 12.6). Clara was able to see another explanation for the creation of her difficulties besides her suspicious appraisal of events in her current surroundings. The formulation looked at how earlier experiences had led to the development of beliefs and rules, and from there, an upsurge of unhelpful and threat-related beliefs that were exacerbated by physiological arousal, information-processing changes, and safety behaviors.

Core Beliefs and Prejudice Metaphor

The therapist used the prejudice metaphor (Padesky, 1993a; see Figure 12.7) to help Clara understand how her thinking about others was maintained. Clara identified with this model and began the process of an alternative "filing cabinet" to assimilate information and develop an alternate, more helpful belief set about others.

Progress, Lifespan, and Termination Considerations

Clara continued to engage surprisingly well in the therapeutic process. She and her therapist identified a number of other factors that played a significant role in her life—namely her voices, beliefs about her sister, and past experiences. However, she remained adamant that she did not want to explore these further and address them with the therapist. It is likely that Clara's issues of distrust still prevailed to some extent and prevented the discussion of the factors that she believed awarded her some safety and specialness. Additionally, Clara viewed these as helpful and did not want to

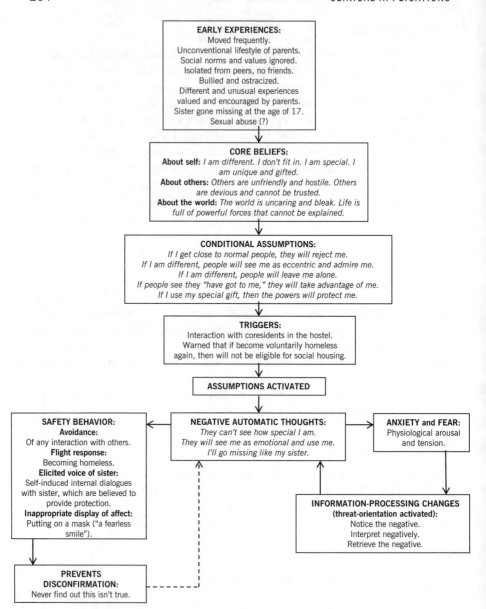

FIGURE 12.6. Clara's developmental cognitive formulation diagram.

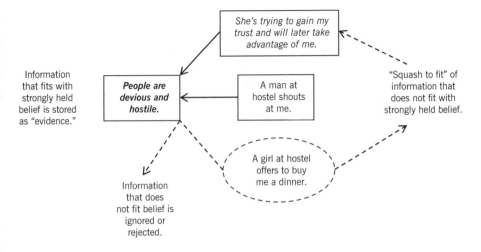

FIGURE 12.7. Prejudice model of one of Clara's core beliefs. Based on Padesky (1993a).

discuss them for fear that they may be lost. The therapist did not press this issue further, out of respect for Clara's autonomy and protection of their collaborative alliance.

Over the course of therapy, Clara became significantly less anxious, and her belief conviction that others were out to get her reduced considerably. She became able to tolerate other residents in the hostel and was able to attend the weekly meetings most weeks. She was awarded a tenancy toward the end of her therapy and moved quickly into a one-bedroom apartment in a large complex. Initially, she experienced an increase in anxiety and belief that other residents were plotting against her. However, the therapist worked with Clara to formulate her emotional response and manage the desire to flee from her new home. This led to a series of behavioral experiments designed to test her cognitions that focused on strategies of approaching other residents as opposed to avoiding them. This proved effective in reducing Clara's conviction in her suspicious beliefs and anxiety levels. Furthermore, she developed a more regular interaction with an elderly neighbor. Clara agreed to walk this neighbor's dog daily and eat lunch with the neighbor on a Sunday. She did not endorse that the neighbor was in any way devious or hostile but was prepared to admit that the lady's old age mediated in some way against her suspiciousness.

Clara attended 30 sessions, choosing to end therapy once she began to feel settled and less anxious in her new apartment. She continued to dress in a military style but over the summer months was prepared to remove her jacket and boots (she had never done this before), and at the end of therapy was contemplating allowing her elderly neighbor to cut her hair. Clara reported that her neighbor would suggest this most times that she visited. Thus, at the conclusion of therapy, it appeared that she had productively used the therapeutic relationship and succeeded in reducing her subjective experience of threat. She reported substantially lower anxiety levels, and had begun to form a relationship with a neighbor in her new building, which was not characterized by suspicion and mistrust. Both Clara and her therapist remained confident about her ability to maintain her tenancy and have planned to use her therapy blueprint to support her learning. Clara agreed that she would return to therapy in the future, should she feel that her stability was at risk.

SCHIZOID PERSONALITY DISORDER

The main feature seen in individuals with schizoid personality disorder (SPD) is lack of, and indifference to, interpersonal relationships. There is a pervasive pattern of detachment from social relationships across all contexts. Such individuals often present as withdrawn and solitary, seeking little contact with others and gaining little or no satisfaction from any contact they do have, regardless of its focus. Clients with SPD often spend the majority of time alone and choose to opt out of any activities involving contact with others.

Individuals with schizoid personalities also present with marked restriction in their display of affect. They are likely to appear slow and lethargic. Speech, when present, is frequently slow and monotonic, with little expression. Such individuals rarely show changes in their mood, despite external events. The mood they do present is generally moderately negative, with neither marked positive nor negative shifts. Any social occupations are solitary. Persons who are schizoid are not given to the development of close relationships of either a sexual or platonic nature.

It is important to stress that such symptomatology lies on a continuum of experience, as do the beliefs behind presenting features. Individuals who are "loners" may be considered schizoid only when such traits are unhelpful, inflexible, and cause the person significant problems in their life or affect. High levels of introversion do not constitute SPD, unless the key feature of indifference to relationships is also present. To warrant a diagnosis of SPD, the context of inflexibility to make life adjustments is necessary, leading to distress for the individual.

Derek, a 36-year-old unemployed man, spends much of his time alone in his apartment, listening to the radio or reading books. He goes to church daily, slipping in just after the morning service has started and leaving just before it ends to avoid having to speak to the vicar or members of the congregation. Derek presented to therapy with increased anxiety and low mood. On initial presentation, Derek avoided eye contact and spoke only minimally to answer questions. His motivation to attend therapy was illustrated by his request that the therapist "gets his family to leave him alone and let him be" as their attempts to make him attend family functions were causing him extreme distress and anxiety. In addition, Derek spoke about a heightened sense of the futility of life and his concerns that his oddness meant that nothing could change. It appeared that such beliefs were leading to his increased feelings of low mood.

Clinical Signs and Symptoms

DSM-5 diagnostic criteria for SPD (American Psychiatric Association, 2013) specify a longitudinal pattern of detachment from and indifference to interpersonal relationships accompanied by considerably limited range of expressed emotions in social situations as primary diagnostic features. As mentioned above, there is little interest in, or reward gained from, interactions with other people. The individual with SPD is not usually distressed by the absence of relationships, but may be distressed by pressure from others such as family members over their lack of involvement. Similar themes appear to be the focus of ICD-10 criteria for the diagnosis of SPD (World Health Organization, 1992) but there is also mention of a limited capacity to express either positive or negative feelings toward others, an excessive preoccupation with fantasy and introspection, and a marked insensitivity to prevailing social norms and conventions.

Research and Empirical Data

Research dedicated to individuals with schizoid personalities is scarce, perhaps because of the relatively uncommon occurrence of this disorder within a general population. Indeed, studies report the prevalence of SPD as ranging from 0.7 (Samuels et al., 2002) to 4.5% (Ekselius, Tillfors, Furmark, & Fredrikson, 2001). In general, studies tend to highlight a problematic low internal consistency of the construct of schizoid personality. For instance, literature reviewed by Mittal, Kalus, Bernstein, and Siever (2007) reported Cronbach alpha coefficients ranging from 0.47 to 0.68. Other studies have been affected by insufficient sample size for conducting statistical analyses (Farmer & Chapman, 2002). Additionally, Fagin (2004) argued that people with SPD rarely come to the attention of mental health services, unless their social isolation, self-neglect, and bizarre interpersonal behavior cause significant distress to them or to their family. In such cases, a relative might bring an individual who is schizoid to a therapist expressing concerns about the person's disengagement from family life. Thus, considerable avoidance of mental health services might be one of the obstacles to the utilization of empirical research among those with SPD.

Differential Diagnosis

SPD and Delusional Disorder, Schizophrenia, Paranoid Personality, and Mood Disorders with Psychotic Features

An individual with SPD describes a rationale of disinterest and vague distrust behind his or her avoidance of others as opposed to a clear series of beliefs regarding the malevolence of others that may be seen within psychotic disorders, or are characteristic of paranoid personality.

Withdrawal from others is often witnessed prior to the development of a psychotic disorder. When such diagnoses are present, to give an additional diagnosis of SPD, the personality disorder must have been present before the onset of psychotic symptoms and must persist when the psychotic symptoms are in remission (American Psychiatric Association, 2013). It is important to note that if SPD is unrecognized, an individual may be considered to be displaying negative symptoms of schizophrenia rather than disengagement due to either disinterest or a range of safety behaviors designed to avoid negative responses from others.

SPD and Avoidant Personality Disorder

Both SPD and avoidant personality disorder display a lack of close interpersonal relationships and engage in many solitary activities. However, the difference can be elicited by questioning an individual's desire for such relationships. Persons with avoidant personalities will avoid such relationships due to their fear of rejection and criticism. Those with SPD may also fear such criticism or rejection, but will not desire these relationships, and consequently, this self-enforced solitude appears less problematic for them.

SPD and StPD

Decreased levels of social interactions are present in both SPD and StPD. However, people with schizotypal personalities hold odd beliefs and perceptual experiences, magical thinking and behavior, and unusually individualistic appearance. Those with SPD present as aloof, detached, and unremarkable in appearance. Subclinical psychotic symptoms are absent in those with SPD.

SPD and Autism Spectrum Disorder

There may be great difficulty in distinguishing between SPD and mild-level autism spectrum disorder, as both display severely impaired social interaction, stereotyped behaviors, and interests. It may be that a comprehensive history is what lends most information to the differential diagnosis. Autism is usually apparent in early childhood, but schizoid traits rarely appear until middle childhood. Furthermore, while presentation is similar, the literature remains clear that these disorders stem from completely different etiologies, with a clear implication for neurodevelopmental factors within autism spectrum disorder, and an explicit psychological foundation within SPD.

Collaborative Strategy

As therapy is by its very nature an interpersonal event, it is likely that a person with SPD will have difficulties in engaging in a collaborative therapeutic relationship. Individuals' beliefs about themselves and their interactions with others will impact the therapeutic relationship as they do other interpersonal interactions. Those with SPD rarely seek treatments of their longer-term difficulties, but should they engage, it is only for a brief period of work, often to tackle heightened levels of psychological distress brought on by a change in their environment. Once this immediate difficulty appears resolved, therapy rarely extends on to revision of the underlying cognitive factors.

On questioning in therapy, it appeared that Derek was ambivalent about participating in the therapeutic process. Not only did he see the problems as stemming from the fact he has "no personality or character" but he remained extremely fearful that therapy would lead him to discover more flaws in his personality and highlight his sense of inadequacy. He also described meeting the therapist weekly as "painful," a process he was adamant that he would dread. Therefore, the therapist needed to engage Derek in discussion of the advantages and disadvantages of attending therapy versus the advantages and disadvantages of not attending therapy. Only when likely advantages appeared to outweigh potential disadvantages in the short term, was Derek able to willingly engage in the therapeutic process. Importantly, the therapist and Derek negotiated a very short contract of sessions for each stage of therapy that gave Derek a perception of greater control over the process and a feeling that he could easily disengage.

Collaborative Problem and Goal List

It may also be difficult to negotiate a collaborative problem and goal list with a client who is schizoid. With respect to the individual's problems, it is important that the therapists are able to listen to what clients are saying and ask them to specify what element of their experience is problematic *to them*, as it may differ markedly from what the therapist expects the problematic area to be. The nature of the profession of psychotherapy is such that it is unlikely to attract anyone with schizoid tendencies, and therefore, a common ground in perception of goals appears unlikely. Hence, if therapists begin to speculate appropriate goals for schizoid-type difficulties, they put themselves in risk of being completely "off the mark." Consequently, a therapist and a client who is schizoid can become involved in an unhelpful process of pursuing cognitive interventions with conflicting goalposts, which might result in the client's eventual disengagement from therapy. Furthermore, the development of SMART goals might not be achievable, as any concrete interpersonally oriented tasks might trigger further increase in anxiety and avoidance, thus resulting in possible disengagement.

Derek's problem list included not working, boredom, being teased by his family, having no one "on his side," and feeling on edge and low. When attempting to set a goal list for each of the problems, it became apparent in sessions that this was difficult for Derek, as he perceived himself as "always being this way." Derek found the process of goal setting extremely challenging and the therapist had to resist the temptation to suggest goals on many occasions. Eventually, and with much guidance, Derek developed the following goals: to help his father out in business, be able to better fill his time, for his brothers to respect his lack of friends, find one person with whom he can discuss difficulties over the Internet, worry less and feel less anxious, and feel better about himself.

Problem Maintenance and Developmental Formulation

In individuals with SPD, a set of early experiences involving peer rejection and bullying are often present. In addition, the individual has often experienced being seen as different from the closer family unit, or in some way diminished in comparison with others. As a result, they have come to view themselves as different in a negative sense, others as unkind and unhelpful, and social interaction as difficult and damaging. Consequently, a set of rules or assumptions may develop to provide "safety" means for such individuals, leading them into a lifestyle of solitude and lack of engagement.

Derek was one of three brothers born to a plumber and his wife. The family was outgoing and physical, and Derek's two brothers had followed in their father's footsteps, one working directly for him and the other dealing in hardware in the plumbing trade. In contrast, Derek had been a shy and timid child and was teased mercilessly at school. Since childhood he had been a solitary person more interested in study rather than playing football with his father and brothers.

When Derek was young he was called "a square peg in a round hole" and was often told by his father that "He must have been switched in the hospital." Throughout his life, Derek had tried to become involved in sports or the family business, but his efforts were often met with comments as to his ineptitude and he eventually gave up. His only regular outing was to his local church, which he attended despite the anxiety it afforded him. On being asked about this, Derek replied that his beliefs about God, heaven, and hell meant that because he was "half a person" and had an "ugly personality," his church attendance saved him from a "forever of purgatory." In recent months, due to his parents' retirement and the impending marriage of his younger brother (his older brother was married with two children), his mother had attempted to "pull the family together again." This appears to have exacerbated Derek's anxiety, emotional distress, and lowered his mood, based on his beliefs about his difference, the futility of his effort, and the negative outcome of this increased interaction with his family.

Derek decided that he would like to work on his anxiety as a first goal of therapy. On exploration of this anxiety, a maintenance formulation was generated (see Figure 12.8). Based on the collaboratively conceptualized understanding of Derek's anxiety, it seemed to have been maintained by his pervasive avoidance of and disengagement from interpersonal interaction, which prevented disconfirmation of negative perceptions of social situations.

Despite his ambivalence about therapy, Derek was very open about his familial history, past experiences, and what he thought about himself and, as a result, it was easy to collaboratively generate a developmental formulation of Derek's difficulties, depicted in Figure 12.9.

Derek felt that this was a good summation of his difficulties. The therapist and Derek discussed which specific thoughts he would need to change to enable some reduction in his problematic symptoms. Derek felt

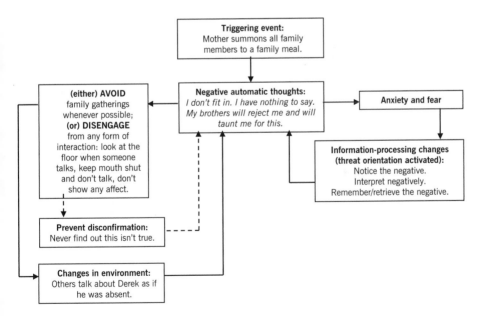

FIGURE 12.8. Derek's problem maintenance formulation diagram.

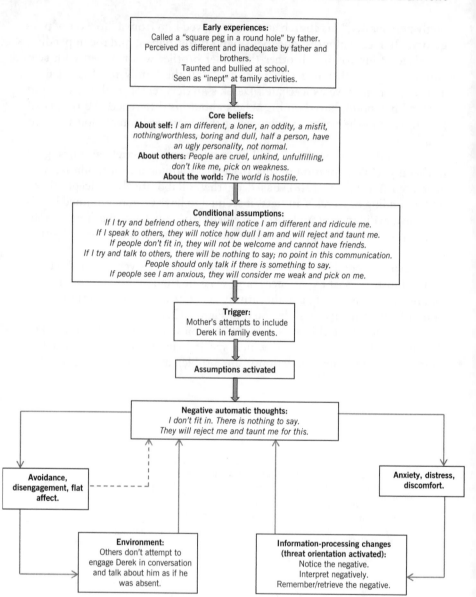

FIGURE 12.9. Derek's developmental cognitive formulation diagram.

that addressing his belief that others may taunt him as a result of his "odd-ness" was likely to be the most effective route to a reduction in his anxiety. In addition, Derek and his therapist felt that he needed to work on some of his assumptions, such as "If I talk to others, there will be nothing to say and no point in this communication," which seemed central to the mainte-nance of his difficulty.

Clinical Application of the Intervention

Derek and his therapist planned a series of behavioral experiments (fol-lowing verbal reattribution to challenge this premise) to find out whether others recognized his anxiety and would taunt him for his interpersonal difficulties. Another series of behavioral experiments looked at Derek's use of flat affect and disengagement as safety behaviors, following his belief that if others noticed his anxiety or his "oddness shining through" they would attack him verbally. Derek and his therapist devised an experiment in which he would drop his safety behaviors (avoiding all eye contact, gaz-ing at the floor, and hiding all facial expression) and see whether he was ridiculed and taunted. This was done following verbal reattribution (con-sidering the evidence and generating alternative explanations) that reduced his belief in being derided from 90 to 25%, affording him the possibility of entertaining other possible outcomes and engaging in the experiment.

Reframing Core Beliefs

Despite his certainty earlier in therapy that he did not want to look at his beliefs about oddness, Derek later decided that these may be central to his distress and may need to be addressed. Derek proposed "I can be normal" as an alternative core belief that he would like to hold. Derek was social-ized to prejudice metaphor as a way of explaining the mechanism by which information-processing changes could maintain negative self-beliefs despite the availability of evidence to the contrary.

The therapist asked Derek to collect data (as homework) that fit with "I can be normal," using a positive data log. Guided discovery questions included the following: "Is there anything that you have done today that seems to suggest that you are normal or that someone else would view as a sign that you are normal?" and "Is there anything that you have done today that, if someone else did it, you would view as a sign that they are normal?" The data collected was then used to help Derek rerate his belief in "I can be normal" on a weekly basis. Evidence that Derek used to sup-port his new belief included talking with another customer in the line at the supermarket, being able to engage in cognitive therapy, cooking dinner for his mother, and saying a friendly hello to a neighbor. At this stage of therapy, Derek reduced the frequency of his sessions, completing much of the work alone while attending therapy for guidance.

Progress, Lifespan, and Termination Considerations

As Derek was often ambivalent about therapy, considerable time in session was put aside to discuss this issue. During each review session, Derek and his therapist would look at his goal list and evaluate progress with respect to each objective. Joint decisions were then made as to whether the goal had been met. If so, was there another goal that would be useful for this area? If not, was the goal still appropriate and achievable? If so, should they still work toward it, and if not, should they choose a new, more appropriate goal? The therapist and Derek discussed inviting his mother or other family members into the session to help him plan or challenge his concerns. However, Derek felt that while he had become able to tolerate the therapy sessions, this would seem overwhelming and unhelpful at this time.

Derek's ambivalence about therapy was evident throughout his participation. Even when therapy was in progress and could be considered successful, the negotiation of new therapy goals always needed to be preceded by a review of the advantages and disadvantages of continuing the therapeutic process. Plans to end therapy were made with Derek once his central goals of being less worried and feeling better about himself had been achieved. Therefore, prior to discharge, work focused on planning to end therapy and consolidate and strengthen Derek's conviction in the new, more positive and helpful belief. Furthermore, a blueprint was generated to reinforce helpful work that had been completed and provide a conceptual framework for Derek to continue his recovery in his agreed direction.

COMMON CHALLENGES AND CLINICIAN SELF-CARE

While this is an unlikely group to seek help, the previous examples show that high levels of anxiety and interpersonal problems, which may threaten employment, housing, and family functioning, can lead such individuals to seek help. However, this does not mean that they are able to engage. Their limited understanding of their range of psychological difficulties and their avoidance of interpersonal proximity means that engagement in therapy remains a challenge throughout. Work can be halted, time and time again, while the pros and cons of therapy are again revisited as this ambivalence about engagement and collaboration is in itself resistant to change. The ongoing ambivalence of these clients can be frustrating and therefore, supervision and a firm retention of a guided discovery approach is necessary to ensure that the individual remains at the helm of his or her recovery.

CONCLUSION

While there are many differences among paranoid, StPD, and SPD, it appears that all of these subscribe to the view that they are different, unlikable, and unable to fit into the social world, and that interpersonal relationships should be avoided. However, the rationales behind such decisions differ accordingly to a belief set specific to the particular disorder—that is, because others want to hurt them (paranoid), others don't care or don't appreciate their uniqueness (schizotypal), or others are cruel and rejecting (schizoid). Because of such unhelpful appraisal of interpersonal activities and social situations, the development of a collaborative and trusting therapeutic relationship is particularly difficult with these individuals. Hence, addressing this through the means of guided discovery needs to be the initial focus of therapeutic work, which will eventually provide a safe place to test these beliefs and an opportunity for *in vivo* modeling for the development of future interactions.

CHAPTER 13

Passive–Aggressive Personality Disorder (Negativistic Personality Disorder)

Gina M. Fusco

Life just seems incredibly unfair.
—"CONTRARIANS" (Rasmussen, 2005, p. 277)

Christina is a 44-year-old single Caucasian female who presented for an urgent evaluation after having made veiled suicidal statements to a colleague. Christina made the statement after having received a negative employee evaluation from her supervisor. The negative review was the result of the many difficulties Christina had at the small real estate firm where she was attending an innovative employee orientation and training program. Difficulties included staff complaints about her irritability, lateness, and frequent arguing based on no real issues, creating and causing "pseudoturmoils" (Harper, 2004, p. 293). Colleagues described her as cynical, moody, and sullen. Christina repeatedly raised questions about policies, and then debated the answers given. When inquired how she would do things differently she would sarcastically respond, "You're the supervisor, you tell me." Although she confirmed to attend, Christina frequently was a "no-show" at open house sales events, claiming a "miscommunication" had occurred. Any area of ambiguity became fertile ground to eschew responsibility. When confronted about frequent lateness, she would say, "You don't understand" and quipped to her supervisor after arriving late on a rainy day, "I don't have an SUV like you." Her colleagues complained about her belittling and devaluing comments that included "They're just lucky," and suggestions that they used unscrupulous tactics.

Christina's supervisor noted inconsistent performance including failing to hand in her competency exams. When compared with her successful training cohort, Christina testily snapped, "They already had the answers." Christina rebuffed her supervisor's offer to assist with preparing for a re-examination by saying, "Thanks, but don't treat me like a child." In response to her few client contacts, Christina retorted to her supervisor that she already had a plan to increase productivity, stating, "I leave messages . . . they'll call me when they're ready." When pressed about her behavior, she responded with verbal sparring, stating that if her supervisor had responded to e-mails and questions faster, perhaps they wouldn't be in this situation. She felt terribly misunderstood and unappreciated, and reveled in the fantasy of when her supervisor would finally recognize and acknowledge her talents.

Historically, Christina experienced a lonely childhood filled with confusing, rejecting, and mixed messages. Her memories were focused on feeling sad, angry, resentful, and frustrated. After her parents divorced when she was 2 years old, she spent little time with her mother. Compounding this rejection, Christina received painful postcards from faraway exotic places in which her mother mockingly exclaimed, "Miss you!" Hoping to win her mother's favor, she did not react or respond, but rather, suffered throughout her childhood years in saddened and simmering silence. She struggled through high school and enviously recalled her peers chatting excitedly about college, but never responded to the school's requests to discuss her own ambitions. Social situations and relationships with boys were unsuccessful. Along with chronic problems with teachers, supervisors, and rules in general, she had few friends and little outside interests. Unable to maintain steady employment, she believed no one understood or appreciated her, lamented the great misfortune and unfairness of her life, and had absolutely no idea why things were the way they were.

CLINICAL SIGNS AND SYMPTOMS

The patient with passive–aggressive personality disorder (PAPD) typically presents for treatment as a result of complaints by others when he or she is unable to finish tasks, complete assignments, or meet expectations (Freeman, 2002; Ottaviani, 1990). An authority figure, legal mandate, or supervisor in a vocational role may instigate the referral due to the individual not meeting deadlines, following directions, or dissolving morale among other employees. Partners, spouses, or family members may also pressure the individual to contribute to the home, children, or a relationship. Demands may be to get a job, enroll in a course, be responsible for child care, or do something at home (Stone, 1993a). Responsibilities such as paying bills, responding to requests for additional information, and difficulties with other persons perceived to be in positions of authority (e.g., physicians, therapists, bill collectors, officers, professors) cause ongoing problems. Contradictions, frustrating ironies, and tension-laden sparring are constant. Everyday expectations, which when met create a reasonable and predictable life, become a series of crises, confirmation of one's misfortune, or an embattled ground of conflict, further alienating any who offer help or support. Others may seek treatment as a result of symptoms related to a comorbid condition, such as depression or anxiety. Distressful automatic thoughts such as "It's not fair," "Good things don't last" (American Psychiatric Association, 2000, p. 790), and "I won't do what they say" derived from powerful underlying core schema can influence depressive, negative, and irritable moods that impact self-esteem, functioning, and interpersonal relationships.

The diagnostic criteria for PAPD have progressed from a conglomerate of oppositional behaviors directed toward authority figures to incorporate a more dimensional definition, negativistic personality disorder (NegPD; American Psychiatric Association, 2000; Millon, 1969, 1981) to the subsequent relegation to the "other specified personality disorder" category within DSM-5 (American Psychiatric Association, 2013). Skodol (2012) noted that the initial DSM-5 draft revision proposed that the DSM-IV-TR Appendix personality disorders would not be included as specific disorders, but rather be defined as a significant impairment in personality functioning with specific traits describing the most remarkable features. In the final version, DSM-5 does not list PAPD as a disorder, but does specifically reference PAPD within the description of the "other specified" and "unspecified" categories. Included in these categories are personalities that meet the criteria of a personality disorder, but do not meet criteria for any current specific personality disorder (American Psychiatric Association, 2013). Similarly, within ICD-10, PAPD is included within the category, "other specific personality disorders" (World Health Organization, 2010). Wetzler and Jose (2012) write in their comprehensive historical review of the disorder, "How is it that a syndrome which used to be hugely prevalent 65 years ago is now not officially recognized at all?" (p. 675). Criticisms that included the narrow-focus situation-based criteria, high comorbidity, low prevalence rates and reliability, and little research "do not appear entirely justified" (Wetzler & Morey, 1999, p. 53), and "evidence suggests that PAPD as a disorder is no less valid than most other [personality disorders]" (Wetzler & Jose, 2012, p. 674). Similarly, McCann (2009) notes in relation to NegPD and [obsessive–compulsive personality disorder], "The longevity of these psychopathological constructs points to their utility" (p. 686), and Gunderson (2010) concludes when considering deletion of disorders, limited research does not equal limited utility. The question of whether the construct represents a specific disorder remains, and consistent with PAPD's exclusion from DSM-5, many researchers do not support its resurrection as a disorder.

Both diagnoses of PAPD and NegPD are included in empirical studies and reviews. In practice, shared constructs include a general pattern of resistance and interpersonal difficulties including feelings of being misunderstood or unappreciated (Sprock & Hunsucker, 1998). Specific characteristics of PAPD form a pervasive pattern of antagonistic neglect of external demands for the individual's adequate social and occupational performance. Evidence of this passive resistance and oppositional style includes persistent, deliberate procrastination; resistance to authority; argumentativeness; protests; and obstruction. Deadlines are nearly impossible to meet, and missing them is frequently externalized so that the missed deadline may be blamed on "forgetfulness," unreasonable demands, or the "authorities" having unrealistic expectations, or even a lack of "fairness" in setting deadlines to begin with (Ottaviani, 1990). The largely passive nature of these resistant behaviors or "calculated incompetence" evokes tremendous frustration in others, straining personal, social, and vocational relationships (Wiggins, 1982, p. 213). Worsening the situation, the individual with PAPD may solicit others' help and guidance, all the while thwarting and sabotaging the suggestions given.

Significant social impairment is evident in the entitled, inconsistent, angry, and contrary interpersonal style of patients with PAPD. Their ambivalence becomes evident when they seek out others, then refuse engagement through an active or passive stance, such as being a "no-show" after confirming attendance. Ambivalence within the therapeutic process is evident through obstructionism, defiance, procrastination, verbal sparring, and treatment noncompliance.

Clinicians can easily recognize the core features of PAPD as a chronic unwillingness to fulfill expectations (Wetzler & Morey, 1999), beyond simply being angry about a life situation (Ottaviani, 1990). As the diagnostic term implies, the patient with PAPD expresses hostility through a covert or passive medium of argumentativeness, cantankerousness, refusal to conform, and irritability. Patients who are passive–aggressive also present as sullen, moody, and ambivalent (Millon, 1969). Malinow (1981) states, "The term itself, passive–aggressive, is ambivalent and suggests paradox" (p. 121). Millon's (1981; Millon & Davis, 1996) description of the active ambivalent defines and embodies the vacillating nature of the patient with PAPD. On one hand, the patient wants someone to take care of him or her and make life gratifying. On the other hand, he or she does not want to lose autonomy or freedom, and he or she resents the direction and power of those in authority or those on whom he or she depends. Trapped somewhere between this intense dependence and demand for autonomy, the patient with PAPD experiences an exquisite anguish of never feeling content or satiated, creating a "stalled life." It is this ever-present lack of content-ment that can emulate symptoms of an ill-tempered depressive as defined by Schneider (1958). The pervasive skepticism of those with PAPD have a narcissistic flair in that life's woes and negative turns are somehow con-nected and directed toward the patient with PAPD, and external demands are predictably viewed as a personal affront and are therefore offensive to their sense of entitlement. Millon and Grossman (2007) note " the wasteful nature of ambivalence" and the rejection of meeting expectations required to fulfill goals blocks and impedes achievement of progress (p. 286). Stone (1993a) indicates the pervasive negativism of PAPD is self-defeating, and due to its very nature becomes self-fulfilling. Benjamin and Cushing (2004) capture this self-sabotaging perpetuating dynamic: "To resist perceived coercion and punish the perceived coercers, the [passive–aggressive] devel-ops the strategy of winning by losing" (p. 49).

RESEARCH AND EMPIRICAL DATA

Little empirical research has been completed with PAPD as the primary focus despite the encouragement of further study as indicated within Appendix B in DSM-IV-TR (Czajkowski et al., 2008). However, this may largely be due to the restrictive criteria of the original PAPD diagnosis (McCann, 1988; Millon, 1993), and its subsequent inclusion within the DSM-IV-TR "personality disorder not otherwise specified" (PDNOS) cat-egory (McCann, 2009). Prevalence rates may actually be higher than indi-cated. Morey, Hopwood, and Klein (2007) suggest the extensive use of the PDNOS category in practice may be related to patients meeting criteria for personality disorders that are no longer included. As an example, Verheul, Bartak, and Widiger (2007) found that among 1,760 psychotherapy refer-rals, PDNOS diagnosis was the second most frequently diagnosed person-ality disorder, and would be the most frequent if co-occurrence with the 10 official personality disorders was allowed (consistent with DSM-IV-TR definition). McCann (2009) indicates that despite difficulty in establishing a concise prevalence rate as there is tremendous variation in the literature (0 to 52%), PAPD warrants continued existence. Recent studies (Rotenstein et al., 2007) have shown that NegPD was evident in 3.02% of 1,158 psy-chiatric outpatients with the authors concluding that their study provides "weak-at best" support for the validity of the diagnosis (p. 40). In another study, females scored higher than males (a small difference) on measures of PAPD in a large community sample of over 18,366 adults (Furnham & Trickey, 2011). Sprock and Hunsucker (1998) found that when a sample of clinicians described patients with PAPD and NegPD, males more frequently met PAPD criteria, while women more frequently met NegPD criteria. To avoid gender bias, the authors suggest NegPD as a broader concept.

Historically, the first study to specifically address PAPD was completed by Whitman, Trosman, and Koenig (1954). The authors examined a total of 400 outpatients where the PAPD diagnosis was the most frequently occurring personality disorder. Those with PAPD broke contact or terminated treatment after one return visit more frequently than any other personality type. Characteristics of PAPD were assessed in a longitudinal study of psychiatric patients (Small, Small, Alig, & Moore, 1970). From the 100 probands selected, patients who were passive–aggressive were more often male, and represented 3% of the total (3,682 subjects). At follow-up after 7 and 15 years, compared with 50 matched controls with other psychiatric diagnoses, the passive–aggressive group was still "in the process of completing their education and had not yet qualified for other than casual employment" (p. 975). Small and colleagues (1970) noted several common attributes among the patients with PAPD at both intervals including alcohol abuse, interpersonal strife, verbal aggression, emotional storms, impulsivity, and manipulative behavior.

More recently, studies have been completed to either validate the diagnosis or examine its characteristics. Joiner and Rudd (2002) concluded negativistic features had incremental validity compared with other personality disorders when measuring the specific forms of distress and impairment evident with clinical disorders among a sample of outpatients who were suicidal. Vereycken, Vertommen, and Corveleyn (2002) investigated the personality style of three groups of young men enlisted in the military in Brussels. The groups consisted of those with no identified mental health issues, and two groups identified as having acute and chronic authority conflicts. Chronic authority conflict was frequently associated with PAPD (28 of 41 patients) and was not associated strongly with other personality disorders, providing some evidence that PAPD is a distinct diagnosis. A relatively high incidence was reported by Fossati and colleagues (2000), based on a sample of 379 in- and outpatients, where 47 patients (12.4%) received a DSM-IV PAPD diagnosis. Of those with PAPD, 89.4% received an additional personality disorder diagnosis, with a significant correlation with narcissism. The authors therefore conclude that PAPD may be more of a subtype of narcissistic personality disorder than a distinct personality disorder.

Bradley, Shedler, and Westen (2006) examined the defining features and distinctiveness of the personality disorders within the DSM-IV-TR appendix. A national sample of 530 psychiatrists and psychologists were asked to illustrate a psychological portrait of a patient by sorting descriptive statements into eight categories, then rating the extent to which the patient met criteria for each personality disorder. The results indicated that only the PAPD diagnosis was distinct from other disorders. Hopwood and colleagues (2009) concluded that the construct of PAPD was demonstrated to be unidimensional, internally consistent, reasonably stable, and most similar to Cluster B personality disorders. Similar to prior studies (e.g., Fossati et al., 2000), Hopwood and colleagues also concluded relationships with narcissistic and borderline personality disorders.

DIFFERENTIAL DIAGNOSIS

Currently, if a patient meets criteria for PAPD, the diagnosis is formally categorized within the "other specified personality disorder" category (American Psychiatric Association, 2013). Although many patients present with behaviors considered to be passive–aggressive (e.g., tardiness, treatment noncompliance, and resentfulness), the patient with PAPD approaches life and all its challenges in this same pattern. These clinical signs are not just reactive and transient behaviors. They are chronic, inflexible, and maladaptive personality traits. It can be difficult to complete a diagnostic interview due to the patient's often confusing, evasive answers. For example, a patient who is asked a direct question such as "Is the sky blue?" answers in a truthful but cantankerous way: "Not where I'm sitting." Simple innocuous questions become fodder that pique suspiciousness. For example, "Did you make here it okay?" to which the patient may say, "Why?" This can lead to tangential discussions defining particular words or constructs yielding a frustrating puzzle of incomplete answers laden with inconsequential details. Interactions can quickly become argumentative as the patient poses additional questions that demonstrate resentfulness at being asked to supply an answer (external demands), such as "How is this important?" Fighting a subordinate or dependent position, the patient retains autonomy by avoiding direct answers and therefore does not acquiesce to the authority figure.

Unlike the depressive style of the individual with PAPD, the individual with depression has more self-deprecating and hopeless thoughts, is more likely to blame him- or herself for misfortune, and exhibits a negative view of the future. Depression is possible in the patient with PAPD, so evaluation for associated high-risk behaviors such as suicidality, homicidality, or substance abuse should not be overlooked. Studies have demonstrated those with PAPD show an elevation in impulse levels (Perry & Körner, 2011); a significant association with alcohol, marijuana, and substance usage (Cohen, Chen, Crawford, Brook, & Gordon, 2007; Corbisiero & Reznikoff, 1991; Hopwood et al., 2009; Podolsky, 1970); migraines (Manlick, Black, Stumpf, McCormick, & Allen, 2012); attention-deficit/hyperactivity disorder (Cumyn, French, & Hechtman, 2009); negative childhood experiences (Hopwood et al., 2009); aversive parental nurturing (Johnson, Cohen, Chen, Kasen, & Brook, 2006); borderline, narcissistic, and paranoid personality disorders (Czajkowski et al., 2008; Hopwood et al., 2009); mood disorders, hopelessness, and suicidality (Alnaes & Torgersen,

1991; Joiner & Rudd, 2002); and childhood abuse in women (Davins-Pujols, Perez-Testor, Salamero-Baro, & Castillo-Garayoa, 2012). In addition, anxiety disorders may be present (Johnson, Cohen, Kasen, & Brook, 2006). Anxiety symptoms are likely to present during times that directly challenge the patient to be assertive, respond to an external demand, or when forced to choose a specific course of action. The hypervigilance associated with anxiety serves to guard against and anticipate the demands of others (Rasmussen, 2005).

Narcissistic and borderline characteristics are quite similar and may overlap with PAPD. Narcissism is manifested in the individual's considerable focus on his or her unique plight and misfortune, attitudes of grandiosity and entitlement, and potent inability to empathize with others. Differentiation can be made between the two disorders as those with narcissism typically are more active and directly aggressive, and if in disagreement with an authority figure or external demand, will not hesitate to assert dominance. The individual with PAPD vacillates in his or her response to authority figures between defiance expressed as biting and quarrelsome interactions, and attempts to "mollify . . . by asking forgiveness or promising to perform better in the future" (American Psychiatric Association, 2000, p. 790). Millon and Davis (1996) write that although patients with borderline personality also demonstrate severe ambivalence and vacillation, borderline personality disorder is more severe in terms of cognitive polarities, shifts in affect, and behavioral impulsivity. To assist with differential diagnosis of PAPD, Kantor (2002) suggests considering behaviors that may be obscured by other disorders, behaviors that are not considered classic PAPD symptoms (e.g., teasing), the underlying dynamics related to the behavior, and information obtained from a thorough history.

CONCEPTUALIZATION

Strongly held, powerful schema will dictate that direct assertion is potentially catastrophic. This is due to believing a loss of autonomy is risked through disagreement, rejection, or refusal from others. Thus, to avoid being controlled and ever resentful of authority, patients with PAPD respond to external demands in a passive, provocative, and indirect manner. Pessimistic and fearful of assertion and confrontation, the patient with PAPD is enveloped within a pattern of self-defeat. This pattern starts and stalls its way through life creating a path of "unfinished business" (Wetzler & Morey, 1999, p. 57). Stone (1993a) writes, "They may refuse to work, stage impasses, refuse stubbornly to progress in any direction, etc.—all of which ultimately defeats their own cherished hopes and ambitions" (p. 362). Coveting others' successes and progression through life, they spurn and reject those very same opportunities. Intense negative mood states related to activated polarities of dependence and opposition create a minefield of unpredictable responses. Reactions may be caustic and oppositional, or alternatively helpless and dependent. If directly confronted about passive behaviors, typical responses are incredulous resentment while proclaiming innocence and justification. Some responsibility for his or her dilemmas may be evident, but the patient will construct counterarguments to nullify any positive suggestion or idea, such that no lasting beneficial change occurs (Stone, 1993a).

The cognitive profile of the patient with PAPD includes core beliefs, conditional assumptions, and compensatory strategies that are consistent with negativism, ambivalence, resistance, resentment, envy, an unwillingness to meet expectations, and an overarching goal of retaining autonomy. Core beliefs such as "No one should tell me what to do!" "To conform means I have no control," and "No one understands me!" can effect and contribute to negative moods, and in response, lead to associated maladaptive behaviors. Automatic thoughts reflect unrelenting pessimistic skepticism colored with an "anticipation of dissatisfying outcomes" (Harper, 2004, p. 282). The skepticism that is prevalent is similar to those with paranoid traits or disorder (McCann, 2009) and pervades how they perceive themselves, others, and the world and all its challenges. Rasmussen (2005) writes, "They look for the negative in situations, and they typically find it" (p. 279). The desire to be in favor with those for whom they may be dependent or seek acknowledgment is in direct contradiction to their belief that to remain autonomous they must circumvent or resist complying with rules or expectations. To manage this ambivalence, independence is maintained through passive behavior that does not directly confront or challenge the authority. They retain control and autonomy by avoiding conflict and potential disapproval. The vacillation and ambivalence between accommodation and opposition is unremitting and creates powerful affective responses that include anger, guilt, and frustration (Harper, 2004). Vacillation can often evoke empathy from others or trigger an angry response leading to contrition and self-deprecation. As others support and provide affection, the pattern of ambivalence is reinforcing as it produces certain awards and avoids some discomforts (Millon & Grossman, 2007).

Core Beliefs

Christina's core beliefs and related dichotomous automatic thoughts emanate themes of wanting to be cared for, yet resisting external control (e.g., "Help me to know what to do," "No one should control me," and "To conform means I have no control"). Compliance is synonymous with a loss of control, freedom, and autonomy. This difficulty or conflict with accepting influence from others is a fundamental aspect of the intense ambivalence that creates such social impairment. Passivity or superficial compliance is the means of maintaining distance from the demands of a person or situation. They often view themselves as long-suffering and unrecognized for their unique contributions. Table 13.1 lists typical core beliefs.

Conditional Beliefs

Conditional beliefs of individuals with PAPD support superficial compliance and magnify their personal means of handling situations as the best, obvious, and most unique way. Thus, successful management of a situation requires shallow acquiescence, and covert insertion of the "better" PAPD approach. Table 13.1 lists typical conditional beliefs.

Christina's conditional belief that if she was elusive and indirect, she would be seen more favorably was demonstrated by her passive behavior in response to leads for potential clients. She believed that house hunters would view her unavailability as a signal that she was a highly desired commodity, and would therefore seek her out when they were truly ready to buy. She could not understand why her supervisor couldn't understand her reasoning, reflecting the conditional belief "If I do what I think is right, then others will be convinced it is right." By telling others she was attending open-house events (but not showing up), immediate confrontation would be avoided and eventually the wisdom of her ways would be acknowledged and recognized. Her supervisor's negative evaluation was a complete surprise, and she remained oblivious to the consequences of her actions.

Compensatory Beliefs

Compensatory beliefs of patients with PAPD largely include themes of remaining in favor of the authority figure by superficially conforming. However, if superficial conformity becomes problematic, they turn to the belief that an extreme injustice has occurred. They are convinced that they are not being recognized or appreciated for their unique and special contributions, nor are others capable of understanding them. They can evoke hostile responses from others due to their persistent complaining and defeatist worldview (American Psychiatric Association, 2000). There is a narcissistic quality to their compensatory strategies that can almost appear as a protective mechanism to avoid or avert rejection. However, the intense rage that accompanies these beliefs somewhat contradicts the notion that these beliefs are protective in their function, but rather the result of a narcissistic injury. Table 13.1 lists typical compensatory beliefs.

Christina's compensatory beliefs consisted of distorted ideas related to her perceived rejection by her supervisor. The rejection was not, in her mind, caused by her insubordination or low productivity, but rather was due to her supervisor's inability to acknowledge and recognize her unique ideas. She expressed intense anger, disappointment, and frustration at her

TABLE 13.1. Core, Conditional, and Compensatory Beliefs

Core beliefs

"No one should tell me what to do!"
"I can't depend on anyone."
"To conform means I have no control."
"Expressing anger may cause me difficulty."
"Rules are limiting."
"People do not understand me."
"Others should not question me."
"People will take advantage of me if let them."

Conditional beliefs

"By resisting demands, I remain independent."
"If I follow the rules, I lose my freedom."
"If someone knows information about me, I am vulnerable."
"If I depend upon someone, I have no say."
"If I do what I think is right, others will be convinced it is right."
"By not asserting myself directly, I stay in favor with others."

Compensatory beliefs

"I must circumvent the rules to remain free."
"I must not follow the path of others."
"I will superficially go along with others to avoid conflict."
"I must assert myself indirectly so that I will not be rejected."
"I do not receive the credit I'm due because others can't appreciate me."
"I have unique means of doing things that few understand."

supervisor's inability to see her creative means of performing her job. The greater the supervisor's pressure for compliance, the more entrenched she became in her convictions. She was intensely resentful and undermining of her "lucky" colleagues who received recognition. As others achieved goals, she became even more convinced that she was being overlooked and neglected, which led to subsequent interactions rife with bitter remarks and pervasive complaining.

KEY TREATMENT GOALS

The ultimate goal of cognitive therapy for the patient with PAPD is to understand how the pattern of ambivalence impacts and effects current relationships, mood, and self-esteem, with treatment progressing to work on the associated passive–aggressive behaviors that isolate and cause alienation, discontent, frustration, and feelings of being misunderstood (Rasmussen, 2005). Work includes creating a more balanced and realistic appraisal of situations that typically generate negative feelings and behaviors. Treatment success will be indicated by improved social interactions and related functioning, such as a reduction in work-related issues, appropriate assertiveness, and an improvement in mood. Meaningful treatment goals based on the formulation of cognitive behavioral therapy include:

1. Patient selection and direction of treatment goals with an agreed-upon goal list. Frequent checking in with the patient will counter passivity and activated beliefs of being controlled. It will be important for the therapist to remain consistent and empathic as the patient vacillates between engagement and rejection of the therapist.
2. Build social interaction, anger management, and assertiveness skills. Patients with PAPD often demonstrate an acerbic, passive, and argumentative stance that alienates others.
3. Learn to monitor and identify emotional states. Creating a list with associated physiological states can help clarify feelings.
4. Learn to monitor and identify maladaptive automatic thoughts and beliefs that contribute to negative mood states and passive–aggressive behaviors.
5. Evaluate cognitive distortions and underlying beliefs related to themes of control, ambivalence, and autonomy that lead to distressful emotional responses such as anger and sadness, and passive–aggressive behaviors that include argumentativeness and oppositional stances.

Setting specific treatment goals, however, can be quite challenging as the patient's defensive posture is often communicated through brash provocative responses that may include trying to prove the therapist incompetent (Benjamin, 2003). Empathically exploring the patient's point of view and distress can help to define goals and build rapport (Robinson, 2005). As an example, Christina's provocativeness and superfluous need for clarification created a tug-of-war as the therapist attempted to probe details about her referral as they worked toward setting goals:

THERAPIST: Thank you for completing those forms. I understand your colleague is with you?

CHRISTINA: She's not my colleague per se.

THERAPIST: Oh, I had thought that you work with her?

CHRISTINA: Well, we work in the same office, but she doesn't do what I do.

THERAPIST: I understand that she was concerned about you.

CHRISTINA: What do you mean by concerned?

To build rapport and set goals, the therapist emphasizes Christina's employment concern and distress as the focus of treatment, and prompts her to identify specific problems that were contributing to the current difficulties. With education about the cognitive model, Christina can learn how her thoughts and beliefs are influencing her depressed, irritable mood and low self-esteem. By learning to monitor for cognitive distortions that include polarized statements such as "I won't be told what to do" juxtaposed with "They should help me" create opportunities for appraisal and assessment of the validity of these thoughts, and can lead to more balanced emotional and behavioral responses. Consistent monitoring, particularly during situations that involve meeting an expectation or an obligation, can help to clarify the ambivalent and vacillating nature of underlying beliefs that influence and generate anger and sadness and illuminate the overdeveloped strategies of resistance and control.

COLLABORATIVE STRATEGY

Collaboration is an essential component to treatment with the patient with PAPD, although the core beliefs will present unique difficulties in a cooperative therapeutic exchange. Stone (1993b) writes, "Many quit treatment (a passive–aggressive act in itself) before any positive changes can occur" (p. 308). As the primary strategy is to resist the dictates of an authority figure, the patient may believe that the therapist is trying to tell him or her what to change, and how he or she should go about it. They may respond in an angry despondent manner alluding to the therapist's incompetence, and counter with statements such as "Yes, but . . . ," consistent with Yalom's (1985) description of the "help-rejecting complainer." It is therefore imperative that the patient becomes actively involved and collaboratively responsible for the direction and focus of the treatment process. This requires ongoing diligence with checking in and soliciting feedback to ensure that the patient remains empowered, thereby countering activated core beliefs of control and opposition. If the patient assumes that the therapist is controlling the session or demanding compliance, the patient will passively resist the process including feigning compliance, "forgetting" homework, not showing up, or canceling the session.

As a means to establish collaboration and a sense of patient empowerment, the therapist emphasized Christina's *unique* perspective in understanding and clarifying treatment goals that included the identified work-related issues that would be most beneficial. As Christina began to participate in setting goals for each session, she became receptive to prioritizing the items and agreed to create a list. Written lists were signed by both the patient and the therapist to assist in collaborative treatment planning. In this way, if the core belief of being controlled became activated, evidence to the contrary was produced. For example, the following potential treatment goals were listed: improving work relationships, examining Christina's contribution to the situation, improving social skills and building supports, examining origins of depressive symptoms, anger management, alcohol use, and identifying long-term posttreatment goals. By encouraging the patient to choose what she wished to work on, the therapist not only challenged the very passivity that caused problems but encouraged an assertive approach to the setting of the agenda and related goals. Any distortions related to the therapist attempting to control the process could then be identified and encouraged to become a more adaptive assertive response, such as asking for further clarification of the patient's goals or related feelings.

Through a consistently empathic and supportive approach by the therapist, and with increasing self-awareness of her thoughts and emotions, Christina began examining her ambivalence, family-of-origin patterns (Benjamin & Cushing, 2004), and what she brought to current relationships or the "wounds and debts from her past" (Thomas, 1994, p. 214). When exploring core beliefs through guided discovery, themes of control were pervasive. As she began to understand the polarities of her wanting and needing authority figures (mother, supervisor) to care for her (dependence) contrasted with the protective stance of not wanting to be controlled (opposition), Christina gained insight into the reenactment of her pattern of anticipatory disappointment and cynicism based on the defeatist belief that her needs could never be met, and if they were met, would not last long. She saw that there was no middle ground where she could at the same time feel cared for, yet remain autonomous. Her polarized and ambivalent beliefs led her to argue, or disregard rules to protect her autonomy and prevent control from others. However, as a means to remain and continue to gain favor with authority figures, she superficially complied when in reality she continued in her own way resisting requests and demands. Ubiquitous through her belief system were themes of victimization and unfairness: being taken advantage of and misunderstood, and that no one should tell her what to do. With an empathic and accepting stance, the therapist responds by providing the consistent support needed to facilitate working through the ambivalence with the overarching goal of creating balance and consistency.

CLINICAL APPLICATION OF THE INTERVENTION

There are several tactical strategies that can facilitate success of other technical interventions throughout treatment for PAPD, as follows:

- *Manage conflict and confrontation with motivational interviewing.* The core features and beliefs of the patient with PAPD is ambivalence between beliefs that "being controlled by others is intolerable" versus "I need authority to support and protect me" (Beck, Freeman, & Davis, 2004, p. 40). As a means to maintain and protect autonomy, strategies that include resistance, opposition, sabotage, and passivity are overdeveloped. Alternatively, to meet dependency needs by courting or garnering approval from authority figures, intimacy, assertiveness, activity, and cooperativeness strategies are underdeveloped (Beck et al., 2004). Christina portrayed this fundamental conflict of dependency versus opposition by frustrating others—that is, wanting to be close, and then responding with rejection. In a dependent manner, she sought answers from the therapist, but when she was redirected to encourage self-discovery and examine her own needs and to consider more concrete goals, Christina's responses vacillated between contriteness and impatience. In response, the therapist must be able to identify the defiance, while importantly, remaining empathic and not overwhelming the patient with intense confrontation. Beck and colleagues (2004; Beck, Freeman, & Associates, 1990) note that the therapist must avoid challenging dysfunctional beliefs, behaviors, and motivation to change too aggressively so as not to activate compelling schema and the related automatic resistance to maintain control and autonomy. To help manage confrontation and resistance, a motivational interviewing (MI) approach can encourage deeper exploration that begins with the therapist resisting trying to "fix" the patient, and continues with a consistent conveying of curiosity in trying to understand the patient's motivation. Fully listening and providing reflective statements that demonstrate an accurate understanding of the patient's perspective creates an attitude and atmosphere of acceptance. Specifically, MI techniques include utilizing open-ended questions, affirmations, reflective listening, and summaries (OARS). In sum, rather than pushing and pressuring, acceptance and empathy actually creates the pathway to change (Rosengren, 2009).

To further reduce conflict and manage confrontation, the therapist can empower the patient by revisiting agreed-upon goals and commitments. Throughout the therapy, the patient is supported in asserting his or her selection of treatment goals and therapy direction (autonomy) by a non-rejecting empathic authority figure (dependence). This balanced approach creates a new experience for the patient: one that encourages adaptive assertion to the authority figure without the threat of rejection. Rosengren (2009) writes, "We must create an atmosphere in which they can safely explore conflicts and face difficult realities . . . by being empathic and communicating that empathy" (p. 10). This atmosphere creates the fertile ground for the therapist to elicit and reinforce change talk, or statements that are indicative of motivation to change. Highlighting and emphasizing change talk can lead to the exploration and activation of change, and the subsequent learning and practice of alternative and adaptive responses (Rosengren, 2009).

At times, Christina was aware of the effect of her bitter and antagonistic interaction style on others, however, discussing actual areas to change was frequently met with ambivalence. Building the treatment alliance through the use of OARS, MI strategies are uniquely suited to address ambivalence and aim to empower patients to view themselves as the source of their own solutions (Martino, Carroll, Kostas, Perkins, & Rounsasville, 2002), and understand their motivation that "lies within and help them to recognize it" (Rosengren, 2009, p. 10). The therapist elicits, remains attuned, and emphasizes change talk, promoting the patient's self-reflection and consideration of the discrepancies between reaching goals and current behaviors. In effect, the therapist empowers the patient to explore his or her motivations, and as the author of his or her story, assume responsibility for change, or not to change. By emphasizing Christina's primary motivation to remain employed and improve relationships, a balance is created between dependence (having the therapist determine the goal) and opposition (remaining steadfastly opposed to change). The therapist reinforces and reflects statements that acknowledge the impact of her negative interaction style to be self-limiting and defeating, ultimately preventing improvement with interpersonal interactions (Nett & Gross, 2011). With greater receptivity to discussing change, the use of the downward-arrow technique to review evidence that change is beneficial, and a related cost–benefit analysis that considers the advantages and disadvantages of changing, produces further clarification that to meet Christina's primary goals of retaining her job and relating better to others, some level of change needs to occur. This change begins with learning to self-monitor reactions (particularly emotional material initially), and interactions with others. Keeping in mind Christina's ambivalent and contradicting beliefs, the therapist frames the building of social skills as a mechanism that will enable her to assert and communicate her needs in a respectful and adaptive manner that will facilitate connections with others. Role-playing exercises that practice appropriate assertiveness and interpersonal exchanges can help demonstrate more adaptive modes of behaving and reacting. By empowering Christina throughout therapy, core schema related to control are mediated; change does not equate to acquiescence, but rather, is a result of a self-determined path to meet self-selected goals.

• *Discuss anger.* A most fundamental emotional problem of the patient with PAPD is maladaptive reactions of anger, hostility, volatile expressions, and, in particular, resentment. In treatment of these emotions, therapists need to initially assist patients with PAPD in being aware of and identifying their cognitive and emotional states, leading to an examination and management of their ideas of "righteous revenge" and the means planned for getting back at others they perceived to have been rewarded with unfair recognition and validation. Associated themes such as "They should be punished" or "No one really understands" should be identified and assessed (Ottaviani, 1990). This may be difficult as it requires patients to focus on their own performance and behaviors rather than on their perceived mistreatment from others. This exploration will likely activate narcissistic beliefs of superiority and entitlement that frequently co-occur with PAPD. If so, strategies of treatment with narcissistic personality disorder may prove helpful. With continued focus on overall motivation and treatment goals, a related cost–benefit analysis that considers the ineffectiveness of both managing anger passively and impulsive hostile reactions can lead to an understanding of healthier and more adaptive responses. The demonstrated benefit of having examined the relationship between core beliefs and their associated emotional responses will be further reinforced through the successful navigation of interpersonal interactions.

• *Avoid power struggles.* Covert expressions of resistance to therapy or the therapist may include being silent; rationalizing failures to comply with treatment recommendations; responding to confrontation increasingly with feelings of shame, humiliation, resentment, and blame; increasing passive resistance to therapy and change that includes oppositional behaviors and purposefully failing or becoming more symptomatic; increasing the amount of help-rejecting complaining and anger toward the therapist and the therapist's apparent inability to help; and talking about or suggesting other treatments or consultations with different therapists (American Psychiatric Association, 1989). Therapists might feel very frustrated and wonder whether the client is testing their competence. To help reduce power struggles, remaining focused on the patient's motivation can help to promote patient empowerment and self-determined direction (Rosengren, 2009). However, therapy boundary conflicts are quite predictable and prudently addressed early in the therapy. Clearly written rules for scheduling, billing, and time frames of treatment should be reviewed and a collaborative agreement established. When the client challenges these boundaries, for example by showing up late, it is extremely important to assess for automatic thoughts such as "Nobody is going to tell me when to arrive or what to do." This provides ample *in vivo* opportunity to explore these beliefs and their potential implications and alternatives. For example, the therapist can work with the patient to express a more direct means of asserting their preferences (e.g., requesting a different session time; Ottaviani, 1990).

• *Maintain consistency and empathy.* Throughout treatment, the therapist must remain consistent, objective, empathic, and not become enveloped in the patient's internal battle of "Help me/screw you" perceptions (Beck et al., 2004, p. 357). His or her caustic interactions can prove to be tiring and at times are offensive, with persistent ambivalence causing starts and stops. As the patient slowly becomes more comfortable (dependent) with suggestions from the therapist, underlying ambivalence can cause an erratic shift, leading to a rejection or setback of the treatment process (oppositional). The therapist needs to be consistently empathic, encouraging self-direction, empowerment, and choice while accepting and working through the ambivalence within a supportive and validating relationship. Although it can appear that such patients revel in their misery, they experience great discomfort, angst, and sadness in their plight. Rather than personalizing the patient's negativism, the therapist can remember to also conceptualize these actions as learned maladaptive behaviors (Beck et al., 2004), and that the patient experiences a life of chronic discontent (Harper, 2004).

Specific Techniques

Assertiveness Training

Assertiveness training can help patients with PAPD make covert expressions of anger overt and more functional (Hollandsworth & Cooley, 1978; Perry & Flannery, 1982). When the patient with PAPD struggles with impulse control and querulous reactions, therapeutic interventions that include relaxation, increasing frustration tolerance, decreasing distress, and considering the impact of reactiveness to others can be helpful in reducing emotional upset so that other more effective or adaptive means of communicating can be practiced. Negative affective states (e.g., irritability or dysphoria) and cognitive distortions and beliefs ("If I say no to the authority figure, they won't care for me") that are related to superficial compliance may indicate situations where healthy assertive skills would be beneficial. Learning appropriate assertiveness with effective and respectful communication helps the patient to retain autonomy with less threat of rejection from the authority figure, and less subsequent collateral damage from complaining, resentfulness, or argumentativeness. In Christina's case, assertion training was successfully used as a means for her to express disagreement with her supervisor's selection of a mentor, and to further request an alternative individual of Christina's choosing. Within the treatment session, the therapist was sure to allot time for feedback as to the direction that the therapy was going, and to solicit any changes that Christina felt they needed to make. This provided ample opportunity to practice appropriate *in vivo* assertion of any disagreements with the therapeutic process in a positive, structured way. In response, the therapist provided a balance between consistent limits (e.g., length of sessions) and receptiveness to Christina's requests (e.g., topics for the agenda).

Self- and Other Monitoring

Those with PAPD often have difficulty in describing their inner experiences, instead favoring a great focus on others' behaviors. Poor metacognition, or the ability to reflect upon, identify, and reason with mental states (Dimaggio et al., 2011) and alexithymia prevents the patient from being able to not only identify changes in his or her mood but what his or her mood and feeling state actually is (Nicolo et al., 2011). An inability to clarify and identify feelings makes establishing cause–effect connections among thoughts, feelings, and behaviors difficult. With a tendency to generalize interpersonal experiences in a maladaptive way, treatment therefore needs to "progressively promote awareness of mental states" (Dimaggio, Attina, Popolo, & Salvatore, 2012, p. 157). Early monitoring may be more beneficial when centered on learning, identifying, and categorizing one's emotional states (self-orientation) rather than moving quickly into narratives and the content of interpersonal interactions (Nicolo et al., 2011). To promote awareness, Dimaggio and colleagues (2011) suggest helping patients recognize that any arousal shifts they experience are actually emotional states and that these states are associated with specific physiological changes. Creating lists to help identify and differentiate these states is formalized with related terms, definitions, and clarification. Identifying how anger, disappointment, and other emotional states actually feel (e.g., physiological reactions) provides a valuable gateway to associated automatic thoughts and underlying core beliefs. The use of the technique of thoroughly describing autobiographical episodes or situations in detail can help to obtain descriptions of the thoughts and feelings that occur specific to that situation, rather than accepted generalized statements or perceptions. When idiosyncratic experience is emphasized, subjective states are clarified (Dimaggio et al., 2011), which help patients to realize and "take a critical distance" from their core beliefs (p. 73). As increasing awareness occurs, ongoing monitoring in session and between sessions of distorted thoughts related to being controlled or deprived such as "Nothing ever works out for me," "I never get what I deserve," or "How dare they tell me how to lead my life?" (Millon & Grossman, 2007) can allow for the patient to assess these thoughts as a means to prevent mood changes or becoming sullen (or hostile).

Specific prompting and monitoring for mood changes with high-risk material including suicidality is important throughout the therapy. Monitoring and collaboratively exploring appraisals and comparisons with others that may reflect a distorted view of how they "have it easy," "are lucky," or that "I'm treated unfairly" can create a more realistic interpretation of situations, ultimately leading to a more adaptive and healthy interaction style. Exploring shared experiences and commonalities with others to offset narcissistic beliefs of one's uniqueness can lead to a positive impact on social interactions. Homework assignments with a clearly understood rationale should include documenting and collecting automatic thoughts, particularly after experiencing an intense emotion. To encourage compliance with these assignments, thought recording should be presented as a "no lose" assignment (Ottaviani, 1990). The assignment allows for a connection between thoughts and feelings, and it can also identify areas related to depression or anxiety. Monitoring for associated offensive and mordant interpersonal reactions including posture, voice inflections (e.g., yelling), body language (e.g., pointing), eye contact (intense vs. avoidant), or use of biting words (Prout & Platt, 1983) can improve interactions. Monitoring others for signs of taking offense or disinterest (loss of eye contact, eye rolling, body posture change, verbal cues, leaving the room, etc.), can help to signal if individuals with PAPD are interacting in a disrespectful way. Self- and other monitoring is an important aspect of building social skills and communicating and remains a priority throughout therapy.

Social Skills and Communication Training

Impaired social and communication skills are vital treatment targets with PAPD. Interactions of the patient with PAPD are fraught with negativism, poor boundaries, and sarcastic, prickly exchanges. A controlling style that attempts to engage the therapist in a cynical assessment of the world alternates between garrulousness and churning silence. Conversely, patients with PAPD frequently lack good listening skills, reciprocation, or sensitivity to feedback or influence from others. For Christina, lack of connectedness and difficulty with social relationships was due in part to her poor perception of interpersonal cues. Social skills training helped Christina better understand the concept of interpersonal boundaries, warning signs from others that she may be violating their boundaries, and how to express herself in a respectful manner. Lists were made collaboratively identifying what good interaction skills might include and subsequently which areas she wished to develop, such as communicating a disagreement in an appropriate and nonoffensive manner. Communication skills practiced in session assisted her to make more "I" statements, pause for responses, maintain appropriate eye contact, and answer with fewer lengthy and detail-ridden sentences. Homework assignments included engaging in conversations with colleagues and practicing not raising her voice, pausing before responding and examining whether her response could be interpreted as offensive, and pausing for others to respond. Possible alternative responses were examined and later role-played in session.

PROGRESS, LIFESPAN, AND TERMINATION CONSIDERATIONS

For the patient with PAPD, progress can be slow. The patient may vacillate between pleasing behaviors and hostile reactions to the therapist. Core beliefs about control and resistance to plans, following the suggestions of others, or general compliance with structure can be easily reactivated.

Situations that place the patient under the direction of an authority can trigger the control–resistance schema and quickly thwart any therapeutic process gained. Throughout treatment, the therapist will need to consistently elicit collaboration as the patient will "attempt to pass responsibility for progress to the therapist" (Carlson, Melton, & Snow, 2004, p. 250). It is not uncommon for the patient to disregard treatment gains, and to even abruptly terminate despite progress. Incremental goals aimed at increasing general everyday functioning that impacts quality of life can provide reinforcement for continued commitment to therapy and lasting change. As new skills are learned that may cause anxiety, anxiety-reduction skills may be needed. With frequent crisis and turmoil that is later minimized, the therapist is challenged to remain steady and aware of his or her own reactions. Through empathic exploration, the patient can experience a relationship that does not respond, reject, or push him or her away providing the safety and room to experiment, grow, and change.

Passive–aggressive behavior exists along a continuum and across the lifespan. Millon and Davis (1996) suggest that highly contradictory parenting contributes to the development of PAPD. Carlson and colleagues (2004) write that the family system, rife with hierarchy, creates opportunities in which passive–aggressive behaviors form a working defense within power struggles. Children with oppositional defiant disorder share many qualities of the adult with PAPD (Carlson et al., 2004; Fusco & Freeman, 2007a; McCann, 2009), however, Rey, Morris-Yates, Singh, Andrews, and Stewart (1995) concluded that there was not a longitudinal link between the disorders. PAPD has been shown in a sample population of adolescents to be associated with risks of violence (Johnson, Cohen, et al., 2000) and to be diagnosed more frequently with age (Johnson, Cohen, Kasen, Skodol, & Oldham, 2008), with symptoms tending to abate with age (Gutierrez et al., 2012). Segal, Coolidge, and Rosowsky (2006) note that for the aging individual, one's changing role suggests a transference of passive–aggressive behaviors from an occupational context to family, caregivers, or medical professionals who may become a more active influence. The authors suggest that of all disorders, with increased dependency that comes with aging, PAPD becomes the most apparent. With a greater dependence on caregivers, providers, or institutions, expectations of medical compliance such as taking medication consistently, or attending follow-up medical appointments, can activate core dysfunctional beliefs related to control (Segal et al., 2006).

Patients with PAPD can be proactively helped to manage the risky situations that could predictably activate old schema by listing and role-playing ways to handle these challenges. Follow-up visits to review their behaviors or problem areas are also helpful in retaining productive ways to manage difficult situations. Other modalities such as group therapy (with careful consideration) have potential benefits for maintaining progress, supporting the schema modification, and consolidating new skills if the patient is willing to become involved.

COMMON CHALLENGES AND CLINICIAN SELF-CARE

PAPD characteristics of negativism, ambivalence, resistance, unwillingness to meet the expectations of others, and an overarching goal of retaining autonomy create significant challenges to a productive therapeutic alliance. Common challenges include the highly comorbid nature of the disorder including suicidality, substance abuse, and depression. Consistent assessment of these areas is vital, including a thorough review of active and current treatment from all providers including prescribing physicians and medications (including over-the-counter medications). Medication regimens may activate ambivalence associated with core beliefs related to control, which may lead to nonadherence or medication abuse. Referrals to marital and family therapies can support individual gains, while group therapy can create opportunities for increasing interpersonal skills. Strong limits and boundaries surrounding suicidal statements and working crisis plans are needed to ensure ongoing monitoring of safety. For example, the patient may allude to suicidality or provide an indirect response rendering the therapist unsure of the patient's stability. Ambivalence can indicate risk, so careful assessment is required. Powerful activation of core beliefs related to control can be especially evident for those mandated for treatment (Yanes, Tiffany, & Roberts, 2010). Thus, mandated treatment requires diligent efforts to promote patient control and choice where possible. The clinician needs to be ever aware of his or her own responses, reactions, and related stress in the context of demeaning, devaluing, and passive–aggressive behaviors. Robinson (2005) writes that the therapist as an authority figure will be treated with both envy and contempt, and "Countertransference can be quite marked" (p. 416). Benjamin advises that the management of countertransference is a key factor in the development of collaboration (1993), as Millon, Grossman, Millon, Meagher, and Ramnath (2004) indicate "Negativists are impressively frustrating" (p. 554). Advocacy groups can be enlisted to potentiate support for the patient and assist family members and treatment teams who may become frustrated or fatigued. Professional peer support, supervision, and consultation are integral to providing appropriate treatment. Ongoing self-care such as monitoring stress, health, and anxiety will be important for the therapist, to notice small warning signs such as personal complaining, sarcasm, and/or negatively anticipating sessions, and take steps to maintain the objectivity and well-being needed to work effectively with this disorder.

CONCLUSION

Although the PAPD diagnosis no longer formally exists as a specific disorder within DSM nomenclature, therapists can indicate the personality pattern that includes general resistance, feelings of being misunderstood or unappreciated (Sprock & Hunsucker, 1998), and passively expressed hostility such as a refusal to conform, argumentativeness, and irritability within the "other specified personality disorder" category within DSM-5 (American Psychiatric Association, 2013). Often presenting with interpersonal difficulties, the patient with PAPD is enveloped in a pattern of self-defeating and vacillating behaviors that are generated from schema that alternately oppose and depend on authority figures. Ensnared between intense urges for dependence and autonomy, the individual with PAPD often leads a life of discontent, and has ongoing struggles in meeting the demands of everyday life. Persons with PAPD have high comorbidity and often experience depression, anxiety, and difficulties modulating their anger. Because of their high ambivalence, evaluation for high-risk behaviors such as suicidality, homicidality, and substance abuse should not be overlooked. Cognitive therapy treatment goals include creating a more realistic appraisal of situations that typically generate negative feelings and behaviors, and to understand how relationships, mood, and self-esteem are impacted by ambivalence. Therapists can create an empathic stance with the use of MI approaches, helping the patient to resolve his or her ambivalence through consistency, support, and exploration. PAPD-related core beliefs and associated behaviors that include resistance, unwillingness to meet the expectations of others, negativism, and a potent need to retain autonomy are significant challenges in building a collaborative, productive therapeutic alliance. Therapists must remain aware of their reactions, as the patient with PAPD may be caustic, rejecting, and brittle. With a commitment to self-care, professional peer support, supervision, and consultation, the therapist can maintain the objective and accepting stance needed to effectively help patients with PAPD.

CHAPTER 14

Narcissistic Personality Disorder

Wendy T. Behary
Denise D. Davis

Jon, a successful analyst for a large financial institution, was prompted to therapy by his wife Stacy's ultimatum: "Get professional help and we will see, or else we are done." At intake, Jon was bitterly preoccupied by his sense of personal injury and unjust treatment: "How dare she intrude upon my work life" and "invade my privacy?" Evidently, Stacy had discovered a number of adult pornography sites stored in his web history on their home-office computer, with many hours logged-in—at times when he was supposedly "working" from home. She also learned that his late nights at the office were actually spent enjoying happy hour(s) with young, adoring, female coworkers nearly two to three nights a week. In therapy, he was indignant about being the "one" who had been "threatened" to get help, especially since "Stacy was clearly the one with mental issues." He immediately asserted his motives that (1) he only agreed to come in so he could calm her "hysterical mind" and (2) reclaim his right to sleep in his own bedroom, and then perhaps (3) when "she comes to her senses" he would be shown some appreciation for the "pretty roof" he kept over her head.

When asked whether he could imagine the hurt that Stacy might have felt when she discovered the lies . . . feeling cut out of his world . . . concerned about his distraction from their family . . . Jon replied, "She just doesn't understand that all men behave this way. It's no big deal. She is just insecure." When asked, "Jon, if this is truly no 'big deal,' then why didn't you share this part of your life with her?" he became annoyed, rolled his eyes, and smugly retorted, "That is a ridiculous question." He just didn't know he had to *ask permission* for a little *down time* at the age of 49, especially given how hard he worked to provide a charmed life for his wife and two children. When queried about his appearing irritated by the "question," he dropped his gaze, pursed his lips, shut down, and began vigorously reinforcing the crease in his perfectly pressed pants. When asked about what part he felt he played in their marital conflict, he simply said, "Hey, nobody's perfect . . . but I am a great catch."

This overtly arrogant yet fragile presentation illustrates classic features of narcissistic personality disorder (NPD). It is difficult to embrace the arrogance, easy to feel intimidated by the power challenges, and tough to elicit collaboration, unless there is some form of leverage. In this case example, the leverage is high because Jon actually does not want to lose his wife and family.

CLINICAL SIGNS AND SYMPTOMS

Persons with NPD typically seek therapy because of social ultimatums, material reversal, or other threats of humiliation such as loss of work status (perceived or actual) or disciplinary sanctions, perhaps related to irresponsible, exploitive, aggressive behavior or abuse of power; loss of a relationship with a partner or child; or adverse outcomes such as suspension of driving privileges or other penalty born from entitlement-driven, "the-rules-don't-apply-to-me" violations of the law. Less frequently, they may explore therapy as a form of self-display, seeking attention and admiration and generally lacking any substantial agenda for change.

According to DSM-5 (American Psychiatric Association, 2013), NPD is a pervasive, inflexible, and maladaptive pattern of inner experience and behavior focused on inflating and protecting self-esteem, with deficits in empathic or egalitarian relationships and adaptive personal development. NPD occurs in 0–6.2% of community samples, with 50–75% of those diagnosed being male (American Psychiatric Association, 2013). Other co-occurring disorders include mood disorders, especially with hypomania or dysthymia; anorexia nervosa; substance-related disorders, especially related to cocaine; and other personality disorders, notably histrionic, borderline, antisocial, and paranoid personality disorders. NPD may be underestimated as a co-occurring disorder because it is difficult to pinpoint in the context of other signs, symptoms, or gender expectations.

Clinical signs of NPD include behaviors and statements that appear self-aggrandizing, competitive, and convey expectations of special treatment, along with minimal insight. These individuals complain about others, minimize their own problematic behaviors, and fail to show reasonable care for the feelings of others. Their stance may be a blend of guarded and pompous, presenting themselves as a "fascinating" case, but seldom copping to any regret, remorse, or role in problems, if they acknowledge problems at all. The person who is narcissistic confidently solicits notice of their achievements, material assets, physical attributes, and social influence. However, this display of alpha-level confidence is actually a rather brittle compensatory shield against beliefs of inferiority, unlovability, defectiveness, and shame. Other important clinical signs can be detected in their lapses and distortions of social reciprocity. The person who is narcissistic compulsively seeks appreciation, yet fails to appreciate others, and tends to compete and "one-up" instead, dominating anyone who threatens his or her turf. Charming demeanor may be marred by arrogant outbursts, heartless remarks, or insensitive actions such as butting in to take control, or acting demanding and self-important. Judging others is an automatic behavior, with cutting insights a form of self-empowerment and social entertainment.

When faced with limits or critical feedback, people with NPD may flip from charming mode to nasty bully mode, turning defensive, providing further clinical signs of the disorder. They may subject certain people to daily harangues of overblown disapproval, lecturing, ridicule, or random micromanagement. The entertaining, powerful, seemingly confident facade of people with NPD may easily draw others in, until they realize their role is to stoke the narcissistic energy with continuous applause and approval. Over time, significant others see a stark contrast between the well-tended public impressions and their personal experience of an emotional void with the person with NPD.

When others set reasonable expectations, or attempt to confront the person with NPD about his or her difficult behavior, he or she shows little concern, or becomes stubbornly defiant. Because persons who are narcissistic gravitate to positions of power and use verbally aggressive tactics to assert their upper hand, it is hard, if not impossible, for others with limited leverage, especially children or employees, to event attempt to negotiate with them. If someone persists in holding the person with NPD accountable, this triggers an agitated state of critical, punitive thoughts toward self and others. Because looking bad or feeling bad are both intolerable, the person with NPD will defensively punish others with blaming, detachment, and stonewalling, rather than accommodating their needs. If a spouse or significant other becomes fed up enough to leave the relationship, the person with NPD is apt to cling tenaciously to a noble role of a hurt, mistreated, and abandoned party.

Clinicians using the Young Schema Questionnaire (Young, 2006) may find not only high scores on items related to entitlement and frustration intolerance but seemingly false negatives regarding self-worth and feelings of connection–acceptance. This is in stark contrast with positive responses regarding early unmet emotional needs of unconditional love and acceptance that may be detected during the assessment interviews. Although individual scores on the most common self-report instrument, the Narcissistic Personality Inventory (Raskin & Terry, 1988), may be high enough to meet its inclusive criteria for narcissism, debates continue about reliable factor structure, with researchers proposing two to seven possible factors (Ackerman et al., 2011). In conceptualizing variants of clinical narcissism, there is strong support for a comingling of two primary manifestations: one of a purely spoiled and dependent (grandiose) narcissism (Miller, Campbell, & Widiger, 2010) merged with the fragile, vulnerable type (Behary, 2012, 2013; Young, 2006).

DIFFERENTIAL DIAGNOSIS

It is important to note that the traits of narcissism can also characterize highly successful individuals (American Psychiatric Association, 2013, p. 672). Nevertheless, one should not presume that high success rules out the possibility of NPD. According to our cognitive and schema therapy models, narcissistic traits can progress from successful adaptation to maladaptive personality disorder when there are exaggerated beliefs; hypertrophied modes; and overactive, inflexible strategies that cause functional impairments. Features of other personality disorders that may overlap with NPD include the exploitive and callous disregard of antisocial personality disorder, or the attention-seeking of histrionic personality disorder. However, persons with NPD tend to be more fixated on seeking appraisal that elevates them above others, rather than attention or emotional support per se. In addition, grandiosity is a persistent feature of the self-concept of the person with NPD, not a function of more transient mood states, as is the case with mania or hypomania.

RESEARCH ON NARCISSISM AND SELF-ESTEEM

Persons who are narcissistic characteristically report moderate to high self-esteem on various self-report measures (Baumeister, 2001). Self-esteem in general is frequently, but not always, based on successful competition and positive self-evaluations (Neff, 2011). Successful competition involves limbic arousal, activation of the dopamine system, energizing emotions, and reward-seeking behavior (Gilbert, 2010; Gilbert et al., 2008). Bursts of self-esteem from successful competition are reinforced by feelings of superiority, well-being, cultural approbation, appraisal of worth and status, and perhaps material rewards. But this can also lead to obsessing over the implications of (possible) unsuccessful competition with regard to self-worth (Kernis, 2005) and may reflect dopaminergic hyperreactivity to reward-predicting cues that create a bias toward activating certain schemas and modes (Treadway, Chapter 4, this volume). Loss of esteem and its link to contingent rewards is a threat that activates hypervigilance, narrowing of attention, and anxious preoccupation. Such rumination can increase vulnerability to depression and diminish self-concept clarity (Kernis, 2005). This cycle affords little or no emotional resilience when dealing with personal limits or adverse events because there is no adaptive coping mechanism other than further pursuit of competitive advantage (Neff, 2011). A maladaptive alternative is to cognitively inflate the self-image, and protect it with a confirmatory bias. Across a broad range of contexts, individuals with an inflated self-image tend to create and maintain a positive illusory bias in which they solicit positive feedback, avoid self-concept change, place uncomfortable demands on others, remain vigilant of and highly reactive to self-evaluative threats, and deal with dissonance via hostility and aggression (Baumeister, Smart, & Boden, 1996).

A positive illusory bias in self-image has been linked to aggressive behavior, interpersonal deficits, undesirable traits, and peer rejection among adults (Colvin, Block, & Funder, 1995) and hospitalized youth (Perez, Pettit, David, Kistner, & Joiner, 2001). Bullies have been shown to overrate themselves on academic and interpersonal skills and endorse unrealistically high self-esteem (Gresham, MacMillan, Bocian, Ward, & Forness, 1998). Furthermore, narcissism is positively correlated with dominance and hostility (Raskin, Novacek, & Hogan, 1991), as well as grandiosity, exhibitionism, and disregard for others (Wink, 1991). In a population incarcerated for violent offenses, high levels of narcissism and NPD were identified as risk markers for violence against family members, particularly when combined with a history of abuse within the family of origin (Dutton & Hart, 1992). The readiness of persons who are narcissistic to behave aggressively toward others appears to be mediated by specific ego threats such as criticism or perceived insult (Baumeister, Bushman, & Campbell, 2000; Bushman & Baumeister, 1998). Narcissism may also be a risk factor for suicidality, particularly when comorbid with bipolar and substance use disorders (Links, 2013), and/or when manifest in military personnel (especially members of specialized mission groups as they transition out of a military role (Bourgeois & Hall, 1993) and in older individuals who blame themselves for falling short of their extreme self-expectations (Heisel, Links, Conn, van Reekum, & Flett, 2007). In an epidemiologic survey, participants who met criteria for NPD were highly cormbid with bipolar I disorder, substance use disorders, and anxiety disorders, and were more likely to be single across all categories (separated, divorced, widowed, or never married; Stinson et al., 2008).

Although there is a correlation between the rise of social media and a progressive increase in college students' narcissism scores over the past two decades (Twenge, Konrath, Foster, Campbell, & Bushman, 2008), there is no evidence of a causal relationship. In fact, developmental theorists note that personality is fairly well formed prior to any age-appropriate interaction with social media (Bergman, Fearrington, Davenport, & Bergman, 2011). Although such social attractions may act as conditions for exacerbating the personality of a well-prepped little prince or princess, it is more likely that development of narcissistic personality has more to do with the early original network of acceptance and responsibility that is learned in interactions with parents and caretakers. With the *everyone-gets-a-trophy* movement of recent times—with educators, coaches, and parents seeking to install invincible self-esteem in their children—rewards become necessary symbols of self-worth. The potential downside to such good intentions is that children are left feeling insecure and vulnerable, without the persistence or humility needed for the real *try–try-again* and *give-and-take* world, or the ability to calibrate self-esteem in a larger context of noncompetitive self-worth. With social media expanding as a culturally normative and even primary platform for connection and influence (Prinstein, 2014), further research is needed to track potential interactions between such media usage and the development of sociocognitive schema for identity and personality (Lloyd, 2002). Such research may be able to investigate the possibility of origination and/or perpetuation of early maladaptive schemas and conditioned cognitive biases correlated with excessive use of social media platforms for interpersonal connection.

CONCEPTUALIZATION

The observable personality of the person with NPD is characterized by beliefs about superiority in relation to others and externalizing behaviors, both of which arise from overcompensating schema modes. Although difficult to see, the core dysfunctional belief is that "I am inferior, defective, weak, and unimportant, unlovable, and alone." This belief, along with the intense emotional and physiologic distress it carries, is embedded in a network of core early maladaptive schemas (EMS; Young, Klosko, & Weishaar, 2003), including *defectiveness/shame*, *emotional deprivation*, *failure*, and *mistrust* (Young et al., 2003). These EMS are formed by experiences that pose a challenge to intelligence, specialness, control, or safety, swamping the individual with poorly integrated feelings of powerlessness, loneliness, anxious arousal, and frustration, and giving rise to the overcompensating schema modes that form his or her observable personality. Severity of the personality compromise toward narcissism depends on the extent to which compensatory attitudes of superiority ("I am a rare and special person," "I am different from and superior to others," and "Others need to know how unique I am, so I can inspire them") have become overdeveloped in their self- and world schemas.

Maladaptive, overcompensating schemas of the person with NPD are *insufficient self-control, entitlement, approval seeking,* and *unrelenting standards.* Maladaptive schema modes are understood as constructed states—conditioned reactions to schema triggers, or as *default states of being,* designed to shield the person with NPD from feared emotional experience associated with the EMS, and thus serve a primary coping function. The *insufficient self-control* schema refers to maladaptive self-soothing and self-stimulating behaviors for discomfort avoidance. *Entitlement* schema refers to exploitive, self-aggrandizing, unempathic, and bullying patterns, and the *approval seeking* and *unrelenting standards* schemas reflect a constant striving to achieve attention, superiority, and hyperautonomy (Behary, 2013; Young, 2006). Mode refers to the activation of the schema complex, with certain predominant behaviors, attitudes, emotions, and response biases toward aggression such as bullying, blaming, showing off, spouting anger, or becoming consumed by competitive striving. The person with NPD might also flip into a detached self-stimulating (coping) mode, engaging in one or more of the following: substance use, sexual encounters including Internet pornography, excessive working, gambling, intemperate social media and web surfing, or overspending. Even simply being without attention can trigger underlying EMS and the subsequent maladaptive coping modes in the person with NPD. Schema modes are self-defeating when they perpetuate that which the person with NPD is actually attempting to avoid—that is, showing off and acting entitled to appear special and to hide underlying feelings of inadequacy perpetuates negative judgments and rejection from others who eventually find the person who is narcissistic to be off-putting, self-absorbed, and overbearing.

Development of a core EMS of inferiority and compensatory superiority can be traced along the following pathway. Beginning with the biological vulnerability of a sensitive/shy or impulsive/aggressive temperament, the child's personality is impacted by caregivers who use them for self-gratification, either overcompensating for the child's insecurities or demeaning them, or both. Instead of learning to accept and master normal and transient feelings of inferiority, weakness, self-consciousness, or uncertainty, the developing child views these experiences, both natural and learned, as profound threats to be defeated and avoided. In addition, the child doesn't receive much empathy, see it modeled, or have it taught by key caretakers. Instead, there is preoccupation with social reflection and protection of pride at any cost. This leads to self-absorbed focus on performing in a way that meets parental needs and creates a reinforcing public image and denial of emotional "weakness." Finally, life expectations are calibrated to grandiose levels, with some measure of enabling that reinforces the youth's growing concept of special entitlement. The message is that it doesn't matter what you do, how you feel, or who is affected, as long as you keep up appearances.

Both cognitive and schema theory propose that the interplay between temperament and environment (natural inclinations combined with noxious ruptures that occur in childhood and adolescence) explain the development of narcissism along a spectrum. Thus, the bedrock that gives rise to NPD is frustrated early unmet emotional needs, due to lack of unconditional love (child is unappreciated unless serving the parent's needs), overemphasis on performance/achievement/materialism (doing/having vs. being), lack of boundaries, poor social modeling/instruction (for empathy, discomfort tolerance, reciprocity, kindness) and dismissive/discouraging reactions to the child's innate interests and emotional expression. The ability to regulate emotions via normal levels of negative affect tolerance, compassion, and respect for the rights of others is significantly underdeveloped.

Persons who are narcissistic often organize their lives around *unrelenting standards* and approval seeking (EMS), using tangible assets or dominant social rank as a source of self-worth. Thus, this patient believes that "I must be the best to prove my worth to others, and they have to notice." Such proof is found in some competitive measure such as community influence, income level, physical attractiveness, material trappings such as the "best" car or the "right" neighborhood—even the "right" spouse, personal awards, job title or office location, exclusive associations, or even just having more friends than anyone else. Consumerism can play a big part in this relentless compensatory cycle of acquiring the best because it is something people can notice and it provides material reward. Such unrelenting standards manifest at all socioeconomic levels, not just the top, and may include many variations of "next-door narcissists," each constantly striving for competitive status within their own frame of reference.

Underlying *failure* schema frequently includes the fear-based conditional assumption that "If I'm not the best, then I'm inferior." Looking bad, feeling bad, or facing failure are all perceived as fundamental threats to self-worth, and trigger extreme anxiety, embarrassment, and shame. Persons with NPD are highly prone to personalize anything that hints of devaluation, and will automatically switch into coping mode and act in defensive ways. Failure schema along with entitlement can also manifest in a refusal to work, compromise standards, or even try when it would be far more adaptive to do so, to ward off activation of the *defectiveness* schemas. Without a guaranteed fabulous outcome, they refuse to make an effort. This may be especially evident among the more purely spoiled/dependent type who, with little tolerance for frustration, remain stuck in avoidance coping and don't take on the due diligence necessary for change, much to the consternation of those around them, including therapists. They demonstrate a poor sense of reality concerning payoffs, believing that tiny efforts should produce big results, and may insist "I've done everything I can to help myself; I just can't do more."

Jon, whom we introduced earlier in this chapter, grew up believing he was a "great athlete" and a very good-looking "boy genius," making him superior to less athletic and average-intelligence people, and entitled to special privileges. His mother doted on Jon's "resumé," providing private coaches and tutors in every flavor. She took great pride in "her special gift" as a mom whenever he delivered the goods—trophies, awards, and perfect scores. Jon had no recollection of affection or even playful times with mom or dad. Showing any vulnerability or emotional neediness was either blatantly ignored or firmly admonished as "silly" or as "a sign of weakness," except during times when mom was lonely or depressed, and "she needed" hugs from him. Jon's dad was primarily consumed with excellence in performance from his handsome son, declaring that he was "not working this hard to end up with a mediocre return on his investment." When friends and family would get together socially, Jon was always the centerpiece–performer, the shiny show-and-tell object for his parents' glowing egos. This third-person bragging about his this-or-that accomplishments was his limited means for feeling appreciated and connected to his parents, even though he always carried the shaky sense that it was more for their benefit than his.

In his preteen years, the poorly prepared and socially awkward Jon was a target for teasing and bullying, mostly for his "annoying" and "quirky" behaviors with his peers. Friendships came in high school and mostly in the sports arena, where he was a fierce and capable competitor. Academically, good grades came relatively easily. On occasion, when he struggled or did not perform as well as expected, his mom was quick to blame it on the teacher or coach, and did almost anything to guarantee her son a stellar outcome, even if it meant doing the work for him. As a teen, Jon had some trouble with drinking, fights, and undermining authority, but mom was quick to the rescue, getting him off the hook with few consequences.

Jon's good looks, sterling resumé, and well-rehearsed charming (albeit cocky) demeanor became his winning ticket. There was no such thing as "good enough" in Jon's world, and his life would be characterized by always needing to have more, be the best, and not sit still . . . lest he become "bored"—or, perish the thought—"boring."

A schema conceptualization presented in Table 14.1 summarizes the relationship of Jon's early experiences, maladaptive beliefs, and coping modes, and how these patterns influence his current problems.

Detecting the Overcompensating Modes and Assumptions

As noted, the core schemas that embody inferiority/unimportance/loneliness are not usually manifested overtly; instead the world sees outward "masks" of smug, superior attitudes that derive from secondary overcompensating, or avoidant schema modes that compromise the personality toward narcissism. The following are several of the most recognizable modes.

TABLE 14.1. Schema Case Conceptualization for Jon

Childhood data

- Parents were emotionally inattentive and unaffectionate, offered conditional praise for extraordinary achievements—attention was paid (mostly third person bragging) for his academic and sports performance and other competitive endeavors.
- Was told it was a weakness to need emotional attention, affection, and support.
- Possessed above-average good looks, athleticism, and high intelligence, and therefore was entitled to do whatever he wanted without consequences.

Hypothesized temperament

- Sensitive/shy

Core schemas: emotional beliefs

- Defectiveness/shame: "I'm not lovable or special just for being me; I have to prove myself to be special."
- Emotional deprivation: "I cannot rely on others for support or affection; I must become completely autonomous and not need anyone."
- Mistrust: "People only act nice to you because they want something from you; I must be wary of other people's motives at all times."

Assumptions: secondary schemas (masks of core emotional needs)

- Unrelenting standards: "I must be smart, good-looking, and successful to be special and superior."
- Entitlement: "I deserve special treatment and should not have to follow the same rules as others"
- Approval seeking: "I need people to admire me to know that I matter."

Coping modes:
self-aggrandizer/detached self-soother/demanding parent/lonely child/healthy adult

Overcompensating self-aggrandizing mode: *Robust default mode of the narcissist.*
  1. Acts entitled and becomes critical when he does not get his way.
  2. Seeks attention/adoration from other women and from work affiliates.
  3. Complains or blames others when challenged or frustrated.

Avoidant detached self-soothing mode: *Activated when alone, in the absence of attention.*
  1. Disconnects emotionally from partner and family.
  2. No real intimate connections.
  3. Pornography/alcohol.
  4. Workaholic.

Demanding internalized parent mode: *Activated when others try to get emotionally close or when the lonely child is experienced.*
  1. Not permitted to have emotional needs—"They are the weaknesses of average folks"—will cause him to lose his edge and become average and unimportant.

(continued)

TABLE 14.1. *(continued)*

Lonely/shamed child mode: *Often stowed away from awareness.*
1. Feels lonely and insecure.
2. Needs affection and unconditional love.
3. Feels shame when not measuring up or fitting in, especially vis-à-vis his peers.

Healthy adult mode: *Somewhat accessible (intellectually) at treatment onset, but gets overpowered by other modes.*
1. Able to show affection and unconditional love for his own children (at times).
2. Can occasionally observe his own self-defeating patterns and the impact on loved ones but dismisses them swiftly and flips into his aggressive mode, making excuses to avoid feeling the shame of the insecure and inadequate child mode.

Therapy relationship

The therapist shows up like a *real* person (who is also an expert) to generalize interpersonal experiences to real-world interactions of the person who is a narcissist by:
- Empathically confronting self-defeating modes.
- Setting limits with aggressive bullying modes.
- Emotionally strengthening the healthy adult mode (via modeling behaviors, skills building, and reparenting attunement) within the limits of the therapy relationship to meet the frustrated unmet needs of the lonely and insecure child.

The All-Knowing Mode: "Let Me Tell You How It Is."

We all tend to believe our personal thoughts, but the person with NPD maintains a stance of absolute authority, and may be compelled to lecture others on "the truth." Although his or her wit, knowledge, or insight can be dazzling at times, he or she is also judgmental, opinionated, and dominates conversations, lacking respect for thoughts and opinions of others. If the person who is narcissistic seeks an opinion, it is must be from a top expert, although expertise is often loosely based on perceived status. "Superior" people have superior judgment, even if the matter at hand is far afield from their skills (e.g., a media celebrity can give financial advice—without any professional credentials). Without sufficient limits, interpersonal dominance can lead to boundary violations of all sorts, as persons who are narcissistic dictate orders ("I know what's right for them"), become angry if others don't capitulate, and may abuse positions of power.

Jon was quite irritated that his wife did not back him up in the legal dispute surrounding his driving-under-the-influence charges. "I know how much alcohol I can handle and I am the best judge of my own competence. These low-rung cops just love to get a guy driving a great car; it makes them feel like big shots" was his take on the situation.

The "Very Important Person" Mode: "I Have Special Rules."

A key assumption that maintains entitlement and insufficient self-control is that there are two sets of rules: normal and special, and the person who is narcissistic believes "My rules are special." "Special" rules can lead to extraordinary recklessness and dismissing or actively distorting evidence of risk, even when overwhelming, because of the firm belief in being an "exception." "This can't be happening to me," is the refrain when exception fails, and the person with NPD must be held accountable because the crime is too heinous to sweep away. When faced with limits, persons with NPD may persist in believing that they won't have to adapt, like other "lesser" people. Normal expectations may be resisted or resented, based on the belief that "It should be easy for me, and I should not have to make that effort." The patient stays tenaciously stuck in blaming other people and circumstances, choosing detached self-stimulation rather than make realistic or empathic adjustments or compete for work he or she considers beneath his or her station.

A related "very important person" (VIP) assumption is that "Because I'm special, I should get what I want." The person with NPD will simply take the best seat, biggest steak, or choice bedroom; dominate entire conversations with personal concerns; and command excessive portions of a family budget, without consideration of the emotional impact or fundamental grasp of an egalitarian social system. Sometimes the concept of male privilege is exploited to this end, as the "head of the family" has a long history of being privileged to such entitlements. If others question the basis of this privilege, they may be subject to retaliatory punishment.

Jon believed that given his "gifts" and well-earned stature, he was entitled to his *boys-will-be-boys* curricula and other self-indulgences. "I don't understand . . . I pay big taxes in this community. I should not be expected to pay such outrageous penalties for enjoying a couple of gin and tonics after a long hard day in the city. I mean really . . . nobody died." He was incredulous to his wife's "lack of appreciation" and thought it entirely reasonable to punish her by canceling their family vacation and scheduling a solo trip abroad for himself.

The Trophy Mode: "Image Is Everything."

Public image is the primary platform where the compensatory unrelenting standards of the person with NPD are transacted, with the key assumption that "Image is everything, and without it I am nothing." In truth, image is a shield that protects against fears of inferiority or shame. Checking and maintaining *the* image is a paramount concern, as persons who are narcissistic are always vigilant to being on display. Regular doses of laudatory feedback are "needed" as a magic elixir, and vigilantly contrived *in vivo* or in imagination. They compare themselves with celebrities, and fantasize approbation from the whole world, even deities. One patient who is narcissistic stated quite confidently: "God admires me."

Persons who are narcissistic also project their image preoccupation onto significant others (spouse, child, friends, employees), with the imperative "They have to make me look good." Perplexing double binds may arise out of this for significant others. If they fail to perform as expected, they may be ridiculed or punished. On the other hand, if they succeed, it may trigger the competitive mode of the person with NPD. They are often expected to flaunt their talents and accomplishments on command in social situations to make the person with NPD look good to others, in a way that feels awkward, uncomfortable, and demeaning.

Jon and Stacy arrived late for a marital session, pulling up in Jon's expensive sports car, which he illegally parked in a space for the disabled. Their session focused on Jon's unremorseful reactions to Stacy's feelings of hurt, betrayal, and mistrust; along with Stacey's admission of a life pattern of "pretending" to be okay with everything asked of her while silently suffering. Stacy described how for years she subjugated herself to Jon's criticisms and demands that she be the "Barbie Doll" perfect partner who he married. He snidely encouraged her to get breast implants and a tummy tuck after giving birth to their second child, which she did, only to become the object of the boastful praise and ogling admiration from her gin-soaked husband and his colleagues at work-related social events.

The Invincibility Mode: "I Don't Have Weaknesses."

Absolute self-confidence and self-control is the perceived gold standard for power and optimal personality among persons who are narcissists, representing a blend of unrelenting standards and entitlement. Strong, powerful people are believed to be free from pathetic emotions. Sadness, remorse, guilt, uncertainty, grief, frustration, and the like are viewed as personal weaknesses, and therefore useless, or worse, signs of inferiority, to be squelched immediately. On the other hand, expressed anger and self-admiration are construed as signs of self-confidence. When frustration is encountered, the person with NPD is likely to fly into a tantrum or rage, or flip into detached self-soothing with food, drugs, alcohol, or other stimulating distractions. Conditional assumptions may include the notions "If I need something, I need it *now*." Persons with NPD may be extremely reluctant to discuss emotions lest anyone see this chink in their armor. On the other hand, recapitulation of what they dislike, what made them angry, and what's wrong with the world is a common pastime, reifying their sense of power and control.

The Bully Mode: "My Way or the Highway."

Bullying and counterattacking are also pernicious social behaviors common to the *entitlement and impaired-limits* schema. Triggers are idiosyncratic, but converge on themes of self-image threat or entitlement demands.
Evaluative comments are predictable threats that, if not precisely flattering,
activate the defensive bully. Disagreement or assertiveness may trigger a
wounded narcissistic "blowup." Even in benign situations, persons who are
narcissistic have a tendency to intrude and treat other people like puppets.
This can escalate quickly if the other party resists, with the person with
NPD saying, "You'll do it right (my way), and give me what I need, or be
replaced!"

Sadly, narcissism is a risk factor for many psychologically destructive
and even physically violent outcomes, with elevated risk if there are comorbid antisocial features. The person with NPD engenders psychologically
destructive situations when proffering gossip and judgment, shunning, publicly humiliating others, or undermining their competence. Making threats
of implied violence to scare the challenger ("You'll be sorry. You don't know
who you're dealing with!"), or engaging in overt acts of physical violence to
punish are, unfortunately, a possibility. All too often, these machinations
are effective in intimidating others to submission and securing a reputation
as the tough, not-to-be-messed-with top dog.

Detecting Avoidant and Detached Self-Soothing Modes and Assumptions

The Fairy-Tale Mode: "I Can Have or Be Anything I Want."

The pursuit of fame, ideal romantic love, extraordinary success, power—
both overt and covert—and various forms of excitement help persons with
NPD escape dreary reality. Some gravitate toward material possessions
and become emotionally fused with their "stuff." For others, exceptional
achievement is the narcissistic supply, and they may even appear to care
little for material things but keenly value performance accolades. Dreams
of high-stakes career moves, athletic prowess, cosmetic transformation,
trophy date (or spouse) collecting, charitable recognition, or immersion
in celebrity culture can all be seductively escapist. Excitement is the lure,
and even minor opportunities for the limelight, brushes with glory, or
daydreams of admiration will suffice. Such ventures may come dressed in
noble robes ("I'm saving the world! I'm doing this for us!"), yet remain
oddly detached from the feedback of loved ones ("You've checked out. I
can't take it."). The pursuit can be hypomanic (and destructively costly),
but tends to be more sustained, and even more compulsive, than mania.

Big dreams, lofty goals and pleasant diversions are not the culprit per
se, but rather the detached, self-soothing avoidance that distorts personality, relationships, and major aspects of normal development (i.e., living in

a heady fog). Even at high levels, the person with NPD is prone to becoming stuck in a fantasy, avoidant mode, followed by anger and blaming the world, creating a vicious cycle with underlying failure schema. A pernicious pattern of detached self-soothing follows, as the person with NPD escapes into highly stimulating, gratifying indulgences that are ultimately destructive, including gambling, drinking, drug taking, pornography and other sexual acting out, or limitless consumption of ordinary pleasures (eating, shopping, TV, entertainment, social media, etc.), despite the pleas and despair of significant others (when they find out about it).

KEY TREATMENT GOALS

Key treatment goals include helping the person with NPD to (1) recognize maladaptive coping modes and weaken their predominance; (2) build affect-regulation skills, emphasizing tolerance of transient frustration, imperfection, and normal emotions; (3) increase respect and empathy for others' feelings, limits, autonomy, and delay of social gratification; (4) increase attunement to natural talents and strengths, and non-contingent self-worth; and (5) increase role involvement and appropriate reciprocity. All of these goals serve the purpose of building a more functional or healthy adult mode for defining self and relating to others in a less defensive, competitive way. Healthy adult mode is not intended to be a homogenized, ideal personality (e.g., "I need to transform Jon into a humble, repentant, buddha-like individual"), but rather a mode that incorporates reasonable awareness and adaptive, prosocial and emotionally responsive strategies, with internalized self-worth. This ambitious agenda represents a composite of potential treatment goals, and may be only partially achieved, depending on the therapist's ability to manage a genuine and sturdy posture amid the aggrandizing, avoidant, and bullying modes by the person who is narcissistic, and the necessary leverage (meaningful consequences for narcissistic behaviors) to enhance a willingness to collaborate. Treatment success may be determined by evidence of adaptive emotional self-care, flexible standards, respectful social impulse control and reciprocity, and role engagement, depending on individual needs.

Jon agreed to work on the following two goals in therapy: (1) stabilize his family connections for the longer term, and (2) identify his deeper, life-long emotional needs and compare different ways to meet them.

COLLABORATIVE STRATEGY

Collaborative challenge is to be expected as a function of this disorder, and requires a more direct, strategic approach than many therapists instinctively want to use, much less know how to execute. Patients who are narcissistic may flatter and/or critique the therapist's office décor, location, credentials, experience, age, looks, attire, or ability to understand his or her very special status, and maneuver for special treatment from the very outset. Such behavior can feel both seductive and threatening, triggering emotional arousal that disrupts the therapist's professional comportment. It is important to spot behaviors indicative of self-aggrandizing, idealizing, demeaning, or any atypical evaluative comments as possible indicators of narcissism. Such comments are notable for deviation from the kinds of comments or requests typically encountered across a range of patients. For example, patients may frequently comment on the pleasant view from the therapist's office window. The patient with NPD, however, covets the view and evaluates the window as a measure of the therapist's status. Being attuned to one's own reactions is crucial, as narcissistic challenges should not be construed as a front-end issue to be resolved so that therapy can proceed. Confronting these moment-to-moment interactions again and again, as the patient with NPD moves among angry, haughty, envious, passive, avoidant, demanding, or vulnerable is the nuts-and-bolts work that *is* the therapy. Collaboration is shaped slowly with patients with NPD, through reminders of therapeutic leverage and empathic confrontation.

Patients who are narcissistic often enter treatment in an "anticontemplation" state, with a stance opposed to personal change (Freeman & Dolan, 2001; Freeman, Felgoise, & Davis, 2008). In essence, they believe "I'm fine the way I am; I do not need to change myself; I just need someone to make me feel better." When a well-intentioned therapist tries to pinpoint targets for change, in the manner typical with symptomatic disorders, the patient with NPD may use any excuse to opt out, to avoid triggering the core schema of *defectiveness/shame*. The primary therapeutic goal at this point is to ease through any early ruptures while also gently moving the patient toward contemplation, and this may recur at later points as well. From the outset, the patient with NPD will likely seek admiration for special qualities (and feel disappointed if the therapist doesn't continuously offer it), but resist exploring feelings of inadequacy, embarrassment, and loneliness, or pressing problems with fractured relationships. He or she may persist in rehashing lengthy narratives that extol his or her virtues and inventory the shortcomings of others and the world.

To successfully engage the person with NPD, one must provide praise and support for his or her strengths, courage, and vulnerability and notice (like a healthy parent) ordinary niceties and thoughtfulness as these behaviors emerge over time. The therapist should listen carefully, ask a limited number of thought-provoking questions, provide warmth through supportive observations, and initiate empathic, confrontational interpersonal feedback for maladaptive behaviors as they occur, on the spot. The person who is narcissistic is accustomed to vying for superlative praise for "extraordinary," "unique," and "superior "performance: this being his or her learned expectation—to gain worth and relevance—he or she must win the top recognition. A *schema therapy* approach explicitly frames the therapist's stance as a limited reparenting agent, a "good parent," offering genuine praise and appreciating "ordinariness"—working to meet the early unmet need for unconditional love and acceptance, and build the internalized sense of self-worth. This nurturance may be the easier part for most therapists; more difficult is the empathic confrontation needed to set limits on undisciplined, disrespectful, or impulsive behaviors and reactions, when appropriate, and to remind the patient with NPD of the losses at stake if he or she abandons therapy.

To override the guarded suspicion of the patient with NPD feeling "used" or "manipulated" for the therapist's gain, the therapist needs to be a credible expert and also provide genuine, constructive feedback, free of technical jargon. This is achieved by a stance of appropriate self-disclosure of personal reactions to the patient who is narcissistic—as they arise in the moment-to-moment experiences in the therapy relationship. Disclosure should be relevant to the patient's problem behaviors, such as criticalness toward others, self-absorbed approval seeking, and other off-putting behaviors like bragging, competing, or not listening, and goals such as cheering for others or treating them with respect. Such empathic therapeutic self-disclosure is a complex skill, one that requires adequate training and practice (illustrative dialogue below). Psychotherapy trainees should be liberally and supportively supervised, as treating this disorder requires integration of multiple clinical competencies. Practicing clinicians may want to use case consultation for role-play practice of empathic confrontation of clients as needed.

CLINICAL APPLICATION OF THE INTERVENTION

During assessment and early conceptualization, it is useful to (1) address any immediate crisis or destructive behavior, (2) focus on symptomatic disorders, and (3) collaboratively map broader goals to modify maladaptive schema through guided discovery, behavioral experiments, and relational interaction. Specific clinical interventions blend psychoeducational, cognitive, experiential, and relational methods.

Psychoeducation

Brief psychoeducation about the interplay of temperament and experience may help soften skeptical attitudes about the "hokey pokey" agenda of psychotherapy. The main idea to impart is that experience is imbedded in memory and implicitly retrieved, so that under seemingly familiar conditions, reactionary impulses, based in temperament, are automatically deployed to protect against any perceived threat to emotional stability. This brief educational input on interpersonal neurobiology, and how we all react from internalized protective mechanisms, helps to normalize the defensive reactions of persons who are narcissistic, and mitigate underlying shame attached to possible exposure of "ordinary emotional weakness" or beliefs about being "trapped" or "used" for the therapist's own gain.

Brief psychoeducation on the concept of schema modes as systemic patterns of thoughts, beliefs, feelings, reactions, and behaviors is also essential. This sets the stage for collaborating on initial cognitive interventions, such as collecting information on various schema modes, labeling these with the patient's own terminology, and having a contrasting cognitive concept of the healthy adult mode, to address the goal of weakening the predominance of maladaptive modes.

Cognitive Intervention

Various cognitive strategies can then be deployed to modify different schema modes in service of the treatment goals. For example, Jon used an activity schedule to track activation of his self-aggrandizing and detached modes, and noted key thoughts and reactions (his and others). He became more aware of his distorted beliefs about superiority and worth connected to success (e.g., "I need to be extraordinary or I am mediocre, worthless"), and his reliance on competitive comparisons for self-esteem. This helped to frame his need for an internal source of self-worth, and led to an experiment to see if persistence and flexibility in his goals (slowing down a bit, taking more time for healthy activity and recreational time with his family) could provide an alternative, less stressful way to demonstrate self-esteem and build self-worth. Although not quick or easy, in time it was clear that this was a more satisfying existence, it supported his goal of stabilizing his family life, and he began to view it as worthwhile. This experiment also helped to shift his investment in perfectionism.

Another valuable cognitive strategy for a person with NPD is constructing dialogues between his or her different schema modes. This exercise creates an *in vivo* experience of combating highly distorted beliefs and assumptions while keeping a collaborative alliance between patient and therapist. It also provides some measure of the relative growth of the healthy adult side versus the demanding unrelenting side; or the grandiose and defiantly detached side; or the lonely, unlovable child side, as treatment progresses. In this activity, the therapist acts as a gentle guide, setting up the exercise, attending to affect, and prompting the deepened exchange. Role plays and empty-chair methods are generally used to create the dialogue, so there is less chance of a lapse into power struggle or argument.

The therapist can participate as much as needed to engage the patient's activity, and then gradually withdraw as the patient generates both sides of the dialogue. Depending on patient response, structuring of the exercise might happen all at once, or it might have to be gradually shaped over repeated efforts.

One very helpful cognitive tactic in the schema dialogue is to ask about *messengers* from experience, such as "Where did you get the message that you should be entitled to special treatment without any consequence for crossing a boundary?" Although the therapist can ask this question directly, it may be far more effective when the client, in a role play of the healthy adult mode, asks this of his or her grandiose side. This helps link the dots between life experience and current maladaptive behavior, and opens the door on considering alternative perspectives (e.g., "My rules are the same as other people's rules").

When dealing with envy or anger over frustrated entitlement, another helpful cognitive strategy is to take advantage as a given, and assess the costs and benefits of realistic coping. For example, Jon believed that "There are some people who can enjoy a couple of gin and tonics after a hard day's work and actually be perfectly competent to drive themselves home safely, despite a certain blood-alcohol level; these people should have separate laws." The therapist agreed that, yes, it would be nice if there were chemical formulas to detect such capacities for safety, and special separate laws for certain (entitled) people (slightly smirking). However, given that the chances are low that this will happen, we still need to cope with this frustrating reality. The costs of getting arrested are high, not to mention paying hundreds of hard-earned dollars in various fines, insurance increases, legal fees, and having a record, or the expense to have it expunged. If the therapeutic rapport is sufficiently well established, the therapist may choose to explore the reasoning behind beliefs of entitlement (When and how did you get the message about special rules?), gently exploring the meaning associated with surrendering the entitlement. What is realistically lost? What might be gained by accommodating the rule? How hard could it be? Jon agreed to try a few self-restraining changes, including avoiding alcohol during the week. Possible benefits were fewer headaches and mood changes, more involvement in his children's after-school activities, and more affection from his wife.

Experiential Methods

Experiential, emotion-focused strategies, such as mindfulness practices and guided imagery are extremely helpful in weakening predominance of maladaptive modes and building affect-regulation skills. Imagery is particularly useful in mapping out the evolution of schema modes, identifying frustrated unmet needs within the early narrative, and rescripting noxious and depriving memories. Imagery can also act as a means for recasting biased emotional beliefs, imbedded in neural networks that inform current reactions to the environment. In this imagery work, the unmet needs of the lonely child and burdened adolescent receive a caring response from the patient's healthy adult self, first, through the imagination, and then by way of helping the healthy adult create more satisfying and emotionally genuine connections in his or her current world. Emotionally focused behavioral role plays and role reversals can be used to strengthen adaptive schema modes for social competencies. This might include generating empathy for others, discerning boundaries, such as when to stop competing, talking about oneself, drilling others into submission, or finding the words to express remorse or gratitude. The therapist's role in these experiential exercises is one of a facilitative guide to the patient's role-play of different modes rather than a directive scriptwriter. As the lonely and unlovable little girl or boy begins to experience more unconditional acceptance and love from the therapist and the healthy adult side of the patient, as well as others who are genuinely capable of still caring for the goodness that dwells beneath surly swells, exaggerated emotional reactions to situations that require reciprocity, waiting, accepting criticism, or tolerating frustration may attenuate and the person with NPD becomes more flexible.

Mindfulness practices and self-compassion training are useful for building internal affect regulation skills, addressing frustration intolerance and perfectionism as well as awareness of self and others. Loving-kindness exercises may be especially helpful to connect the person with NPD with a sense of common humanity and non-contingent self-worth (Neff, 2011), providing an alternative to reliance on competitive comparisons and unrelenting standards for self-esteem.

Empathic Relational Feedback

Perhaps the most important clinical tool is intermittent use of empathic relational feedback or confrontation of maladaptive interpersonal behaviors on the spot, when they occur in session and the mode is active. This method of relational feedback is intended to deepen awareness of pernicious, maladaptive cycles that can, indeed, be changed by the person with NPD. Often this includes limit setting and directing attention to the need for reciprocity or frustration tolerance (and the downside to immediate gratification or filter failure). Feedback is *always* delivered in a genuine, understanding, and supportive manner. A variation of this method includes relational feedback from an empathically resonant listening stance. For example, Jon's therapist picks up on bullying counterattack behavior when he complains about Stacy's reaction to his lapse of accountability, and says the following to him:

"You know, Jon, if I were Stacy, I would be very upset, too. And what a shame because I think there was actually something important that you were trying to tell her. Didn't you want her to know that you miss her too, and you care about her feelings? But instead, your angry bully mode fired off and attacked her for expressing disappointment when you arrived home 2 hours late."

This was followed with role-reversal imagery to generate greater empathy for Stacy's experience.

To provide empathic feedback competently, the therapist must be self-attuned, able to understand how others might respond to the same interaction, aware of the patient's vulnerable core, and grounded in a helping mode that is both compassionate and insightful about treatment goals for this specific patient. It is important to manage one's arousal, and not to misconstrue confrontation in aggressive terms.

Homework

Written and audio flash cards can structure useful homework, maintaining a transitional connection between sessions and the therapy relationship. The therapist writes or records a brief customized message, offering praise for courageous emotional work in the therapy session, for growth in accountability or empathic awareness, and offers instructional reminders for practicing mindful awareness exercises, for refuting distorted belief patterns, or anticipating glitches that may occur during the week—schema-activating conditions—or to practice and execute interactions with partners and important others that were role-played in session.

Although Jon came to therapy begrudgingly, he was willing to mollify Stacy's ultimatum to seek help. In the first session, the therapist established a trustworthy and credible presence by sharing some honest feedback. When Jon launched critical comments her way (crooked picture on the wall, terrible whirring sound of the ceiling fan, "impossible" to find the building address, incompetent staff), she asked him to imagine if others might feel hurt or put off by such comments, if they were not trained to understand the psychological makeup of someone like him. Of course, she took a deep breath and steadied herself before offering this statement in a calm manner. Grounded in her awareness of his vulnerable side, she empathically shared her hypothesis that he was given an early message to do and say as he pleased without regard for "silly and weak" emotional reactions. She asked him to imagine how this self-expressive style might be aversive to others; how they may tolerate but feel uncomfortable with him, and try to avoid him whenever possible. This honest, open (and brave) discourse cultivated a safe enough atmosphere to allow (1) empathic confrontation, as just described; (2) limit setting for his interruptive style and cynicism; and (3) leverage reminders of what he stood to lose if therapy was aborted. By Session 2, Jon agreed to an initial 10–12 sessions, with an option to continue. In a short time, he came to look forward to the sessions as an opportunity, not as a threat of weakness, shame, or loss. Stacy's reactions of appreciation and admiration for his commitment and emotional sharing reinforced his participation.

The following dialogue illustrates the use of empathic confrontation of Jon's self-aggrandizing stories about triumphs at work and his best-of-the-best material world, and connects him to deeper, unmet emotional needs.

THERAPIST: Jon, I know that in the world of your parents it was critically important to entertain your mom by being clever, extraordinary at school, and thankful for your handsome physical appearance that you "inherited from her." For your dad it was much the same, adding the athletic prowess to those great expectations. I also know that these assets can be extremely useful in business. But in the world of relationships, these traits, while admirable, can become tiring and boorish. They are like an endless one-way street where it's only about you, and void of human vulnerability—being naturally imperfect people who are also lovable and good, who give and take, who care about each other's needs, and celebrate each other's triumphs, taking turns in so doing. It's not your fault, though. You were not prepared for the world of interpersonal connection and intimacy. But it is your responsibility, if you are willing to accept it, and if you want to be truly loved and cared for by those who matter to you most.

JON: Okay, but this is therapy and it's not supposed to be about you, it's supposed to be about me!

THERAPIST: Touché. And while you are correct that this relationship is different from others, it is still a relationship—one that honors the right for honesty, safety, and respect, but has distinct limits. It actually best resembles a parenting relationship, whereby I can offer my care to little Jon and together, your healthy adult side and I will guide his emotional growth and understanding of human relationships and help him to gain (and to give) the love, acceptance, and respect he needs. I am very proud of you and your achievements, and I can even easily get caught up in your remarkable storytelling, but because I understand the "hiding places" of little Jon, and the exclusive pathways to specialness that he was taught, I can best provide you with feedback when I see you switching into one of those modes in the here and now. Do you feel the part of you that may be trying to steer clear of the uncomfortable emotions that we agreed to look at today in imagery?

JON: (with a bowed head and the fidgety fingers of a frightened child) Well, I just thought you might want to know how hard it was for me to secure that deal and how much the dough will mean to Stacy. I don't know any other way of being important to her. Pretty pathetic, huh?

THERAPIST: It's not *pathetic* at all. It's actually sad knowing that you never feel the right to turn the switch "off," to just "be," to take in the love of your family without having to bring home a "new toy." It's all you know, Jon. And yes, of course I want to hear about it, especially given how important it is for you as a means of feeling worthwhile. I just don't want to abandon the important feelings that reside deep within this story—you know, *little Jon.*

JON: I know, I know. "Him" again. Sometimes I just don't see how all of that past stuff really makes a difference in the present. I mean, it feels good to me in some crazy way, but you can't really change the past, and besides, I didn't have it that bad, really.

THERAPIST: Our past informs our present. (*smiling*) You didn't come up with these ideas and behaviors at the age of 49. We cannot change what actually happened to you, but we can change the way it has become organized in your mind and the automatic way in which it still shows up in your life. It's not about blaming your parents. It's about meeting the needs that weren't adequately met so you can share that precious *little you* with the world, without always having to dress him up so perfectly.

JON: That would be nice for a change. (*Sighs deeply, as he looks down at the photo of a shy little Jon—show-and-tell trophy in the perfectly pressed suit, feigned smile, sandwiched between his mom and dad at the annual bring-your-family-to-work event.*)

To help Jon to see what he was "up against," an experiential chair exercise was used to identify different defensive modes and the strength of each. As Jon moved from chair to chair, he expressed the feelings, beliefs, and, in some cases, demands of the mode he occupied at that moment. For example, while in the lonely and unlovable child mode, Jon longed for acceptance and the chance to be cherished without contingencies, but in the bullying/critical mode he was reminded that these longings were for losers and weaker persons without ambition; in invincibility mode (hyperautonomy and power), he denied having any problems, and assailed his wife to be a stronger and more appreciative partner and "get over this crap" (commanding control). In the fairy-tale mode (wishful thinking), he disappeared into a bubble, daydreaming of grandeur, and striking a disconnected intellectualistic posture, becoming invincible and proclaiming that he really didn't have emotions and didn't need people for such things. In his trophy mode (approval seeking), he went on and on about his professional achievements, artistry with words, charismatic way with people, and idealization of success. Finally, in his healthy adult mode (with the help of the therapist), he was able to look upon this quagmire and quickly figure out that the distributions were off. He was up against a fiercely constructed armor that (ironically) kept him unprotected, burdened, and ultimately defeated—perpetuating the very thing that he was fighting to avoid: feeling unloved and unworthy. Nothing would ever be good enough, and this was the story of his life . . . until now.

Jon completed 50 sessions of treatment over 20 months, some of which included sessions with Stacy. During the last several sessions, he and his therapist made a list of things to remember from therapy. These included keeping close contact with his lonely little boy, taking clear risks in sharing emotions honestly and courageously and, being an accurate spokesperson for the vulnerable side of himself when hurt or frustrated. He used reminders to pay attention and listen, find common ground with the people at work, show empathy for Stacy and interest in her life as well as that of others—fondly now referred to as "sharing the stage"; and pay better attention to his own physical health. His termination was flexible, in that the plan was to follow up, as needed, for support as he encountered new adaptive challenges on the road ahead.

PROGRESS, LIFESPAN, AND TERMINATION CONSIDERATIONS

Normal adolescent development may include narcissistic self-absorption that will not necessarily stabilize into an inflexible and pervasive personality structure, although some will continue on this trajectory. As life progresses, those who develop narcissistic psychopathology may encounter more than expected difficulty with the normal changes of aging (American Psychiatric Association, 2013). Physical changes in attractiveness, strength, or competitive edge are deeply threatening to the person with NPD, and apt to trigger clinically significant problems, if not full mood disorders. These individuals may also be especially sensitive to perceived loss of status or potency in occupational settings, and adapt poorly to role shifts that others would simply see as part of a progression toward career consolidation or retirement. Such developmental considerations are useful in designing a well-targeted treatment plan for improving the internal coping skills and anticipating predictable triggers for relapse.

Progress can be measured in a number of ways in addition to the standard notion of reducing toxic levels of emotional and behavioral impairment. Of course, we hope to assist the patients who are narcissistic in overcoming dysthymia, chronic anger or hostility, or decreasing the incidence of high-cost self-stimulating behavior, but to terminate without further work would be less than optimal. In addition, we hope for increased flexibility in conceptualizing themselves and others, greater emotional acceptance and expressions of warmth and compassion for themselves and others, more evidence of reciprocal social interactions and other respectful behaviors, and better management of competitive strivings

It may be helpful to maintain contact with patients who are narcissistic on a consulting basis over time, even if sessions do not occur with great frequency. Such follow-up can support functional efforts and adaptive beliefs and note any regression toward self-aggrandizing and detached self-stimulating strategies. Possible challenges or transitions can be anticipated, keeping in mind the developmental tasks likely to be encountered in the intermediate and longer-term future. Collaboratively summarizing useful tools and important ideas from therapy is also valuable. Patients who are narcissistic are difficult to engage and keep in therapy, so it may be that intervention takes place in brief, intermittent consultations over a very long period of time, rather than a single prolonged episode of treatment.

COMMON CHALLENGES AND CLINICIAN SELF-CARE

The defensive characteristics and aggressive features of the patient with NPD can easily activate a therapist's own schemas and counterproductive, defensive responses. Trainees need extra support, due to the complexity of skills required, such as heightened self-awareness, appropriate and genuine self-disclosure, and negotiating the patient's motivation for change. Overall, expectations for progress need to be calibrated to the difficulty of this patient and entrenched compensatory modes. In addition, the duration of treatment may be quite limited if there is no significant leverage or buy in from the patient. Narcissism significantly interferes with collaboration due to the need to impress, avoid emotions, and shift the focus of "blame" to external sources, including the therapist. Patients with NPD feel entitled to special treatment, expect to feel better without effort, and may resent real or implied responsibility. They may lapse into entitled dependence, resist homework, and need to be empathically confronted and guided repeatedly through contemplation of problems and emotional experiences before they will accept any influence from the therapist. Emotional reactions to these clinical aspects of narcissism will significantly challenge the therapist's coping skills, no matter how sturdy. The therapist may feel charmed, seduced, exasperated, or threatened. Any of these reactions suggest some possible threat to the integrity of the treatment and need to proceed with deliberation. It is helpful for the therapist to practice self-therapy and/or seek consultation to reduce the risk of misjudgments or boundary violations and to identify and heal personally vulnerable schemas and modes, and develop stress-reducing tactics geared to the specific issues of the patient. For a pre-session boost of one's empathic and reparenting stance, a quick glance at the patient's childhood or adolescent photograph can be a good reminder that there is a "story" and a vulnerable (often injured) child trapped beneath the prickly, demanding façade about to enter the room.

CONCLUSION

NPD can be severely damaging to interpersonal relationships and successful life adjustment. Persons who are narcissistic rarely give up all of their, albeit maladaptive, protective layers. But, the integrative approach of schema therapy–cognitive therapy can help fortify an awareness of the destructive impact of their defenses, and weaken the intensity of internal ruptures and constructed defenses, allowing access to more adaptive modes and beliefs.

CHAPTER 15

Histrionic Personality Disorder

Mehmet Z. Sungur
Anil Gündüz

Our illustrative patient, Mrs. A, is a 32-year-old unemployed, married woman who suffered from low mood and loss of pleasure about her daily activities. In the first session, she emphasized a few times that she had been seen by several psychiatrists who were not able to understand and help her. She described them as shallow and boring, doing nothing apart from prescribing antidepressant medications, which did not help her. Her expectations of a good psychiatrist was a person who would devote time when she demanded help and be avaliable any time she felt needy. She expected her therapist to see her uniqueness and specialness and emphasized that she particularly disliked the nongenuine initial overcaring behaviors of psychiatrists. She thought they were fake, and that the caregiving attitudes did not last long, diminishing at the end of a few sessions. On many occasions this resulted in her premature drop out from treatment.

Although Mrs. A suffered from low mood and loss of pleasure, she emphasized that her mood was unstable and she could be joyful, fun, and charming on many occasions. She insisted that most of the time, her friends admired her impressive behavior and charm. However, the only person who gave her unconditional care and love was her husband. Despite an unsatisfactory sexual life from the beginning of their 10 years of marriage, she described him as always attentive and faithful to her.

Mrs. A also suffered from some physical symptoms such as dizziness, nausea, palpitations, and fear of fainting, which amounted to occasional panic attacks. This happened particularly following interactions with people whom she described as uncaring, overly critical, and insensitive. She also described some temper tantrums that involved agressive and intimidating behaviors as a response to experiences that she judged as " humiliating, criticizing, and uncaring."

Individuals with histrionic personality disorder (HPD) display excessively dramatic behaviors and show emotional exhibitionism. An intense longing for affection and attention drives their self-centered, seductive, and manipulative behaviors, without consideration of their impact on others. HPD is characterized by a need to be the center of attention, giving others the impression they are continuously performing. HPD signs and symptoms are usually egosyntonic—that is, those diagnosed as HPD often do not recognize that others may perceive their behavior as shallow, excessive, or manipulative, nor do they see themselves in this way. This often leads to interpersonal difficulties, disturbed relationships, and emotional struggles with anger and low mood that they attribute to external causes. The same pattern is displayed to the therapist, which presents therapeutic challenges and pitfalls. Patients with HPD may seem willing to engage in treatment as they seek relationships, but it is not easy to engage them in the treatment as they can be very manipulative, emotionally labile, and easily frustrated and distracted.

CLINICAL SIGNS AND SYMPTOMS

According to DSM-IV-TR (American Psychiatric Association, 2000) and DSM-5 (American Psychiatric Association, 2013), HPD is a pervasive and persistent pattern of excessive emotionality and attention seeking that emerges at early adulthood and presents itself by displaying seductive or provocative behaviors, rapidly shifting and shallow expression of emotions, use of physical appearance to draw attention, and speaking in an impressionistic style that lacks details. The individual with HPD feels uncomfortable in situations in which he or she does not become the center of attention, is easily influenced by others and the environment, and considers relations to be more intimate than they actually are. Being uncomfortable with lack of attention and inappropriate sexually seductive or provocative behaviors have the highest predictive values (Links, 1996).

It is reported that some individuals with HPD believe that other people exist only to serve and admire them (MacKenzie, 1997). Patients with HPD overdevelop the strategies of exhibitionism, expressiveness, and impressionism at the expense of reflectiveness, control, and systematization (Beck, Freeman, & Davis, 2004). Patients who are histrionic tend to be emotionally labile, get easily frustrated and bored, crave excitement, and often have difficulty in concentrating (Millon, 1996). They are also described as needy and dependent with excessive needs for approval and reassurance (Westen & Shedler, 1999a, 1999b).

DIFFERENTIAL DIAGNOSIS

Other Cluster B diagnoses, particularly borderline and narcissistic personality disorder and Cluster C diagnosis such as dependent personality disorder share common features with that of HPD (Pfohl, 1991; Widiger et al., 1991). Individuals with histrionic, narcissistic, and dependent personality disorders all seek attention, admiration, approval, and support from others (American Psychiatric Association, 2013).

However, inappropriately seductive and provacative behaviors are essential signs of HPD. Emotional expressions are shallow and exaggerated, and the patient who is histrionic assumes a deep connection and dependence quickly. Details are not presented in their speech style, expressed emotions are not stable, and self-dramatization is used often. Their symptoms of discomfort at being on the sidelines and low frustration tolerance results in demands for immediate gratification, even if that causes other problems or negative reactions from others.

Patients with HPD and those with borderline personality disorder both display attention-seeking and manipulative behaviors and rapidly changing emotions but patients with borderline personality disorder can be distinguished with their severe and repetitive self-damaging behaviors, feelings of deep emptiness, and intense and inappropriate anger outbursts in interpersonal interactions (American Psychiatric Association, 2013).

Some features of narcissistic personality disorder, such as seeking attention from others, overlap with that of HPD. However, patients with narcissistic personality disorder crave acknowledgment and praise for their superiority and "very important person" (VIP) status, even among their friends. Patients with narcissistic personality disorder have distinct features such as specialness entitlement, grandiosity of self-significance, and severe absence of empathy. Patients with HPD and those with narcissistic personality disorder have a need to draw attention, but patients with narcissistic personality disorder desire acknowledgment of their superiority, whereas patients with HPD desire to be the center of attention sometimes at the expense of being negatively viewed (American Psychiatric Association, 2013).

Individuals with antisocial personality disorder share common features with patients with HPD in the sense that they are also manipulative, seductive, impulsive, and display novelty- and excitement-seeking behaviors. However, patients with HPD are manipulative to attract attention, nurturance, and approval, whereas those with antisocial personality disorder manipulate others to gain power, control, and profit (American Psychiatric Association, 2013).

Patients with dependent personality disorder also seek care, attention, and guidance but they do not display self-dramatization, inappropiate sexually seductive or provacative behaviors, and do not seek being the center of attention (American Psychiatric Association, 2013).

Personality changes due to other medical conditions can be differentiated from HPD as they emerge in response to the effects of other medical conditions (American Psychiatric Association, 2013).

Lack of insight for dramatic and manipulative histrionic behaviors makes the diagnosis problematic because patients do not view their internal experiences as symptomatic (Standage, Bilsbury, Jain, & Smith, 1984). Exaggerated reactions in response to undesired minor life events are not evaluated as excessive by the patients. They may also complain of pressures to continuously perform for others, and report feeling fatigued or despondent about meeting expectations, presenting themselves as a victim of external demands. Patients with HPD frequently have some somatoform disorder, including high comorbidity with conversion and pain disorders, illness phobia, and body dysmorphic disorder (Skodol, 2005).

RESEARCH AND EMPIRICAL DATA

Despite the fairly consistent descriptions of the patient who is histrionic in the psychiatric literature, among all of the personality disorders in the Cluster B group, HPD is the one that the least amount of research has been devoted to. Lack of evidence-based, randomized controlled studies of therapy focusing on HPD leave the clinicians to rely on expert opinions for diagnostic criteria and epidemiological research. No controlled cognitive-behavioral therapy (CBT) -outcome studies have been found for HPD (Crits-Christoph & Barber, 2002). However, a thorough literature search showed the cost-effectiveness of schema therapy in treatment of HPD in one randomized controlled trial (Bamelis, Evers, & Arntz, 2012).

CONCEPTUALIZATION

One of the basic beliefs of individuals with HPD is that they are inadequate on their own and therefore need others for survival. This might be a healthy belief as building relationships is part of the human evolutionary process to prevent isolation. Additionally, many others may have similar thoughts and beliefs about being inadequate on their own. What distinguishes them from one another is the way they respond to these thoughts, and how overdeveloped the responses become over time. People who are depressive mainly ruminate about how they have come to this point and why they feel this way. People with dependent personality look for someone to cling on for care, and become submissive to their caretakers. However, people with HPD do not leave anything to uncertainity and they constantly strive to keep others around them by exhibiting entertaining, dramatic behaviors and putting themselves and their emotions on display, ensuring that their needs for attachment will be met. Believing that constant attention and approval are essential to their survival, they seek approval from others for anything they do. Need for approval comes with fear of rejection. As any sign that might be interpreted as rejection is catastrophized, strong negative emotions are felt even when the people who are rejecting are not significant to the patient. This may lead to a vicious cycle where more dramatic behaviors are displayed through temper tirades, demands, or other aggressive actions when approval is delayed.

People try to make sense of their environment from their early developmental stages to organize their experiences in a meaningful way and function most adaptively (Rosen, 1988). Their interactions with the outer world lead to certain beliefs about themselves and others. The core HPD belief that the person is inadequate on his or her own leads to intermediate beliefs that focus on the need for attention and approval, and corresponding fear of disapproval to compensate for this inadequacy. Beliefs that frame attention as an urgent need include "I must always be able to take other people's attention" and "If I'm dramatic, or charming enough, I can get the attention I need." The attitude that "Rejection or disapproval shows that I am worthless, inadequate, and unlovable" fosters the belief that "Being rejected is terribly humiliating and unbearable." Sensitivity toward the possibility of rejection is activated by the assumption that "If I'm not the center of attention, I am bound to be rejected or abandoned." As these basic and intermediate beliefs are frequently and easily activated in every social interaction, the individual with HPD finds him- or herself "performing" for others on many, if not all, occasions. According to Young, Klosko, and Weishaar (2003), people exhibit three different schema-coping responses when their schemas are activated. They may use "schema avoidance," which involves avoiding people or situations that trigger a schema, such as building superficial relationships to avoid risks of intimacy and rejection. They may choose giving into the schema using "schema-surrender" responses by demanding attention or developing extreme reactions to frustration, such as dramatic, somatically based symptoms (e.g., dizziness, fainting) that express their belief of being unable to function without support. A third way of coping is just doing the opposite of the schema content, called "schema compensation," perhaps by choosing partners who are likely to be highly dependent on them to avoid rejection or abandonment. This gives them a sense of empowerment and control as they believe dependent people will provide unconditional acceptance and are not likely to abandon them (Bernstein,

2005). Mrs. A, introduced in the beginning of this chapter, emphasized on many occasions that she chose Mr. A as her husband as he was the only person in her life who gave her unconditional acceptance and care.

Early maladaptive schemas stem from unmet developmental neeeds such as the need for affection, guidance, and validation (Young et al., 2003). Treatment often requires focusing on early developmental experiences and cognitive restructuring of basic beliefs that emerged as a consequence of past experiences. Certain overdeveloped and repetitive strategies are used to compensate a distorted view of self and others that have emerged as a response to negative developmental experiences including past traumas and disruptions of attachment. Patients with HPD view themselves as impressive and glamorous, others as easily seduced and receptive (Beck et al., 2004), and develop manipulative strategies to obtain their goals of impressing others. Individuals with HPD believe that they can achieve these goals through charm, dramatic behavior, anger outbursts, crying, and sexualizing or other overdeveloped manipulative behaviors (Beck et al., 2004).

Patients with HPD get so involved in their overdeveloped strategies that they fail to recognize their underdeveloped skills in observation and judgment. This reliance on overdeveloped strategies takes them far beyond from what may be effective or functional, and gives rise to cognitive distortions. Emotional reasoning clouds their judgment as they rely on internal emotions and feelings (and automatic thoughts) as evidence for the truth, rather than using external evidence such as objective observation to judge others' reactions to them. Therefore, they keep trying to impress others until they feel assured and satisfied that they have impressed them sufficiently to get the approval and attention they believe they need, and this may result in the characteristic drama. This also explains why they tend to assume that if they feel inadequate, they must be inadequate, and if they feel like they are being rejected, they must be rejected. Dichotomous thinking intensifies their demonstrative attention-seeking behaviors until they feel that they have fully impressed the others. Social interactions that are appraised as "rejecting and humiliating" become a major issue in treatment.

For instance, when Mrs. A called a man on the phone and could not have access, she thought "He is not taking my call on purpose." As a result of this thought, she felt very frustrated and presumed she had been humiliated or at least not taken seriously. This made her more angry and kept her calling until she had access to that person. She initiated the phone conversation by blaming him for being uncaring and insensitive, despite being told that the call could not be taken due to being busy or taking part in a meeting. Being very vulnerable to sense of rejection, she was hardly satisfied with these explanations. She revealed that she gave similar responses to her prior therapists. If the therapist was only a few minutes late to accept her into the session, she expressed her disappointment for waiting and blamed the therapist for neglect and lack of genuine care. If the therapist did not seem to be responding to her accusations, she responded by displaying seductive or aggressive behaviors to impress upon and teach him that she is not a "disposable object." When asked about the consequences of too little attention, Mrs. A said that she needs other people's and especially her therapist's attention to feel safe and happy. Her firmly held belief was that if she is entertaining enough, others won't notice her weakness and will be interested in her.

As the treatment progressed Mrs. A revealed that she had a few affairs with people whom she described as "popular, attractive, and clever," some of whom were her husband's friends. She said that she chose those men to assure herself that she is capable to draw attention from highly qualified men. She believed all men are easily seduced and sought attention particularly from men (including therapists) whom she described as "difficult to be emotionally challenged." When she felt uncomfortable with the amount of attention she was getting, she would send some sexually seductive and provocative messages and photographs. She said that most men were impressed and expressed admiration about her photos, confirming her belief that they could easily be manipulated if she used her beauty and charm.

One of Mrs. A's core beliefs about herself was that she was worthless unless she was noticed, taken care of, and admired by others. She felt overwhelmed by feelings of worthlessness and shame when she felt neglected, believed that she couldn't stand these negative feelings, and might go insane if she didn't do something to reduce the tension. Her emotional pain was only relieved if she could catch the attention and approval of the person whom she felt was disapproving of her. The emotional deprivation schema (Bricker, Young, & Flanagan, 1993; Young et al., 2003) made her believe that her needs for emotional support and nurturance would never be properly met by others, which made experiences of emotional frustration or disappointment intolerably painful. She also viewed the world and others as the providers of the special care that she needed. The self-centeredness schema (Young et al., 2003) made her feel entitled to take or receive the attention and approval needed, without considering its impact on others. She had learned from past experiences that the easiest and most effective way to get attention and feel worthy was by seducing the opposite sex. If sexual provocation did not work, she would display dramatic anger outbursts, crying, and minor self-harm (such as overdosing her antidepressant medications) until she had access to nurturance. This relief was short-lived, but powerfully reinforcing. In the long term, these behaviors led to negative consequences such as losing friends and premature termination from therapies. She acknowledged these long-term negative consequences but stated that she could not control her inflexible and inappropriate behaviors.

Assessment of the origins of Mrs. A's core belief showed that her worthlessness developed at an early age after realizing that her father fully cared about her only when she was sitting on his lap and when she allowed him to touch her face and body. She could never tell whether this touchy behavior was sexual abuse but realized soon that sitting on his lap was an effective shortcut strategy to affection. These were the only times she was the center of attention, as her mother was distant and depressed and her father was very busy with his job. She witnessed her father devaluating and verbally abusing her mother on many occasions. Her mother frequently fainted following heated arguments and verbally abusive behaviors, which prompted extra care from her husband. Her mother spent most of her time in bed, leaving young A and her 4-years-younger sister without a good maternal role model. This led to the reversing of roles where she and her sister had to learn how to take good care of their mom at an early age. She said that she still has images of herself cooking, cleaning, and shopping for the household as a young girl.

Individuals with HPD may show variations of phenemonology and clinical features of the disorder in different cultures. Societies with different cultural heritages differ about what behaviors will be accepted, tolerated, or rejected (Segall, Dasen, Berry, & Poortinga, 1990; Sungur, 2013), and thus problems and strategies to deal with them are not culture free (Bhugra & de Silva, 2007). Physical symptoms such as dizziness, light-headedness, and fainting are seen as more care provoking than emotional signs and symptoms in many cultures. The display of bodily symptoms or somatization generally takes more attention, nurturance, and support than expressing complaints verbally in many collective cultures (Sungur, 2013). Over-self-sacrificing behaviors and continous efforts to please one's family and others accompanied by development of bodily symptoms are generally observed in the past history of many patients diagnosed with HPD in the Turkish culture. Many patients with HPD coming from rural areas exhibit an initial "silent suffering and adaptation period" to negative life circumstances surrounding them, which is then followed by an exhibition of bodily symptoms to warrant attention and care needed from others.

Mrs. A, as a young girl, tried hard to please her mom and dad by taking household responsibilities to compensate for her mom's lack of energy due to her depression. She thought that her efforts were neither appreciated nor noticed and felt helpless until she realized that exhibiting bodily symptoms like her mother might be an effective way to get the attention and support she craved. She also discovered at age 11 that being seductive and attractive could be an effective way to receive care and intimacy after seeing her parents having sex while the bedroom door was half open. She witnessed that her father treated her mom with care and compassion following sex. She revealed that after watching her parents' sexual activities, she got curious with bodily sensations and started touching her genitals, which was followed by mutual genital touching with her younger sister.

To summarize conceptualization, the presenting complaint of Mrs. A was low-fluctuating mood with physical symptoms and some agressive and intimidating behaviors following social situations that she judged as uncaring and/or humiliating. Her developmental profile showed that her mother was distant and uncaring to her children due to her depression and she displayed bodily symptoms to get attention from her husband. Her father also neglected her as he was busy with his work and showed full attention only if young A permitted him to touch her in a way that she could not clearly define. Her parents argued a lot and she witnessed their sexual interaction at an early age. She grew up feeling neglected despite all her efforts to please her family. She developed core beliefs about herself as worthless and unlovable and the outer world as uncaring, neglecting, and rejecting. Her intermediate (conditional) beliefs that were shaped by her basic beliefs emerged as "Being rejected or not being able to get approval shows that I am worthless and unlovable," "I must always be able to get other people's attention," and "If I can display some manipulative and seductive behaviors, I will be noticed and get others' attention." Her basic beliefs were frequently activated in social situations that she regarded as uncaring and rejecting, and this precipitated her compensatory overdeveloped strategies such as exhibiting dramatic attention-seeking behavior that sometimes amounted to showing temper tantrums if she felt not fully noticed and approved. Getting too involved with her overdeveloped strategies to avoid emotional pain prevented her from recognizing her underdeveloped skills, such as building appropriate rapport, empathy, communication, and intimacy skills to establish more healthy and stable alternative ways of getting approval. Fears of no approval and rejection made her vulnerable to any sign that might be interpreted as a lack of attention toward her, which initiated threat monitoring in every social interaction.

KEY TREATMENT GOALS

Collaborative goal setting is a major requirement for successful intervention. It is crucial that the goals be specific, concrete, understandable, and acceptable for the patient. The ultimate goal for patients with HPD is to increase their sense of emotional security and strengthen healthy adult schema. Treatment success may be determined by the patient's ability and capacity to tolerate, to some degree, situations with low approval or attention, and to demonstrate effective communication and social skills involving healthy restraint, more empathy for others, and greater self-confidence in managing interpersonal stresses or other evaluative experiences. There are several component goals that may be part of the case formulation, depending on individual patient needs. These include the following:

1. Increase affect awareness and regulation skills to improve frustration tolerance and allow learning of uncomfortable but healthy new behaviors. The second part of this goal is for the patient to use these skills to reduce the occurance of dramatic display or other aggressive behavior.

2. Test fears about rejection and decatastrophize the extreme ideas about the meaning of disapproval or loss of attention. Sensitivity to these fears may be reduced by separating the idea of "self" from behavior when interpreting outcomes, so that any criticism is connected to transient or changeable actions or situations, rather than personalized as a measure of self-worth. It is also important to build confidence to face realistic experiences of criticism and rejection through assertive defense of self (Padesky, 1997).

3. Improve communication and social skills, including building empathy for others and learning alternative ways to connect with others more directly without drama or sexual acting out. An important component of this goal is to improve the patient's skills for listening and taking data from others and integrating that information instead of relying solely on his or her internal sense of satisfaction through immediate and intensive attention from others. This includes the specific skills of active listening and taking a different perspective, and being a good audience member rather than taking center stage.

4. Increase self-sufficiency, problem-solving skills, and sense of identity with less dependence on others' attention.

COLLABORATIVE STRATEGY

Depending on the goals set with the patient, a wide variety of techniques from challenging thoughts to more experiential ones, such as behavioral experiments, can be used in treatment. However, without good collaboration these techniques are not likely to conclude with a successful outcome. Establishing a collaborative relationship is essential to motivate the patient with HPD to evaluate his or her own dysfunctional strategies and modify them as needed. It may also be useful to meet some of the basic developmental needs of the client while maintaining appropriate boundaries. This can be achieved by offering genuine warmth and emphathy for a client who did not receive adequate nurturing. As treatment of HPD takes some time and dropouts are seen frequently, the primary challenge is keeping these people in treatment. This can be done by maintaining stable and consistent efforts to make them feel understood and accepted while simultaneously keeping them motivated to embrace a treatment approach that requires change.

Often, patients with HPD view the therapist as a powerful rescuer who will make everything better by giving advice and solving the problems on their behalf (Beck et al., 2004; Sperry, 2006) Therefore, they expect an active role of the therapist (Othmer & Othmer, 2002). This fantasy may also motivate an inexperienced therapist to take the powerful rescuer role where he or she provides immediate advice, gives in to patients' inappropriate demands, and makes decisions on their behalf. This may increase the patient's rescuer fantasy, reduce feelings of adequacy, and sustain their original relationship pattern. It also eventually and inevitably leads to feelings of anxiety, anger, self-blame, helplessness, and lack of motivation by the therapist. When the patient perceives reduction of initial motivation and enthusiasm of the therapist, his or her schemas of rejection and worthlessness gets reactivated. This diminishes the quality of the therapeutic relationship and may be followed by premature dropouts and hostility. Indeed, Mrs. A was very angry with the reduction of initial care and attention of her prior therapists, which she blamed on lack of genuine interest and incompetency. She viewed them as witholding and unreliable, which activated her emotional deprivation and rejection/abandonment schemas once again. The therapeutic relationship provides an opportunity to observe schemas in the "here and now" as the patients' schemas and coping responses are activated in the therapeutic relationship (Bernstein, 2005). Empathic gentle confrontation can help the patient see how his or her responses interferes with treatment progress. Collaboration and guided discovery can motivate the patient toward independent problem solving without the therapist taking on the rescuer role.

Erotic transference is another common response that interferes with treatment. This is a mixture of erotic feelings directed toward the idealized therapist that may sometimes be accompanied by feelings of embarrassment and/or anger when the patient recognizes that the feelings are not mutual. The patient may cope with this by increased seductive and manipulative behaviors, which can trigger rejection or exploitation if the therapist is unable to effectively manage this sexualized transference. These transferences need to be handled competently and analyzed in close cooperation with the patient. The therapist must keep clear limits and point out these patterns with gentle confrontation, drawing parallels to the patient's strategies in current life situations. This kind of gentle, empathic confrontation may evoke an understanding of the origins of these behavioral patterns and help patients with HPD give meaning to experiences that seemed embarrassing or meaningless.

Mrs. A stated that her seductive behaviors resulted from the crossing of professional boundaries with one of her therapists, leading to feelings of being exploited and abused. A mutual reconceptualization of the past experiences helped her to see her needs and the dysfunctional strategies she used to fulfill those needs. Her therapist explained that childhood experiences establish core beliefs about ourselves and the outer world and that dysfunctional coping strategies emerge to protect us from danger and perceived threats. This explanation helped her to normalize the process of overdeveloping some strategies and underdeveloping some skills, leading to the reduction of the patient's internal attribution of fault or blame.

CLINICAL APPLICATION OF THE INTERVENTION

Therapist Validation and Psychoeducation

Collaborative treatment requires acceptance, nonjudgmental attitudes, and validation. Validation of painful experiences makes the patient feel understood and accepted. Validation includes a normalization rationale, which again helps the patient give a new meaning to his or her past experiences when looked at from a different perspective. This new perspective may help the patient to give meaning to what seems meaningless.

The therapist validated Mrs. A's basic beliefs of worthlessness by explaining that the core beliefs, such as "I am worthless," are the results of attaching meaning to childhood experiences. He explained to Mrs. A that the way a child thinks may be completely different from the adult way of thinking in the sense that a child has the tendency to think "I am what I am given." Therefore, as a child, Mrs. A had no other choice in evaluating her value apart from assessing how much care and support she received. Her therapist explained that worthless feelings could stem from the lack of care, attention, and appreciation received as a child. She was confused and impressed to hear that this equation of self-worth/value is determined by reactions of significant others in childhood and is expected to change as one grows older and becomes more mature.

Mrs. A was told that when she was a child she would have little choice apart from believing that the adults in her life were the right role models. Therefore, it was understandable that she made sense of her mom's bodily symptoms and took it as a way to attract attention to feel worthy. In other words, as a child's self-worth is determined by the care, love, and compassion received from significant others, it was not surprising that she felt worthless given the fact that her mom was busy with her own problems and her dad was busy with his job. It was also made clear that when the outer world (represented by her parents) is appraised as uncaring, a search for finding new ways to be cared for becomes a reasonable and rational step to take, and that was what she did. Unfortunately, this search ended by discovering dysfunctional strategies to achieve the care and attention she needed. These strategies included exhibiting bodily symptoms; flirtatious and sexually seductive behaviors; dramatic, impressionistic behaviors; and exaggerated expressions of emotions amounting to temper tantrums to feel cared and loved.

Mrs. A was also helped to realize that these strategies were the only ones used to avoid negative consequences of unlovable–uncared–unworthy schemas that were easily and frequently activated. They became more dysfunctional as they were used more intensively due to a lack of other coping skills and strategies. This explanation also helped her realize that she needed to develop new skills.

The therapist also validated the strategies used in childhood based on her intermediate beliefs ("It is terrible to be unworthy and unlovable" [attitude], "I must always be able to get other people's attention to be cared for and desirable" [rule], and "If I'm not the center of attention, I'm being rejected or abandoned"), as these assumptions were constituted to protect her from the negative outcomes of the basic beliefs she had. In short, Mrs. A was told that she used these strategies to avoid emotional pain. This made her feel relieved and she reported that, for the first time in her life, she gave meaning to her persistent approval- and attention-seeking needs.

The therapist also helped Mrs. A find out by guided discovery that the core belief that emerged as a result of childhood experiences was justified at that period of life, but is now less adaptive and less functional due to its inflexible nature. She realized through experiential techniques described later in this chapter that the persistent and rigid nature of the overdeveloped coping strategies used until the present time prevented her from developing more adaptive and flexible alternative strategies. Socratic dialogue and downward-arrow techniques such as asking "What do you think would have happened if you did not display that behavior?" were used. This helped her find out that the frequent use of the overdeveloped strategies to avoid emotional pain were perhaps preventing her from seeing what might have happened if those strategies were not used.

Cognitive Interventions

Within the working therapeutic relationship, the therapist gradually guided Mrs. A to consider other possible explanations for actions and reactions faced in social situations or challenged her existing belief while remaining attuned to her point of view. In this sense, the therapist functioned as an easily accessible source for generating other possible perspectives regarding herself, the outer world, and her interactions (relationships) with others. This facilitated further change as a patient with a personality disorder has no other choice but to see the world only from his or her own particular perspective unless gently challenged. Mrs. A realized that core and intermediate beliefs influenced her perspective of life events, which determined how she thinks, feels, and behaves. After educating the patient about core beliefs and monitoring how they operate by using daily thought records, she was able to see the link among her automatic thoughts, feelings, and behaviors.

The next stage was to help the patient realize that every belief is not neccesarily a truth, and every belief can be tested. Rather than being selective in choosing the data that support the original belief and discounting the evidence on the contrary, it was suggested to gather evidence for and against the belief. During this monitoring process, the therapist introduced the core belief worksheet. Mrs. A and the therapist worked on the old belief that she would be unlovable and worthless unless she became the focus of interest. She was asked to gather evidence for and against the old belief and found that she could still be desirable and worthy even if she did not display her automatic attention-seeking behaviors. Another area that they worked on together was to increase awareness and insight about the fact that even if the worst scenario happened and she was not desired or liked by others, that would not mean that she is unlovable or undesirable. The therapist and patient worked collaboratively to find alternative explanations to interpret others' behaviors without making reference to herself. Despite her efforts, there were times Mrs. A felt that she was unable to change as the therapy progressed. The therapist and the patient discussed the definition of change and challenged the biased belief that only complete change is noteworthy. They came to a mutual conclusion that change is not an all-or-none phenomenon and even a small change may have a significant impact on her relationships with others.

The patient was able to acknowledge her sensitivity to neglect and rejection but despite this acknowledgment intense fear and anxiety arose when she was asked to expose herself to social situations while dropping her overdeveloped strategies. Understanding that her childhood experiences made her so vulnerable, she described herself like a victim. At that stage the therapist validated her painful experiences and expressed how much he regretted that she had to deal with such adversity at an early age. He then discussed with the patient whether she was a victim or a survivor and even if she was a victim in the past, could she change the victim role now and be a survivor by reclaiming her life. This helped her realize that she can live a more meaningful life despite a difficult childhood.

Therapists may also use techniques such as "setting timetables" to postpone patients' ruminations about being worthless and inadequate. They can be helped in learning to postpone ruminations about their past as well as postponing worries about their future. Ruminating and worrying are strategies that are frequently used to avoid emotions that might emerge in response to negative thoughts (Leahy, 2006). Setting timetables can be used to postpone feelings of anger and hatred that may emerge in response to their negative thoughts. Patients could be told to postpone negative feelings and worries until a certain time of the day for purposes of establishing control on what seems uncontrollable. Mrs. A was asked to postpone expressing her strong feelings instead of being overwhelmed and getting carried away by them. Although she found it initially difficult to postpone negative feelings and worries, she interpreted the experience to be extremely helpful as she recognized that she can circumscribe her painful emotions by time frames. This led to a paradoxical effect where she felt no need to engage in ruminations and worries during the time of the day scheduled to express them. She realized that as she succeeded in postponing them until the set time, there might be no need to express them when she was allowed to do so. This paradoxical effect reduced the need to schedule such worry time on a regular basis in the long term.

Experiential Interventions

Experiental techniques such as guided imagery, emotional processing, imagery rescripting (Young et al., 2003), role play, and role reversal were frequently used to reduce the emotional impact of the early maladaptive schemas. They also helped to restructure early memories by reexperiencing them not only at an intellectual level but also at an emotional level. Guided imagery was found to be most effective in challenging the schemas at an emotional level with Mrs. A. When she was asked to close her eyes and relive a past experience in vivid detail, she was able to recall some pivotal developmental events that activated her core beliefs of being unlovable and worthless. She was then asked to close her eyes again to recall a recent event that was annoying for her. This scene also activated the same core beliefs that made her realize that similar annoying experiences make her feel the same way.

The patient's main schemas and coping behaviors became quite evident both for the therapist and the patient during these reliving with the emotional processing sessions. This made her understand the link between the past and the present. Additionally, activation of core beliefs gave the therapist the opportunity to guide her through the image and generate new perspectives to reconceptualize the past experience. This helped Mrs. A to establish new and more adaptive explanations that had not been accessible in the past. Imagery scripting (Young et al., 2003) was used to heal the emotional pain that her maladaptive schemas represented. During imagery rescripting she was asked to close her eyes and recall an early painful experience involving her parents. The goal was to activate a vivid image of neglect and lack of approval and also reexperience her father touching her body with the associated physical sensations, emotions, and cognitions. Immediately after bringing forth this image the therapist briefly described how to alter some of the imagery scenes and change the neglect of her mother and the vague—difficult to interpret—touchy behavior of her father to a more acceptable outcome. She was asked to visualize her adult self today entering the touching or neglect scene to confront her mother and father directly and experience a sense of empowerment. The mastery image was to "rescue" the child from the touching scene by taking her to a safe place and tell her mom assertively that it is young A's right to be soothed, protected, and approved by her. The therapist was cautious not to tell the patient what to do or suggest what should be happening, to increase the level of mastery on the patient's side. The last stage of imagery scripting began following a successful and assertive confrontation with her mom and dad. It involved the adult self interacting directly with the traumatized child in a calm, reassuring, and nurturing manner. The goal was to make the child feel safe, approved, nurtured, and accepted, and the adult to be more able to empathize and feel the child's pain so that the child and the adult self could feel more connected. When it appeared that the child has received sufficient nurturance from the adult, the therapist asked if the adult self has anything else to tell the child before bringing the scene to an end. The adult self replied, saying "You are not inadequate and you are able to handle your life on your own. You do not need to perform to get the approval of others. You are lovable even when you do not try to charm and seduce others."

Postimagery debriefing and processing was conducted by asking Mrs. A's reactions to the imagery sessions, how she felt, and what the experience meant for her. She was confused by the experience but was suprised to see how this imagery work made her feel more sufficient and lovable than she ever felt. Adequate time was given for the patient to gain control over her emotions prior to leaving the session. The imagery exercises were found to be cathartic, helping the patient to release painful emotions. The rescripting helped to modify the meaning of some childhood memories and gain mastery over her passive experiences. This made the memories less painful and helped her to meet some of her developmental needs as the patient felt much relieved after being nurtured by her adult self. She also expressed that she found her own approval to be more important than others' approval to feel desirable and lovable, and lack of others' approval may not necessarily mean that she is unlovable.

Techniques such as role play, role reversal, and reenacting an event helped the patient further to process the past experiences at both cognitive and emotional levels. This helped her understand that it is possible to make alternative explanations for the past behaviors of her parents. Role play and role reversal helped improve her empathy for others by reconceptualizing their behaviors when looked at from a different perspective.

After looking at the major life events that had a strong emotional impact in her life, the patient started seeing how her core beliefs affected the way she felt and behaved through her lifespan. The use of a cognitive continuum helped her to be less rigid and change the polarized (all-or-none) thinking when she encountered data contrary to her perceptions of herself and others. Mrs. A believed that if she was not getting the attention or approval of others, she would be a failure and rejected. Real-life behavioral experiments were conducted where the consequence of staying silent and showing a nonverbal but attentive and caring interest was compared with the consequences of showing dramatic speech, gestures, and behaviors (where she became the center of attention). These behavioral experiments had a significant impact on changing her thoughts and behaviors. At that point she reported that for the first time in her life she felt she was receiving "genuine care and attention" without displaying any manipulative behavior.

Another technique called point–counterpoint (J. Beck, 2011; Young, 1990) was also employed simultaneously with the behavioral experiments when Mrs. A said that she could intellectually see that her beliefs were not functional but emotionally they still sometimes "feel" true. The therapist asked her to play the "emotional" part of her mind, which strongly endorsed the emotional maladaptive beliefs, while the therapist played the rational part. Later on, they switched roles and during this role play both the patient and the therapist spoke using "I" language where every sentence was rephrased in the "I" form (such as saying "I am hurt" instead of saying "You hurt me"). Switching roles provided the patient the opportunity to voice and understand the rational arguments brought forth by the therapist. The therapist used the same emotional reasoning and the same words the patient used during the role play. This helped Mrs. A respond more precisely and accurately to her own specific concerns. A detailed description of this technique is illustrated elsewhere (J. Beck, 2011). Although she initially felt uncomfortable with this technique as she thought the therapist was being critical of her while she was displaying nonverbal gestures, she grasped its meaning later on and developed a more helpful view of the rational and emotional parts of her mind.

PROGRESS, LIFESPAN, AND TERMINATION ISSUES

Patients with HPD have a long history of exhibiting lively and energetic patterns of behavior. Therefore, they generally fear being perceived as dull or boring if they drop their manipulative, attention-seeking behaviors. It is important to clarify to the patient that the goal is not to drop all of these behaviors, but to use them more constructively and establish new and more efficient ways to be appreciated, recognized, and approved by others. It is important to emphasize that seeking approval may be a very positive attribute, as that shows that an individual cares about the perception of others and their feelings. However, to establish a "self-value" dependent on other's approval and appreciation may prevent individual differentation and may lead to a merging of self-identity with the opinions of others. Indeed, when Mrs. A was asked about what she understood about the therapeutic experiental techniques used in treatment, she said, "We can do our best to please others but it is not in our control to make them approve or appreciate all of our behaviors and we need to learn to live with it." However, she was also told that the need for recognition can be achieved to an extent by taking part in competitive situations and other exciting activities. It is important to show that the need to be appreciated can be materialized through efforts to take part in social interactions but by taking a different perspective where the person actively listens and empathizes with others rather than acting as a social director, taking on the role of "prima donna."

Mrs. A was asked to show genuine interest and attention to others' problems without trying to be the center of attention and to compare the extent of approval and appreciation she received this way with that of her routine strategies to get attention. At the end of 2 weeks she reported that despite finding it difficult to listen without showing off, the payoff was that she could see herself being appreciated without extra effort.

Another issue that needs to be handled in achieving progress is the consistent need of patients to bring up their past emotional traumas as a reason for their lack of progress and collaboration. It may be helpful to use techniques such as "imagery scripting" to obtain empowerment in situations where they felt helpless in the first place. Indeed, Mrs. A found this technique beneficial in recognizing that she is a survivor rather than being just a victim. She also realized that she is no longer the helpless little girl who cannot reject behaviors unacceptable for her. In addition, she acknowledged that use of manipulation or seduction is not necessary to get the attention of other significant people.

Little has been written about interventions other than individual therapy in treatment of patients with HPD. Mrs. A's treatment began with individual therapy but couple therapy was added as the treatment progressed. It was necessary to include the husband in the treatment as he gave unconditional acceptance to Mrs. A's dramatic behaviors. Assesment showed that he exhibited dependent personality traits and assumed increased responsibility for the relationship, whereas Mrs. A displayed a more irresponsible role. At times, he became very worried when Mrs. A threatened him with separation or divorce due to his submissiveness, which Mrs. A both liked and disliked. She suffered from lack of emotional sensations and blamed her husband for the lack of romance and the routine, boring marriage. A behavioral systems couple therapy approach helped them overcome the dominance and submissiveness issues in the relationship and balance their investment and commitment to the relationship.

Mrs. A was seen for a total of 61 sessions over the course of 2.5 years. She showed a rapid improvement in her depressive and panic attack symptoms in the early stages of treatment but considerable change in HPD was achieved only at the end of 30 sessions. Fluctuations were witnessed frequently during the progress of treatment but she reported that she felt stable in terms of emotions and behaviors only at the end of 50 sessions. She also reported that she and her husband established a better, more meaning-ful and solid relationship including sexual activities.

Following the 50th session, the therapist started the fading process by spacing out the treatment sessions. This made Mrs. A realize that the rela-tionship that she found very nurturing and providing growth was due to end. A repetition of the dysfunctional histrionic patterns emerged for a few sessions. Mrs. A's fantasies of rescuer and nurturer role given to her thera-pist were revisited. Fantasies of a continuing relationship with the therapist after the termination of treatment were discussed in an empathic manner. She realized that these yearnings were no longer as compelling and unbear-able as before. The therapist and Mrs. A talked about the genuine relation-ships that Mrs. A established recently with others to balance this sepa-ration. Her anxiety peaked in the 58th session when she was confronted gently with the fact that the separation was real and a relationship outside the context of treatment would not be possible. Once again, her therapist pointed out that maintaining further contact would not help increase her sense of self-efficacy and personal growth that she managed to accomplish over the long period of treatment.

Relapse prevention became the main issue of the agenda of the last two sessions. The therapist and the patient discussed fully the specific situ-ations, places, internal states, and other vulnerabilities that might increase the likehood of emergence of the old patterns. The therapist and Mrs. A. worked collaboratively to find answers to "What if?" questions that pro-voked anxiety and worry such as "What if I start wanting to impress oth-ers again?" "What if I start to self-sacrifice again to please and receive approval from others?" and "What if I start believing more in my older beliefs instead of my new perspective?" Role plays and role reversals were done to improve self-confidence. Coping cards were generated for use when she felt overwhelmed. Significant triggers such as interpersonal relation-ships that start the histrionic behavioral pattern were carefully analyzed until Mrs. A felt competent and confident that she could manage future challenges.

COMMON CHALLENGES AND CLINICIAN SELF-CARE

There are many challenges the therapist encounters during the course of treatment of HPD. A good formulation and unique case conceptualization made and shared with the patient is essential to establish an effective treat-ment plan. As new data are gathered, they need to be inserted into the for-mulation accordingly in a competent way. Therefore, the therapist must be flexible enough to modify and refine the initial formulation when required. New data might confirm some hypotheses made earlier and disconfirm others, whereas different hypotheses may be established depending on the content of the new information. Sharing this conceptualization with the patient may initially annoy some patients with HPD but can help the ongoing data gathering process by providing a rationale and understanding of experiences that initially seem irrational or meaningless. Drawing diagrams may help the patient see how to fit subsequent experiences into this overall formulation.

Engagement of patients with HPD in treatment is another challenge as many have difficulty in adherence to treatment and dropouts are commonly seen during the course of treatment. Some patients drop out because they believe that they may be hurt if they reveal themselves. Others think that change might be difficult and threatening, or that they do not need to change. A direct confrontation with such distorted or biased ways of thinking and confrontational exposure to contradictions may result in hostility and loss of rapport. Therefore, accepting and validating past experiences, showing empathy, and effort to give meaning to what seems meaningless may make the patient more motivated and facilitate progress. In the initial stages of the treatment, patients with HPD may be more likely to think "I cannot change" and "It is too late for me." Most of the time this can be dealt with by discussing the definition of change and challenging the biased belief that only complete change is noteworthy. Redefining change within a spectrum and discussing the impact of small changes in altering the quality of life might motivate them to see that small can be beautiful and noteworthy.

Creating and keeping a good therapeutic relationship is a major challenge when the patient with HPD has had negative experiences with a prior therapist(s). Mrs. A had been seen by several therapists whom she found to be shallow and incompetent. Her expectations of a good therapist included a rescuer who will make everything better for her. Transference issues, such as rescuer fantasy and eroticizing and idealizing the therapist. and countertransference issues, such as rescuer role, anxiety, frustration, anger, and risks of exploitation of the patient, should be handled carefully. These issues might lead to fatigue, boredom, aloofness, regret, and self-blame by the therapist if not handled in a competent way (Sperry, 2006). Supervision may be essential to provide feedback and guidelines, even for the experienced therapist.

Straightforward techniques of CBT that are effectively used in symptomatic disorders are not likely to be sufficient in treatment of personality disorders such as HPD. A longer course of treatment that includes additional experiential techniques such as behavioral experiments, imagery scripting, facilitation of self-efficacy, empowerment, and building new skills is apt to be necessary. Sometimes patients are not motivated to develop new skills as they believe that even if they acquire these skills and use them in problem solving, they might still be exposed to the fact that there is no solution.

Nonadherence to homework instructions in between sessions is another challenge. The therapist must work with patients to understand what blocks them from doing their homework. Building collaboration in setting homework might be difficult as patients may be scared to experience negative emotions while doing homework. The therapist must make sure that the patient understands why homework is given and what will be achieved as a result of doing it. This might increase the motivation of patients to do homework. Homework must be specific, acceptable, and attainable in the time available. Sometimes nonadherence may be an indication of hostility toward the therapist or therapy or it might be one way to manipulate the therapist and get his or her attention.

End-point termination issues can be uniquely challenging, as separation anxiety may be triggered by the treatment progress, and may peak toward the end of treatment. Sometimes patients with HPD are afraid of losing the attention of their therapist and thus display their old pattern of attention seeking. Both patient and therapist may be challenged by the termination expectations, the potential for blurred boundaries, and the need to set and keep realistic, functional limits in the therapeutic relationship.

CONCLUSION

In summary, we believe that cognitive therapy for HPD requires empathy, flexibility, acceptance, creativity, and patience by the therapist. More empirical research is required to test the conceptualization provided in this chapter and clarify the effective components of a successful treatment for HPD.

CHAPTER 16

Antisocial Personality Disorder

Damon Mitchell
Raymond Chip Tafrate
Arthur Freeman

The following disguised case example provides a profile of antisocial personality typically seen in an outpatient court-mandated treatment setting: Warren is a 35-year-old male parolee. He was born and raised in a socioeconomically depressed city. Growing up, he had only brief contact with his father, who he described as an alcoholic. His mother, who worked as a nurse's aide, raised him and his two siblings. By his account, his siblings have led stable and prosocial lives. Warren was held back twice in school and dropped out of high school in his sophomore year following a string of suspensions for behaviors such as swearing at teachers, truancy, and fighting. He is currently unemployed and his work history has been unstable, marked by short-term unskilled positions in restaurants, construction, and landscaping. He is divorced and has a pattern of involvement in volatile short-term relationships. He has a 17-year-old son with whom he has had minimal contact. Warren disclosed a history of regular marijuana use going back to age 15, as well as experimental use of cocaine and phencyclidine (PCP). He reports occasional alcohol use but acknowledges that when he does drink, he becomes highly intoxicated. He has no formal mental health treatment beyond a vague recollection of counseling as a child due to his behavioral problems at school. He was first arrested at age 16 and has been in and out of the criminal justice system ever since. His criminal history includes arrests for burglary, larceny, robbery, assault, drug selling, and domestic violence. He served 8 years in prison for an aggravated assault in which he stabbed another man during a drug sale. His most recent offense involved threatening several family members of his now ex-girlfriend after a dispute. When he was arrested for the threatening charge, he had an unregistered firearm in his possession. He served 2 years for this most recent offense and has been on parole for 6 months. Warren is at risk of receiving a parole violation due to a positive urinalysis for marijuana and poor attendance at a mandated anger management program.

CLINICAL SIGNS AND SYMPTOMS: THE ANTISOCIAL CONSTRUCT

There presently exist three recognized conceptualizations of the antisocial construct: antisocial personality disorder (ASPD) as outlined in the *Diagnostic and Statistical Manual of Mental Disorders* (DSM-5; American Psychiatric Association, 2013), dissocial personality disorder in the *International Classification of Diseases* (ICD-10; World Health Organization, 1992), and psychopathy as formalized by Hare with the Psychopathy Checklist—Revised (PCL-R; Hare, 2003). A conundrum for therapists is that these conceptualizations are overlapping but not identical, emphasizing different symptom clusters.

The DSM-5 emphasizes the overt conduct of the patient through a criteria set that includes criminal behavior, lying, reckless and impulsive behavior, aggression, and irresponsibility in the areas of work and finances. In contrast, the criteria set for dissocial personality disorder is less focused on conduct and includes a mixture of cognitive signs (e.g., a tendency to blame others, an attitude of irresponsibility), affective signs (e.g., callousness, inability to feel guilt, low frustration tolerance), and interpersonal signs (e.g., tendency to form relationships but not maintain them). The signs and symptoms of psychopathy are more complex and are an almost equal blend of the conduct and interpersonal/affective aspects of functioning. The two higher-order factors of the PCL-R reflect this blend. Factor 1, *Interpersonal/Affective*, includes signs such as superficial charm, pathological lying, manipulation, grandiosity, lack of remorse and empathy, and shallow affect. Factor 2, *Lifestyle/Antisocial*, includes thrill seeking, impulsivity, irresponsibility, varied criminal activity, and disinhibited behavior (Hare & Neumann, 2008). Psychopathy can be regarded as the most severe of the three disorders. Patients with psychopathy would be expected to also meet criteria for ASPD or dissocial personality disorder, but not everyone diagnosed with ASPD or dissocial personality disorder will have psychopathy (Hare, 1996; Ogloff, 2006).

As noted by Ogloff (2006), the distinctions among the three antisocial conceptualizations are such that findings based on one diagnostic group are not necessarily applicable to the others and produce different prevalence rates in justice-involved populations. Adding a further layer of complexity, therapists will encounter patients who possess a mixture of features from all three diagnostic systems rather than a prototypical presentation of any one disorder. For these reasons, we use the terms "antisocial," "antisociality," and "antisocial patients" throughout this chapter rather than a particular diagnostic label. Although court-mandated or correctional settings may be the most common for the treatment of patients who are antisocial, such individuals are also commonly encountered at substance abuse rehabilitation centers, and occasionally appear in general outpatient psychotherapy or counseling for help with collateral issues (e.g., relationship and vocational difficulties).

DIFFERENTIAL AND CO-OCCURRING DIAGNOSES

A single arrest, even for a violent offense, should not be construed as synonymous with the presence of antisocial patterns. Clinically it is important to distinguish incidents of criminal behavior from the constellation of signs that characterize an antisocial person. Furthermore, it is essential to distinguish criminal behavior that occurs as a consequence of another disorder such as a substance abuse, bipolar, or psychotic disorder from criminal behavior that occurs *in addition to* the symptoms associated with these disorders. For example, a patient with a heroin addiction who does not have significant antisocial patterns may commit larcenies in order to support his or her habit, a pattern that ceases when he or she is clean. In contrast, a patient who is antisocial with a heroin addiction would be expected to engage in a variety of criminal behaviors related to, and unrelated to, his or her addiction. Obviously a substance abuse, bipolar, or psychotic disorder can be co-occurring with an antisocial diagnosis. Such cases are associated with greater symptom severity and lower functioning than patients without a co-occurring antisocial diagnosis (Mueser et al., 2012).

Therapists concerned about the truthfulness or reliability of the self-report of a patient who is antisocial should attempt to obtain relevant documents, such as previous treatment and/or legal records. Collateral information is particularly useful in determining if and how much the patient's perspectives on his or her criminal and other antisocial activities may be distorted. For example, when asked about his experience of incarceration, Warren said that he had generally gotten along well with the correctional officers and had only a few problems with other prisoners, leading to the clinical impression that he had adjusted well to custody. However, a review of his correctional records indicated that he received well over 50 disciplinary reports and spent significant time in administrative segregation.

CONCEPTUALIZATION

Patients who are antisocial are somewhat bewildering in terms of beliefs and cognitions. Their cognitive life could be likened to a mirror image of persons with depressive and anxiety problems. For example, patients who are antisocial are unlikely to harshly blame and judge themselves when faced with criticism, as is common in patients who are depressed. In fact, patients who are antisocial often express little concern for the opinions of others or for how their actions affect others. Nor are they likely to overestimate and exaggerate potential dangers, as is common in patients suffering with anxiety difficulties. Patients who are antisocial have a tendency to underestimate danger, seeking out risky situations precisely because of the excitement they afford.

Criminal Thinking

A valuable aid in conceptualizing the cognitive life of patients who are antisocial can be found in the empirical literature that has developed around the assessment of *criminal thinking patterns* (thinking patterns that facilitate criminal and self-destructive behavior). At least seven criminal thinking assessment instruments have appeared in the literature since the mid-1990s: the Psychological Inventory of Criminal Thinking Styles (PICTS; Walters, 1995), Criminal Sentiments Scale—Modified (CSS-M; Simourd, 1997), Measure of Criminal Attitudes and Associates (MCAA; Mills, Kroner, & Forth, 2002), Texas Christian University Criminal Thinking Scales (TCU CTS; Knight, Garner, Simpson, Morey, & Flynn, 2006), Measure of Offender Thinking Styles (MOTS; Mandracchia, Morgan, Garos, & Garland, 2007), Criminogenic Thinking Profile (CTP; Mitchell & Tafrate, 2012), and Criminal Cognitions Scale (Tangney et al., 2012). Each instrument measures multiple thinking patterns (ranging from three to eight), which have been derived from a variety of theoretical conceptualizations found in criminology and psychology (e.g., traditional cognitive-behavioral therapy [CBT], neutralization theory, psychopathy, and differential association theory). As recommended by Kroner and Morgan (2014), administering more than one criminal thinking instrument can provide therapists with a useful range of potentially relevant thinking targets for intervention.

Looking across all the instruments, the total number of thinking patterns adds up to an unwieldy 37. However, there is a degree of overlapping content in the nature of the thinking patterns measured by the various instruments, and taking this overlap into account reduces the number of distinct thinking patterns to a more clinically manageable 13 (Seeler, Freeman, DiGuiseppe, & Mitchell, 2014). These patterns can be broadly categorized into those that pertain to beliefs about self and others, and those that pertain to interacting with the environment:

- Self and others
  1. *Identifying with, and seeking approval from, criminal associates* (e.g., "I don't have anything in common with people who live a straight life").
  2. *Disregard for others, lack of empathy, lack of remorse, and callousness* (e.g., "There's no point worrying about people you hurt").
  3. *Avoiding intimacy and vulnerability* (e.g., "If I open up to someone, they will take advantage of me").
  4. *Hostility and suspiciousness toward criminal justice personnel* (e.g., "The cops are the real criminals").
  5. *Grandiosity and entitlement* (e.g., "All women want me").
  6. *Seeking dominance and control over others* (e.g., "Nobody can tell me what to do").
- Interacting with the environment
  7. *Demand for excitement and thrill seeking* (e.g., "There is no better feeling than the rush I get when stealing").
  8. *Exploiting and manipulating situations/relationships for personal gain* (e.g., "It doesn't make sense to work full time if you can get on a government program").
  9. *Hostility toward rules, regulations, and laws* (e.g., "Laws are there to hurt you, not help you").
  10. *Justifying, minimizing, and excuse making related to harmful behaviors* (e.g., "If I don't sell drugs in my neighborhood, somebody else will").
  11. *Willfully lazy attitude, path of least resistance* (e.g., "Everything will take care of itself").
  12. *Giving up in the face of adversity* (e.g., "When I don't understand things, I give up").
  13. *Underestimating negative consequences* (e.g., "I'll never go to jail for selling drugs because I know all my customers").

In general, criminal thinking patterns seem to operate at the level of intermediate beliefs, as they are neither as fixed and global as schemas, nor as situation specific as automatic thoughts. An emerging literature on schema-focused therapy for patients with antisocial and aggressive personality patterns may be helpful to interested readers (e.g., Bernstein, Arntz, & de Vos, 2007; Keulen-de Vos, Bernstein, & Arntz, 2014; Sun, 2014). Our focus on the intermediate belief level in conceptualization is not intended to negate the importance of schemas in personality pathology. We focus on intermediate beliefs as a useful starting place for conceptualization and treatment because they can be reliably assessed, and criminal thinking instruments are readily available, free to use, and easily administered and scored.

Interplay of Criminal Thinking across Life Areas

Our conceptualization of Warren provides an example of how criminal thinking patterns may be reflected in criminality and a variety of noncriminal problem behaviors. Although subjected to frequent urinalyses while on parole, Warren continued to engage in recreational marijuana use and tested positive, risking a return to prison. He believed he could "time" his marijuana smoking relative to his appointments so that he would not test positive, and he believed that his parole officer would not violate him for a positive test result (number 13 from the list above). He was noncompliant with his anger management program because he did not think it was necessary to attend since he had already completed one in prison years ago for a prior charge, thinking "You can't violate me for not attending a program I've basically already done" (9 and 13). Discussions around his prior street robberies revealed the belief that he was a uniquely skilled criminal who was too clever to be caught (5 and 13). When discussing the impact of his crimes on others, Warren expressed a marked disregard: "I didn't care. What I needed, they had, and I had to go get it . . I wanted certain things, the finest clothes, the finest jewelry . . I felt sorry, maybe, if I got caught, but as far as the victim, I didn't feel remorse" (2).

Warren's criminal thinking manifested in a variety of ways that put him at risk for recidivism. First, he had little interest in severing ties with his friends who used and sold drugs and engaged in other criminal activities: "We have been tight for a long time" (1). Second, opportunities to connect with prosocial family members were at a standstill because he had severed contact after they declined to provide him with housing after his most recent release from prison. This had been preceded by years of borrowing money without paying it back, and relying on them for shelter and food without thanks. From his perspective, however, his behavior had not been a problem because "They're family, they're supposed to help me out, and they have plenty to give me" (8). Third, he had not taken advantage of educational opportunities in prison, "The education I had from the streets is as valuable and maybe even more valuable than the education other people get from school," and searching for employment was complicated by the fact that he believed the jobs available to him (unskilled) were beneath his capabilities and talents (5). He was reluctant to start at a low-wage job and work his way up, expecting immediate recognition and promotion (5).

KEY TREATMENT GOALS

Other ways in which patients who are antisocial differ from patients with traditional mental health symptoms are in their perceptions of the need for change, and the consequences of *not changing*. Patients who experience depressive and anxious symptoms often perceive themselves as suffering, and they seek symptom relief. The consequences of not addressing their symptoms are more harmful to themselves than to anyone else. In contrast, patients who are antisocial may find their criminal and harmful patterns rewarding and egosyntonic. Their interest in changing such patterns may be quite minimal, even something to actively resist, as they lack the sort of subjective distress that usually motivates personal change. Even when negative consequences arise, patients who are antisocial typically see the locus of their difficulties as external and independent of their own behavior. They frequently view themselves as victims of unfair, prejudiced, or hostile treatment at the hands of individuals or institutions. From their perspective, the problem and need for change resides in other people and institutions and not in their own behavior. The consequences of not addressing their disorder (future criminality and victimization) are more harmful to others than themselves. Thus, although there are many observable signs of antisocial personality, the disorder is asymptomatic in the sense that there is little internal distress or motivation for change.

These differences in perceived need for change and the consequences of maintaining the status quo have significant implications for treatment. First, therapists may have to devote considerable energy toward engaging the patient in identifying treatment goals, much more so than ordinarily required for patients with traditional mental health symptoms. Second, the harm to others and society caused by criminality and victimization means that an overarching goal of treatment should be the reduction of criminal and manipulative behavior, even though such activity may be perceived as rewarding, legitimate, or justified by the patient.

The Risk–Need–Responsivity Model

The identification and the reduction of the risk factors specifically linked with continued criminal behavior have been the subject of a large body of theoretical and empirical work connected with the risk–need–responsivity (RNR) model of offender assessment and rehabilitation developed by Andrews, Bonta, and Hoge (1990). Although the RNR model may be unfamiliar to therapists who have worked in traditional mental health settings, it has been increasingly influential in correctional assessment and treatment. Each component of the model is briefly described below and interested therapists are encouraged to consult Andrews, Bonta, and Hoge (1990) and Andrews and Bonta (2010) for further reading.

The *risk* component addresses the dosage of intervention, and holds that intensity of intervention should be adjusted depending on the patient's risk of recidivism. Higher-risk patients should receive more services than lower-risk cases. The *need* component addresses the target(s) of intervention, and holds that intervention should focus on specific factors linked with a patient's risk to recidivate. The *responsivity* component addresses the interplay between the patient and intervention. Interventions should be consistent with the learning style, ability, and motivation of the patient as much as possible to achieve greater success.

The risk factors most linked to recidivism have been referred to as the "Central Eight" (Andrews, Bonta, & Wormith, 2006) and are presented in Table 16.1. The RNR model draws a distinction between *static* risk factors (those that cannot be changed such as prior criminal behavior) and *dynamic* risk factors (those that can be changed such as current substance abuse). Among dynamic risk factors, a further distinction is made between those that are *criminogenic needs* (those most strongly related to reoffending such as criminal thinking and criminal companions, etc.) and *less criminogenic needs* (those only weakly related to reoffending such as self-esteem, physical health, etc.). Assessment of the Central Eight can be done through clinical interview or the use of a standardized instrument such as the Level of Service Inventory—Revised (LSI-R; Andrews & Bonta, 1995), Correctional Offender Management Profiling for Alternative Sanctions (COMPAS; Northpointe Instituted for Public Management, 1996), or Ohio Risk Assessment System (ORAS; Latessa, Smith, Lemke, Makarios, & Lowenkamp, 2009).

Of the Central Eight risk factors, only one is static (history of antisocial behavior). The remaining seven are considered criminogenic needs because they are subject to changes that can increase or decrease a patient's risk profile for future offending. Two of the seven criminogenic needs are antisocial personality and criminal thinking. The remaining five represent a variety of ancillary problems (e.g., substance use, unproductive use of leisure time) that facilitate criminal and self-destructive behavior. Addressing those ancillary factors along with the patient's criminal thinking are key treatment goals when working with antisocial patients (Andrews & Bonta, 2010; Andrews & Dowden, 2005; Latessa, 2004). The first meta-analysis of correctional treatment found that programs adhering to RNR principles had greater reductions in recidivism, whereas generic programs had a limited impact on recidivism, and incarceration without any treatment or rehabilitation attempts was associated with increases in recidivism (Andrews, Zinger, et al., 1990). CBT modalities were particularly highlighted as effective, a finding that has been replicated in subsequent meta-analyses (Landenberger & Lipsey, 2005; Lipsey, Chapman, & Landenberger, 2001).

Returning to the case of Warren, we consider his standing on criminogenic needs and find that he is at high risk for future criminal behavior:

- *Antisocial personality/criminal thinking.* Warren's thinking patterns associated with criminal and other antisocial behavior are targets to address throughout the treatment process (thinking patterns 1, 2, 5, 8, 9,

TABLE 16.1. Central Eight Criminal Risk Variables

Risk factors	Key aspects
1. History of antisocial behavior	A pattern of antisocial behavior starting in childhood and continuing into adulthood
2. Antisocial personality	Signs and symptoms of ASPD, dissocial personality disorder, and psychopathy
3. Antisocial cognition (criminal thinking)	Attitudes, values, and beliefs that facilitate antisocial and self-destructive behavior
4. Antisocial associates	Close association with, or seeking approval from, antisocial friends; relative isolation from prosocial influences
5. Family/marital	Family and marital bonds that lack nurturance and ignore, reinforce, or model antisocial behavior
6. School/work	Low levels of performance and satisfaction in school or work; negative attitudes toward school/work
7. Leisure/recreation	Low levels of enjoyment and satisfaction in prosocial pursuits; engages in risky activities; enjoyment of antisocial activities
8. Substance abuse	Abuse of alcohol or drugs; positive attitude toward use

and 13). These patterns are also likely to be related to his problems in the other criminogenic need areas noted below.

• *Criminal friends and associates.* Warren is reluctant to sever ties with his former antisocial friends. He has yet to develop a network of pro-social friends who could provide support and modeling. Therefore, one treatment goal for Warren might be engaging in activities to meet and develop new prosocial acquaintances.

• *Family.* His relationship with his family is poor, which is a source of particular concern because in his case, his family members could provide opportunities for prosocial contact and support. Repairing his relationship with his family is one possible treatment goal. Had Warren been highly enmeshed with a family involved in criminal and other antisocial activities, a treatment goal might have been the avoidance of family members and the nurturance of new extrafamilial relationships.

• *Employment.* Warren is unemployed and his attitude toward a job search is not productive. One immediate treatment goal would target his thinking about work with a longer-term goal of involvement in a vocational program to obtain skilled employment.

• *Leisure.* Warren has no involvement in structured prosocial pursuits such as sports, hobbies, community service, or spiritual activities. Because he has significant downtime in his day-to-day life another treatment goal is the development of productive leisure activities.

• *Substance use.* Warren's continued marijuana use is putting him at risk for a parole violation and return to incarceration. An immediate treatment goal would be abstinence from marijuana. On the positive side, Warren has not used alcohol since his release from prison and sees his continued abstinence from alcohol as an important goal.

RNR and Traditional Mental Health Symptoms

Notably absent from the Central Eight are depression, anxiety, low self-esteem, and other common mental health symptoms. These symptoms are related to recidivism, but not as strongly as the Central Eight and are therefore classified as less criminogenic in the RNR model. Focusing on them is unlikely to have an impact on the antisocial patient's future criminality. In fact, a recent study found that for patients with both significant mental health symptoms and criminogenic risks/needs, focusing solely on the mental health components produced limited effects on recidivism (Guzzo, Cadeau, Hogg, & Brown, 2012). Even patients who are antisocial with severe mental health symptoms will require interventions that directly address their criminogenic needs to impact their reoffending. In cases in which the mental health symptoms are particularly severe, alleviating psychological distress is important so that patients who are antisocial can later work on criminogenic needs. However, alleviating distress does not replace the importance of intervention around those factors most associated with future criminality.

COLLABORATIVE STRATEGY

In spite of images from reality television, a "get tough" or "get real" approach with patients who are antisocial is not advocated. Confrontation quickly leads to disengagement and loss of forward momentum. Because of the motivational challenges posed by patients who are antisocial, therapist qualities such as being warm, collaborative, directive, rewarding, and quickly understanding a patient's perspective are perhaps even more critical with this population. In addition, prior to utilizing more structured and directive CBT interventions, effective therapists will take the time to establish a good working relationship, eliciting from the patient his or her motivations for making changes, exploring the impact of antisocial patterns on the patient's life, investigating potential strengths, and delving into what he or she values most. A sophisticated arsenal of engagement skills is a prerequisite for working effectively with this population.

Motivational Interviewing

Motivational interviewing (MI), or adaptations of MI, is an essential skill set in forensic practice. Within CBT, MI has an immediate practical advantage in moving patients toward greater engagement and collaboration and moving therapists away from confrontation, advice giving, and interventions for which the patient is not yet ready. MI is a complex therapeutic style comprising four broad and dynamic processes: treatment engagement, focus, evoking intrinsic motivation, and planning change (Miller & Rollnick, 2013). MI conversations are characterized as nonjudgmental, nonconfrontational, respectful, inquisitive, supportive, and collaborative, emphasizing client autonomy and self-direction. MI practice also uses twice as many reflections as questions, strong emphasis on open questions (rather than closed), and skillful reinforcement of the patient's own reasons for change.

The process of evoking the patient's own reason and means for behavior change lies at the strategic heart of MI. Two terms are relevant to the evoking process: *sustain talk* and *change talk*. Sustain talk involves client counterchange verbalizations that favor maintaining the status quo or not changing (Miller & Rollnick, 2013). In the case of Warren, an example of sustain talk would be "Smoking pot is no big deal, my parole officer rarely tests me." Change talk is any client speech that favors movement toward and commitment to change: "If I decided to, I could stop smoking pot." A predominance of change talk predicts actual behavior change, whereas a higher proportion of sustain talk—or equal levels of sustain talk and change talk—are predictive of not changing (Moyers, Martin, Houck, Christopher, & Tonigan, 2009).

Levels of client change talk relative to sustain talk can be influenced (Glynn & Moyers, 2010), and skillful MI yields increasing levels of client change talk over time. Thus, those practicing MI "key into" client language related to change and facilitate its expression. For many CBT-trained therapists, learning MI involves adding a new lens with which to view patient language. A more complete discussion of incorporating MI into forensic practice can be found in Tafrate and Luther (2014).

Review of Signs and Symptoms

Another engagement strategy is to review the symptom lists with patients (e.g., ASPD, dissocial personality disorder, psychopathy). Antisociality can be framed as a "lifestyle disorder" that develops over time. Individuals usually remain unaware of its signs, and if not addressed, the lifestyle disorder will result in negative long-term consequences (e.g., damaged relationships, vocational maladjustment, financial instability, and incarceration). The patient can be reminded that this is a serious disorder that affects judgment and behavior. Therapy is an opportunity to evaluate potential changes before the damage gets worse. Patients are then asked to review the signs and note the ones that fit, and don't fit, with their own history and patterns. Patients can be asked, "Which of these patterns have you noticed in your life?" Once a pattern is identified, further exploration can follow (e.g., "When did the pattern first emerge?" "How has this pattern negatively affected your life?" "What is at stake if you do not change it?" and "What steps could you take to change this pattern?").

Reviewing signs of antisociality raises patient awareness about important behavioral clusters that may not have been previously viewed as part of a unified problem. One benefit for patients is that seemingly disparate behaviors become connected and seen as part of an overarching theme, helping to make sense of problems in multiple areas of the patient's life. For example, a patient may acknowledge that chronic lying, irritability, and failure to sustain consistent employment have been disruptive experiences in his or her life, but has never viewed these issues as being part of the same problem constellation. It is important to keep in mind that the purpose of reviewing signs is not to label the patient. In fact, we recommend in such discussions with patients avoiding the use of labels such as "antisocial," "sociopath," or "psychopath," not only because these labels may trigger reactance and argumentativeness but also because these labels signify "badness" and evoke distressed emotions that undermine treatment engagement. The objective is to raise patients' awareness of the negative consequences associated with their long-standing and pervasive behavior patterns.

Focus on Strengths and Values

Acknowledging a patient's strengths helps to bring him or her on board with our change efforts. Perhaps the most well known of the strengths-based approaches for patients who are antisocial is the good lives model (GLM; Ward & Brown, 2004). Within the GLM, working with patients who are antisocial to desist from high-risk behaviors (avoidance goals) is conceptualized as only part of the change process; helping them develop behavioral paths to a life worth living (approach goals) is an equally important component. The strategy is to discover competencies, enhance them, and utilize them to reduce risk factors. For example, Warren expressed the desire to use his experiences with the criminal justice system to help at-risk adolescents from his neighborhood stay out of the system. Developing this approach goal for Warren naturally led to volunteering his time in several organizations, which was a more productive use of his leisure time, reduced his exposure to criminal acquaintances, and fostered relationships with new noncriminally minded people.

One important contribution of acceptance-based CBT approaches is a focus on exploring and clarifying patient values (Amrod & Hayes, 2014). In acceptance and commitment therapy (ACT), a distinction is made between goals and values. Values provide anchor points to guide future behavioral choices, helping to reduce choices that interfere with core values and increasing behavioral activation plans likely to lead to a more meaningful life. For example, a patient who is antisocial might have a goal of successfully completing parole, and therefore attend a mandated domestic violence program. That goal might end once parole supervision is completed, while the underlying value of "having positive family relationships" might be pursued in a variety of ways long after supervision ends. Once core values are identified, patients can be regularly asked "What is one thing you could do this week that would be consistent with that value?"

We have noticed in our consulting work a degree of concern among therapists that discussions about core values will be counterproductive because patients who are antisocial may hold values and goals that are at odds with prosocial and healthy change (e.g., being the most respected drug dealer in their city). In actual practice however, patients who are antisocial are similar to traditional patients: they desire opportunities to provide for family, connect with others, have meaningful work, and so on. In the majority of instances, antisocial patterns are typically inconsistent with patient values, and are a reflection of unskilled attempts to meet one's values and cope (albeit unproductively) with the challenges of life. This is not to say that therapists will never encounter patients possessing antisocial values, it is just not as common as people expect. Of course, even with the highest skill levels, therapists will not be effective with all patients who are antisocial. The important point is that prematurely assuming that the majority of patients who are antisocial have inherently antisocial values shuts the door for powerful discussions about what matters most. Although Warren had not been much of a father to his son, this was a source of regret and remorse rather than a source of pride or indifference. This issue was heightened when he recently found out his son had been arrested. One of the values that Warren verbalized was to reconnect with, and help, his son.

CLINICAL APPLICATION OF THE INTERVENTION

Criminal thinking patterns are beliefs that affect choices and behaviors, which if unaltered, ultimately influence one's life trajectory. The goal of

CBT with patients who are antisocial is to alter the thinking patterns behind decision making that results in subsequent harm to self or others, while increasing decisions that lead to productive behaviors, prosocial outcomes, and ultimately a nondestructive life. In this section, we present three strategies to impact antisocial patterns and decision making.

CBT Sequences Focused on Criminogenic Risks/Needs

Conversations, or CBT sequences, can clarify how criminal thinking patterns affect decision making in life areas connected to the Central Eight risk factors. For example, one risk factor for Warren was his continued involvement with peers who were antisocial. Below is a sample CBT sequence that may be appropriate for patients whose decisions are negatively influenced by companions. In conducting CBT sequences, therapists should remember to reflect back patient verbalizations about thinking as well as any change talk that emerges.

F-T-D Sequence: Friend–Thoughts–Decisions

1. Discuss the high-risk FRIEND and the role the friend plays in high-risk behavior.

   "Looking back over the past year, tell me about a relative, friend, or acquaintance of yours who tends to get in trouble with the law or who you think is probably a bad influence on you in some ways. What is it about this person that makes him or her a bad influence or that seems to lead to trouble? What makes it hard to avoid spending time with him or her?"

2. Explore the risky DECISIONS connected with this person.

   "Give me an example of some of the trouble you have gotten into with this person."

   Or

   "Give me an example of something you did with this person that you think was probably bad for you, or self-defeating."

3. Explore the THOUGHTS preceding the risky decisions related to this person.

   "What were you telling yourself when you agreed to [insert incident]?"

   Or

   "What was going through your mind when you went along with [insert person]?"

4. Explore a better DECISION related to avoiding this person's influence.

> "Give me an example of a time when you were able to avoid this person's influence and get out of a potentially bad situation with him/her."

5. Explore the THOUGHTS preceding the better decision.

> "What was going through your mind when didn't go along with [insert person]?"
>
> Or
>
> "How was your thinking different when you [insert positive incident]?"

6. Summarize the contrast in THINKING that leads to the two different decisions.

> "So, summing up the connection between [insert person] and bad outcomes, it sounds like you're thinking _____; while the times you've made better decisions, you're thinking was more like this _____."[1]

Self-Monitoring and Restructuring Intermediate Beliefs

Another strategy is to identify a criminal thinking pattern, one of the 13 from the list presented earlier, that affects the patient's decision making and make it the focus of ongoing self-monitoring and cognitive restructuring. One of the more difficult patterns in the case of Warren is disregard for others (2). It is best for therapists is to present the pattern in nonjudgmental language, as a potential area of exploration. This pattern would be introduced to Warren by saying the following: "Based on our discussions, and the way you filled in the questionnaires, it seems like you have a tendency to look out for yourself and not think about how your actions affect others. I'm wondering if we could take a look at that pattern and explore its impact on your everyday life."

If Warren seems amenable to this exploration, then the Thinking Helpsheet (Figure 16.1) can be introduced and become the focus of subsequent sessions. In Part I, Warren and his therapist would collaboratively discuss how disregard for others has repeatedly led to poor decisions, damaged relationships, and possibly contributed to criminal behavior. In Part II, Warren provides his recollection of one specific occasion where

---

[1]For additional scripts of CBT sequences around criminogenic risks/needs readers can contact Damon Mitchell. We would like to acknowledge Tom Hogan for his contributions in developing CBT sequences.

Part I: To be completed by the practitioner

Thinking pattern:

Part II: To be completed by the client

Identify a situation where the thinking pattern emerged: Specify what happened, where, and who was involved.	Circle the problem area or areas related to the situation.	Immediate thinking: Write a sentence or two that captures what was going through your mind during the situation.	Better thinking: Write down another way of thinking that led you to a better decision or that would have led you in a better direction in this situation.
	Friends and associates Family Substance use Employment or education Leisure or downtime Other: _____	**Thinking:** **Actual decision:** Write down what you ended up doing.	**Thinking:**

FIGURE 16.1. Thinking Helpsheet.

361

the belief influenced a decision. In the third column, he would sum up his thinking on that occasion, trying to capture as accurately as possible his perspective (immediate thinking) at the time. The fourth column provides an opportunity for Warren to formulate an alternative perspective (better thinking), which may have led to a different outcome. In the Actual Decision section, he reviews the original choice (which reflects the influence of the intermediate belief) and then contrasts it with a choice that might have followed if the alternative belief was adopted. Between sessions Warren would be asked to monitor this specific thought pattern around his everyday decision making.

Decision Review

Therapists may also wish to use a structured format for reviewing different problem areas and evaluating the "risk–benefit ratio" of various patient choices. The Decision Helpsheet (Figure 16.2) may be adapted for homework or modified to meet patients' specified needs. This format allows for a wide variety of scenarios for the patient to identify as problematic, assists them in considering possible actions and rating the advantages and disadvantages of each course of action. On top, the patient describes the problem area, including the facts regarding the situation. Some examples, in the case of Warren, might include problematic family relationships, difficulties finding employment, or the risk of continued marijuana use.

Below, the Possible Decisions column is for listing as many options as possible. This column would typically include a mixture of current maladaptive behaviors, as well as more adaptive and socially acceptable alternatives. Options in the Possible Decisions column incorporate the patient's immediate, "automatic" reactions, as well as prosocial choices resulting from discussions between the patient and therapist. Warren's Possible Decisions column might consist of "Avoiding friends who smoke marijuana," and "Trying to come up with activities other than smoking marijuana when I experience boredom." The two adjacent columns consist of advantages and disadvantages of each decision listed. In this section, the therapist assists in generating likely outcomes the patient might not consider. After listing the advantages and disadvantages of each decision, the patient rates the effectiveness of each possible choice on his or her life, using the 0–10 scale (0 being most ineffective and 10 being most effective). Subsequent therapeutic sessions should include ongoing reviews of the behavioral choices listed, along with an evaluation of their effectiveness. Repeated ineffective choices could indicate a need to review and/or revise the previously identified advantages and disadvantages, or identify specific skill deficits that need to be addressed. Alternatively, the patient may need to process his or her continued ineffective choices, as they may result from unrecognized intermediate beliefs.

Describe a current situation that will require a decision.

Possible decisions: List three or four possible decision options.	Pros: Describe likely advantage of decision.	Cons: Describe likely disadvantage of decision.	Effectiveness: Rate likely effectiveness of decision from 0 to 10 (0 = highly ineffective, 10 = highly effective).
1.			
2.			
3.			
4.			

FIGURE 16.2. Decision Helpsheet.

PROGRESS, LIFESPAN, AND TERMINATION CONSIDERATIONS

Both behavioral and cognitive gains are more likely to be maintained if the patient who is antisocial is able to identify emotionally compelling reasons to implement the strategies learned in treatment. Thus, it may be helpful to regularly review with individual patients their small successes along the way to raise awareness of, and reinforce, positive change. In addition, opportunities to enhance prosocial relationships and networks should be introduced and encouraged whenever possible.

A unique aspect of working with patients under court or correctional supervision is the potential lack of input and planning related to termination of treatment. For example, both prisoner and correctional mental health provider may be given no warning about the prisoner's transfer from one institution to another, leading to an abrupt and premature termination of treatment. Similarly, both probationer and outpatient therapist may be given no warning about a revocation, resulting in an unplanned treatment termination. Such endings may exacerbate dysfunctional thinking and behavior patterns. To minimize patient harm and the potential loss of treatment gains, therapists should discuss the possibility of unwanted termination early in treatment and develop a plan, if possible, to counter negative reactions and resume care.

COMMON CHALLENGES AND CLINICIAN SELF-CARE

Whether prisoner or outpatient, the motivation for patients who are antisocial coming to treatment often results from an external source demanding "change." The court, correctional system, family members, or employers may provide the patient with an ultimatum of treatment versus incarceration, denial of parole, loss of a job, expulsion from school, alienation from the family, and so on. Thus, the motivation for change, participation in treatment, and making changes in behavior of patients who are antisocial may be low or oppositional. Unfortunately, a recent meta-analysis found that mandated treatment for offenders was generally ineffective in reducing recidivism, whereas voluntary treatment was associated with reductions in recidivism (Parhar, Wormith, Derkzen, & Beauregard, 2008). This suggests that patients who are mandated can be most successful when they develop an interest in change akin to that of their voluntary counterparts. Therapists should strive to have patients who say they are "forced to be here," come to say they "want to make changes anyway" (Tafrate, Mitchell, & Novaco, 2014).

Just as the therapist must be aware of, and respond calmly and appropriately to, the patient's transference behaviors, the therapist must also monitor for his or her own automatic, and often negative, emotional responses to the patient. For example, the therapist may feel manipulated by a patient who repeatedly misses sessions with questionable or even ludicrous excuses. Posing even more of a countertransference challenge, patients who are antisocial may also attempt to exaggerate or malinger symptoms, hoping to obtain a prescription for a controlled substance, cell change, sympathetic response from the court, and so on. In this latter case, it is most important to separate the identifiable psychological problems and appropriate treatment from the attempted manipulation, while striving to maintain a collaborative relationship. Therapists must keep in mind that collaboration may be 80–20, or 90–10, with the therapist initially carrying the greater burden that brings with it a high level of therapist stress and burnout (Freeman, Pretzer, Fleming, & Simon, 1990).

CONCLUSION

We encourage CBT practitioners not to shy away from working with patients who are antisocial, as it presents opportunities to provide a service that contributes to the safety of our communities, reduce the human suffering caused by criminal victimization, and affords these patients a chance for a more positive future. Although patients who are antisocial may be expected to show little initial interest in treatment, the integration of techniques from MI, review of the losses due to antisocial patterns, and discussion around core values can heighten their awareness of their need for change and direct them toward prosocial behaviors consistent with their own values. Once engaged, we recommend a therapeutic focus on the patient's thinking and decision making around criminogenic risks/needs, as those areas put him or her most at risk for continued antisocial conduct. The ensuing therapeutic process is one of altering the thinking patterns that have facilitated the antisocial behaviors, while encouraging decisions that lead to pursuing core values and, hopefully, a more fulfilling life.

CHAPTER 17

Borderline Personality Disorder

Arnoud Arntz

Borderline personality disorder (BPD) can be characterized by the remarkable instability that pervades many if not all aspects of personality functioning, including relationships, self-image, affect, and behavior. For example, Natasha, a 29-year-old who had been married for several years, sought help after being "too tired" to work for more than a year, lying in bed for most of the day. Her problems seemed to have started with a relationship conflict at work that affected her performance. She started an affair with her boss, despite his engagement to another woman. Natasha ended it when he proceeded with the marriage that he had planned before the affair. She felt strongly disappointed by him and started an affair with someone else. According to Natasha, her boss resented this, gave her work below her former level, and criticized her so much in front of other personnel that she became "burned out." Diagnostic impression after the first interview was an adjustment disorder with mixed emotional features and relational problems. After the second interview, the picture was much more complicated. She described her marriage as characterized by lots of fights and aggressive threats, expressed resentment toward her family, and admitted high use of cannabis and alcohol. She repeatedly said that she found that life had no use and expressed mistrust of other people. When asked what should be done in treatment, her answers were rather vague, such as "I have to feel at home with myself." Although the therapist thought that Natasha probably suffered from high levels of anxiety, sadness, and loneliness, she presented a tough appearance, and it was easy to imagine how this could provoke others to anger.

Noting evidence of further psychopathology, the therapist proceeded with semistructured clinical interviews. In addition to a number of symptomatic disorders, it became clear that Natasha's problems met the criteria of BPD, including many unresolved emotional problems related to her youth and relationships with her parents. The clinician raised the possibility that BPD was the main problem and they discussed the pros and cons of treating her long-standing personality problems. Natasha decided to start with a long-term cognitive therapy (CT) focused on personality problems. She reasoned that something fundamental should be done with the way she felt about herself and other people, and she wanted to emotionally process the painful experiences she had had with her parents.

BPD is a relatively common disorder (1.1–2.5% of the general adult population, usually about 70% women; American Psychiatric Association, 2013; Lieb, Zanarini, Schmahl, Linehan, & Bohus, 2004), with enormous societal costs, comparable to schizophrenia (Linehan & Heard, 1999; van Asselt, Dirksen, Arntz, & Severens, 2007), high risk of suicide (about 8–10% die because of suicide in a 10- to 15-year period (Lieb et al., 2004; Paris, 1993), more than 50 times higher percentage than in the general population (Pompili, Girardi, Ruberto, & Tatarelli, 2005), and considerable impairment in the individual's life. The proportion of patients with BPD generally rises with the intensity of the health care treatment setting, from less than 10% in outpatient facilities to more than 50% in specialized inpatient units (American Psychiatric Association, 2013). Patients with BPD are a burden for relatives, friends, and colleagues, and there is a high risk that they induce psychopathology in their offspring (Stepp, Whalen, Pilkonis, Hipwell, & Levine, 2011; Weiss et al., 1996). Many individuals with BPD are intelligent and gifted people, but their disorder prevents them from developing themselves, and many have troubles finishing education, do not work at all, or have jobs below their capacities. Although BPD symptoms often reduce with treatment, social functioning, societal participation, and quality of life remain long-lasting problems and should be more focused on in treatment (Gunderson et al., 2011; Zanarini, Jacoby, Frankenburg, Reich, & Fitzmaurice, 2009). Relational crises are common, including intense ups and downs in relationships with friends and colleagues. Most patients with BPD injure themselves (60–70%), though this is not unique to BPD, and they often abuse substances, usually as a form of self-medication. Although most patients with BPD seen in mental health care centers are female, male patients with BPD are prevalent in settings like forensic institutions and addiction clinics. Patients with BPD are also heavy users of physical health care facilities (van Asselt et al., 2007). Many seek help because of a crisis or because of posttraumatic stress disorder, depression, or addiction. They should be helped to view their difficulties in the perspective of their personality problems, simultaneously installing hope that these problems can be treated.

Notorious for their angry outbursts and their crises, patients with BPD have a bad reputation in health care, and many therapists are afraid of them. The belief that these people cannot really be helped is widespread. Recent research proves that this view is incorrect. Specialized forms of CT are among the most promising treatment options available. Although CT for BPD is in no way simple, many therapists have discovered that with this framework, treatment of individuals with BPD is a successful and rewarding experience.

CLINICAL SIGNS AND SYMPTOMS

Despite its high prevalence, BPD is often overlooked. When a clear, stable, and autonomous symptomatic disorder is the reason for seeking help, treatment may not be too problematic, though BPD might constitute a risk for treatment dropout (Arntz, 2014; Mulder, 2002). In many cases, however, the main problem is BPD and underdiagnosis constitutes a big problem that results in insufficient treatment.

DSM-IV-TR and DSM-5 describe BPD as characterized by instability and impulsivity. The instability can be evident in relationships that tend to be intense but are often suddenly stopped; in identity, with instability in self-views, ideals, future plans, and moral values; and in affect, with strong emotional reactions, which leads to sudden and strong switches among different emotions. Impulsivity manifests in potentially self-damaging activities that are rewarding in the short term but are engaged in impulsively, like spending, substance abuse, eating, and sex; in anger outbursts with difficulties with anger control; and in suicidal behavior and self-injury. Other criteria involve abandonment fears, with attempts to prevent being abandoned; chronic feelings of emptiness; and stress-related temporary paranoid experiences or dissociation. Five or more criteria need to be met to warrant a diagnosis of BPD. Although this theoretically leads to many possible combinations of BPD criteria, suggesting that patients with BPD differ considerably, the internal consistency of the criteria set, when treated as a dimension, is very high and suggests that the majority of these BPD features relate to one underlying dimension (Arntz et al., 2009; Giesen-Bloo et al, 2010). ICD-10 (World Health Organization, 2013) defines BPD as a subcategory of "emotionally unstable personality disorder" (F60.3). This broader personality disorder is defined as

> A personality disorder in which there is a marked tendency to act impulsively without consideration of the consequences, together with affective instability. The ability to plan ahead may be minimal, and outbursts of intense anger often lead to violence or "behavioural explosions" that are easily precipitated when impulsive acts are criticized or thwarted by others. Two variants of this

personality disorder are specified, and both share this general theme of impulsiveness and lack of self-control.

The subcategory borderline type (F60.31) is defined as follows:

Several of the characteristics of emotional instability are present; in addition, the patient's own self-image, aims, and internal preferences (including sexual) are often unclear or disturbed. There are usually chronic feelings of emptiness. A liability to become involved in intense and unstable relationships may cause repeated emotional crises and may be associated with excessive efforts to avoid abandonment and a series of suicidal threats or acts of self-harm (although these may occur without obvious precipitants). (World Health Organization, 2013).

The overarching emotionally unstable personality disorder impresses as relatively more impulsive and aggressive than BPD defined by DSM-5 criteria and more akin to antisocial personality disorder. The borderline type misses, compared with DSM-5 criteria: stress-related dissociative and psychotic episodes (DSM-5 criterion 9). The agreement between the two diagnostic systems has been found to be limited (NICE, 2009).

DIFFERENTIAL DIAGNOSIS

The usually high comorbidity associated with BPD may complicate diagnosis, especially in determining the primary diagnosis and initial treatment plan. Almost all disorders can be comorbid to BPD, notably mood disorders, substance abuse/dependence, anxiety disorders (especially social phobia and posttraumatic stress disorder), psychotic disorders, and other personality disorders. Because BPD is viewed as one of the most severe personality disorders, BPD is recommended as the primary personality diagnosis and treatment is adapted to address comorbid disorders along with the BPD. Antisocial and narcissistic personality disorders might be an exception, especially when criminal features are present.

Some disorders need priority in treatment when comorbid to BPD. Most prominent are bipolar disorder, severe depression, psychotic disorders (other than transient, stress-related psychosis, which overlaps with criterion 9 of BPD), substance abuse that needs (clinical) detoxification, attention-deficit/hyperactivity disorder, and anorexia nervosa. These disorders should be treated first. These disorders are also problematic because they partially overlap in criteria with BPD and can make the diagnosis of BPD highly problematic. Bipolar disorder, for instance, can be mistaken for BPD, or the other way around. Finally, some conditions can lead to apparent personality changes that are similar to BPD, such as posttraumatic stress disorder and chronic substance abuse (e.g., cocaine).

Structured assessment of both syndromal and personality disorders is perhaps the best safeguard against diagnostic mistakes. Given the high costs incurred by, and suffering of patients with BPD, and the difficult and long treatment, the effort of executing semistructured clinical interviews is minimal.

CONCEPTUALIZATION

There are, roughly speaking, three cognitive-behavioral conceptualizations of BPD: Linehan's dialectical–behavioral view, Beckian formulations, and Young's schema mode model.

Linehan's Dialectical–Behavioral View

According to Linehan's (1993) model, patients with BPD are characterized by a dysfunction in emotion regulation that is probably temperamental. This dysfunction causes both a strong reaction to stressful events and a long time until emotions return to baseline. A second assumption is that the environment of the patient with BPD was, and often still is, invalidating. Denying, punishing, or incorrect responses to emotional reactions of the child are hypothesized to contribute to the problems in regulating, understanding, and tolerating emotional reactions. Later on, patients with BPD invalidate their own emotional reactions and adopt an oversimplistic and unrealistic view toward emotions. Primary targets of treatment are inadequate emotional reactions, notably the poorly controlled expression of impulses and self-damaging behavior, including (para)suicidal behavior. Therapists use a dialectical stance, on the one hand accepting emotional pain (instead of trying to change it), and on the other hand changing antecedents of stress and the way the patient tries to cope with the emotions. Acquiring skills in emotion tolerance and regulation, as well as validating emotional reactions, are central to Linehan's dialectical behavior therapy (DBT). DBT was originally developed to treat (para)suicidal patients, before it was clear that most of these patients would be diagnosed with BPD. Of the specialized BDP treatments, DBT has been studied most often, though not necessarily in the methodological best studies (Stoffers et al., 2012). Effect sizes are on average moderate (Kliem, Kröger, & Kosfelder, 2010).

Beckian Formulations

Early Beckian formulations of BPD stressed the role of assumptions in the disorder. Beck, Freeman, and Associates (1990) hypothesized that a large number of assumptions common to other personality disorders are active in BPD. Pretzer (1990) further hypothesized that three key assumptions are central in BPD: "The world is dangerous and malevolent," "I am powerless and vulnerable," and "I am inherently unacceptable." The first assumption in combination with the second is hypothesized to lead to high levels of vigilance and interpersonal distrust. In addition to hypervigilance, two other cognitive characteristics are assumed to be central to BPD: dichotomous thinking and a weak sense of identity (i.e., a poorly articulated self-schema). The three key assumptions and the three cognitive characteristics are assumed to play a central role in the maintenance of the disorder and are consequently major targets for therapy. For instance, the somewhat paradoxical combination of dependent assumptions (the belief of the patient to be weak and incapable, whereas others are strong and capable) and paranoid assumptions (the belief that others cannot be trusted and are malevolent) are thought to fuel the unstable and extreme interpersonal behavior of the patient with BPD, alternating between clinging to other people and pushing others away out of distrust. Dichotomous thinking contributes to the emotional turmoil and extreme decisions, as lack of ability to evaluate things in grades of gray contributes to the abrupt and extreme shifts made by patients with BPD and should be addressed early in treatment, as soon as a working relationship is established.

Layden, Newman, Freeman, and Morse (1993) further elaborated the cognitive model and suggested numerous other biases and processes and related these to early child development and presumed stagnation of development of patients with BPD. Layden and colleagues (1993) also stress the role of nonverbal elements in core schemas of patients with BPD, which they also link to early preverbal development. Consequently, Layden and colleagues emphasize the use of experiential techniques, notably imagery work, in treatment. Arntz (1994) related Pretzer's (1990) observations to findings of high prevalence of childhood abuse in BPD, suggesting that the way the abuse was processed by the child led to the formation of the key assumptions and cognitive characteristics of the patient with BPD. He proposed an integration of Beckian here-and-now CT with historical work to process childhood abuse and correct pathogenic conclusions from the abuse. In accordance with Layden and colleagues, the importance of experiential methods in treatment of early childhood memories is stressed (see also Arntz, 2011; Arntz & Weertman, 1999). There are few studies testing Beckian CT for BPD. Brown, Newman, Charlesworth, Crits-Cristoph, and Beck (2004) tested CT in an open trial and found moderate effect sizes. Cottraux and colleagues (2009) compared CT with supportive Rogerian therapy, and found better treatment retention and some better effects in CT, but high dropout rates in both arms. Davidson and colleagues (2006) tested whether a limited number of CT sessions added to treatment as usual would have positive effects. On the primary outcome no evidence for this was found, but limited evidence was found on secondary outcomes (4 of 11 outcomes), notably on suicidal acts, and on the Young Schema

Questionnaire (Young, 2006). A cost-effectiveness study did not reveal notable differences between the two conditions in difference in costs versus difference in quality-adjusted life years (Palmer et al., 2006).

Young's Schema Mode Model

The conceptualization of the core pathology of BPD as stemming from a highly frightened, abused child who is left alone in a malevolent world, longing for safety and help but distrustful because of fear of further abuse and abandonment, is highly related to the schema model developed by Young (McGinn & Young, 1996). To understand the abrupt changes in the behavior of patients with BPD, Young elaborated on an idea, introduced in the 1980s by Aaron Beck in clinical workshops, that some pathological states of patients with BPD are a sort of regression into intense emotional states experienced as a child. Young conceptualized such states as schema modes, and in addition to child-like regressive states, he also stipulated less regressive schema modes. A schema mode is an organized pattern of thinking, feeling, and behaving based on a set of schemas, relatively independent from other schema modes. Patients with BPD are assumed to sometimes flip suddenly from one mode into another. As Beck observed, some of these states appear highly childish and may be confusing for both the patient and others. Young hypothesized that four schema modes are central to BPD: the abandoned/abused child mode, the angry/impulsive child mode, the punitive parent mode, and the detached protector mode. In addition, there is a healthy adult mode, denoting the healthy side of the patient.

The abused and abandoned child mode denotes the desperate state the patient may be in related to (threatened) abandonment and abuse experienced as a child. Typical core beliefs are that other people are malevolent, cannot be trusted, and will abandon or punish you, especially when you become intimate with them. Other core beliefs are "My emotional pain will never stop," "I will always be alone," and "There will be nobody who cares for me." The patient may behave like an upset and desperate child, longing for consolation and nurturance but also fearing it. Usually the patient fears this mode, not only because of the intense emotional pain and the reactivation of trauma-related memories and feelings but also because its activation can be followed by an activation of the punitive parent mode. This indicates a severe self-punitive state, during which the patient seems to condemn him- or herself as being bad and evil, deserving punishment. Expressions of negative emotions, opinions, and wishes were usually punished by caregivers, attributing these to character, either explicitly ("You are a bad child") or implicitly (e.g., ignoring the child for days). Threats of abandonment ("I'll send you to an orphan home"), verbal or physical aggression, and (threats of) severe punishments by caregivers are supposed to be internalized in this mode. Typical core beliefs are "You are bad (evil) and deserve punishment," "Your opinions/wishes/emotions are ill founded," "You have no right to express your opinions/wishes/emotions," and "You are only manipulating." Often the patient not only experiences these punishing thoughts but adds punishing acts to them, such as self-injury, damaging the good things in his or her life, and not coming to treatment sessions. Guilt is the prominent feeling. The patient might evoke punishing reactions in others, including the therapist.

One of the other modes the patient (and the therapist!) frequently fears is the angry/impulsive child mode. This denotes a stage of childish rage or self-gratifying impulsiveness that is in the long run damaging for the patient and his or her relationships. Whereas Young, Klosko, and Weishaar (2003) state that patients with BPD typically avoid the experience and expression of anger, the tension of suppressed anger may build up and suddenly be expressed in a relatively uncontrolled way. These tantrum-like states are, according to the model, typically followed by an activation of the punitive parent mode. Impulsive, immediate, need-gratifying behaviors are also attributed to this mode. Underlying beliefs are "My basic rights are deprived," "Other people are evil and mean," and "I have to fight, or just take what I need, to survive." In the model, this mode is not seen as expression of greediness, but as rebelliousness against (perceived) maltreatment—thus as a basically good and understandable state (given the maltreatment patients with BPD experienced as children), though leading to dysfunctional actions.

Although patients with BPD are notorious for their crises and anger, therapists who work for longer periods with these patients have observed that they tend to be detached most of the time. They do not seem to really make contact with others, or with their own feelings and opinions. According to Young and colleagues (2003), they are in the detached protector mode, a sort of protective style the child developed to survive in a dangerous world. This mode is hypothesized to serve to protect against attachment risks (because attachments will be followed by pain, abandonment, punishment, or abuse), emotional experience, self-assertiveness, and development, as each of these signals potential pain and activation of the punitive mode. Core beliefs are that it makes no sense to feel emotions and to connect to others, that it is even dangerous to do so, and that being detached is the only way to survive and to control one's life. Often the patient uses a bulk of strategies to maintain this mode, including cognitive avoidance of feeling and thinking; not talking; avoidance of other people and activities; sleeping, developing, and complaining about somatic discomforts; use of drugs and alcohol; and even (para)suicide. Superficially, the patient may seem rational and healthy, but this is not really healthy because the patient suppresses important aspects of human functioning.

Therapy based on Young's model (schema therapy; Young et al., 2003) aims to reduce the use of the detached protector mode, heal the abandoned/

abused child mode by offering safety and processing traumas, shape the angry/impulsive child mode into healthy forms of assertiveness, expel the punitive parent mode from the patient's system, and increase the strength of the healthy adult mode. Treatment studies have found very strong effects of this model, both in individual, group, and combined format, and very low dropout rates—which is important given the usually high dropout from treatment by patients with BPD (McMurran, Huband, & Overton, 2010).

KEY TREATMENT GOALS

The key treatment goals depend on the possible duration of treatment. With shorter treatments, the goal is usually restricted to reducing the most severe BPD manifestations, such as suicide attempts and self-injury, other forms of self-damaging impulsivity, substance abuse, and so on. Typically many problems remain (even when the patient does not formally meet DSM diagnosis of BPD), thus the patient should be referred for further treatment if the means for that are available.

For a more extensive treatment, the key treatment goals usually include:

1. Reduction of all BPD symptoms (including problems in relation-ships, fear of abandonment, identity problems, emotional instabil-ity, and emptiness).
2. Feeling safe with experiencing and expressing emotions and needs, and with personally connecting to others.
3. Developing a satisfying life on personal, social, and societal levels.

With a time- and objectives-limited treatment, goal setting with the patient can be much easier than with the longer approach. In the latter case, the goals are necessarily global and stated in terms of reduction of the influence of core schemas and dysfunctional strategies and the creation and increase of healthy schemas and strategies. Formulating the latter can be complicated because many patients with BPD have no idea what healthy views and strategies are.

Before treatment proper starts, the therapist should decide as to what treatment he or she wants to offer. On the one hand, a relatively short treatment directed at reducing the most problematic and dangerous BPD problems can be offered. The objectives of such a treatment are a reduc-tion of impulsiveness and self-injury, and perhaps substance abuse, and gaining some control over emotions and insight into the problems, so that the patient is suitable for further psychotherapy. The studies by Linehan, Armstrong, Suarez, Allmon, and Heard (1991) and Brown and colleagues (2004) demonstrated that these objectives are achievable in a 1-year treat-ment. For a real recovery of all BPD-related problems a longer therapy is necessary, during which an intensive personal relationship between therapist and patient (or among group members in the case of group therapy) usually develops. Patients with BPD have such a fundamental distrust of other people, especially when they become intimate with them, and their attachment style is so pathological, that it simply takes extended time to overcome these interpersonal barriers (Gunderson, 1996). Thus, for a real treatment of BPD, time to develop a new secure attachment as a fundamental correction to what went wrong during childhood is necessary. Related to this is the attention that should be given to the treatment of traumatic childhood memories, which also takes time.

COLLABORATIVE STRATEGY

The type of relationship the therapist tries to develop with the patient depends on the duration and goals. With the first option, the therapist should keep a bit more distance from the patient because treatment stops soon and discontinuing treatment when secure attachment just develops can be particularly problematic, and even damaging to patients with BPD. Crisis support should always be provided, but with the first treatment option the therapist does not need to be deeply involved in treatment of crisis. Frequency of sessions can be once or twice a week.

With the second option, on which the remainder of this chapter concentrates, the therapist tries to develop a more personal and caring relationship with the patient. The therapist actively breaks through the patient's detachment, is actively involved in crises, soothes the patient when sad, and brings in him- or herself as a person. Frequency of sessions is initially twice a week—this will foster safe attachment and refresh new insights gained in sessions before it is lost in memory. Compared with most syndromal treatments, the therapist is more directive with content and process, as the patient lacks healthy views to use in Socratic dialogues. Thus, the therapist uses psychoeducation to inform the patient about healthy views on emotions, needs, and relationships; on child development and healthy parenting; and refers to the universal rights of children and adults (e.g., refer to United Nations declarations; *www.un.org/cyberschoolbus/ humanrights/resources/plainchild.asp*; *www.un.org/cyberschoolbus/ humanrights/resources/plain.asp*). The therapist is also more personal and direct, showing more care and interest, as patients with BPD need this. The therapist uses self-disclosure as a powerful means to educate the patient and to make the relationship a bit more personal—when it is helpful to the patient (and not when it is too overwhelming or scaring the patient). Also different from the standard syndromal approach, the therapist tries to meet the needs of the patient within professional boundaries, to directly correct dysfunctional schemas in the therapeutic relationship.

Young and colleagues (2003) called this approach "limited reparenting" by which he referred to the aim to partially repair what went wrong during the patient's childhood.

This approach is highly appreciated by most patients—studies have found higher therapeutic relationship quality reported by patients and less dropout in treatments using this approach. But it can also provoke discomfort in the patient, triggering core schemas, which is good because these can be subsequently addressed in therapy. Thus, this "reparenting" approach is an essential ingredient of treatment. E-mail contact between sessions, and calling the therapist in case of crisis, is encouraged, to promote secure attachment. Personal connection in between sessions refutes the patient's beliefs that there is nobody who really cares and that expression of negative feelings will be followed by punishment or abandonment, and reinforces a secure attachment. Talking, and especially listening, in an accepting way to patients when in crisis is most effective to teach them to tolerate and accept negative feelings. It demonstrates to patients that with such an approach, negative feelings usually calm down. Given a means to reach the therapist in between sessions does not imply that the therapist should be always available, or is omnipotent. In addition to the option of contacting the therapist, a crisis facility should be available, in case the therapist cannot be reached or the patient is unable to calm down when speaking to the therapist.

This approach requires therapists to be able to set limits when the patient goes beyond their personal boundaries. Frustrating the patient by setting personal limits is essential in a reparenting approach, as it is in real parenting, and can be curative, especially when the patient can test negative beliefs about consequences such as "Setting a limit means total disapproval of me as a person" and "Expression of my anger about the limit will be followed by punishment or abandonment by the therapist." There are two important caveats in communicating personal limits to the patient with BPD. One is that the therapist should only address patient behavior and not make character attributions, as caretakers often did. Furthermore, the therapist should give a personal motivation for the limit and not rationalize solely on the basis of institutional or professional rules. For example, the therapist may limit phone responses to certain times of the day due to other personal commitments. The following is an example of a dialogue concerning the communication of personal limits:

NATASHA: This weekend I'll have my 30th birthday party, and I would like to invite you to be there, so that I can introduce you to my husband and friends.

THERAPIST: That is very nice of you to invite me to your birthday party, but I'm afraid I don't want to attend.

NATASHA: Why not? I so much hoped that you could be with me.

THERAPIST: I like you very much, but I want to spend my leisure time with my family and friends.

NATASHA: (*getting angry*) So you are not considering me as a friend? And you said that I could expect therapy to be a very special place, which would evoke deep feelings, and that you would take a special role and care for me? Like a parent toward a child? And now I'm asking you something personal, something that is very important to me, and you just say no. You lied to me! I must have been a fool to trust you!

THERAPIST: You are right, I don't think of you as a friend, though I like you a lot, and I need my time with my family and friends to recuperate. So this is my personal decision, I like to see and work with you here, but I don't want to come to your party.

NATASHA: Jesus, you don't need to repeat that, you don't need to pour salt into a wound. I heard what you said. (*becoming afraid now*) Oh my God, I shouldn't have asked it. I knew it. I knew that you would refuse and resent me for asking such an impertinent thing. I want to go. I cannot stay here. (*Stands and starts to leave the room.*)

THERAPIST: Don't leave, please stay. I see that my refusal is hurting you very much. I also see that you are now extremely afraid that I will hurt you even more because you dared to ask me. Am I correct? Let's talk it over. It doesn't feel good to me if you leave now. Can we try to do that?

NATASHA: (*Sits again and starts to cry.*) Okay, but I feel so ashamed . . .

This approach requires the therapist to tolerate high levels of negative emotions, especially anger directed toward him or her, as well as sadness and despair. Positive emotions directed toward the therapist can be challenging as well, especially lovesickness and other unrealistic expectations of him or her. Consultation with colleagues who work with similar patients is invaluable.

The objectives of the therapeutic relationship are clear, but its application is not without hassles. Though patients with BPD long for a caring relationship, they also deeply fear it, and have serious troubles with tolerating the fears and distrust that are evoked by long-lasting personal and emotionally open relationships. Thus, the therapist should try to balance distance and intimacy and adapt this to the phase of treatment but also actively address the fears and distrust that are evoked by treatment. As Pretzer (1990) stated, "Trust is most effectively established through explicitly acknowledging and accepting the client's difficulty in trusting the therapist (once this becomes evident), and then being careful to behave in a consistently trustworthy manner" (p. 191). Relating the problem to underlying core schemas (or modes, if the therapist uses a mode model) can also be helpful in putting such problems in a new perspective and instilling hope that the problems will be overcome by treatment.

The big problem of dropout risk should be targeted early on. The therapist should be active in keeping patients in therapy, by calling those who do not show up for sessions, asking for (and actively suggesting to break through detachment) the reasons for avoiding therapy, and adapting his or her behavior to what the patient needs. Common reasons for staying away from treatment are related to detaching strategies (not connecting to people, avoiding and pushing away feelings and thoughts about difficulties as ways to survive), fear of being abused or abandoned by the therapist, and self-punitive attitudes ("I don't deserve therapy" and " I should destroy positive things to punish myself"). Such underlying beliefs should be clarified and the patient empathically confronted with the reality that staying away from therapy would mean continuation of pathology and missing the chance to correct the underlying beliefs.

Cognitive therapists who are used to working on symptomatic problems should resist their usual habit of immediately looking for biased interpretations that led to dysfunctional emotions. Instead they can instill healthier schemas for emotion regulation by accepting and validating emotional experience, but discouraging impulsive emotional acts. Through modeling and direct instruction, this will help patients to correct characteristically negative beliefs about experiencing feelings, thinking that their feelings are ill founded, that they are "bad" to have such feelings, that they will lose control of urges to act on their feelings, and that other people (including the therapist) will punish or reject them for these feelings and actions.

A last important relationship technique is empathic confrontation, a confrontational message consisting of three elements: (1) empathic expression that the therapist understands why a dysfunctional strategy is chosen; (2) confrontation with the negative effects of the strategy and the continuation of the disorder if really followed; and (3) explicit formulation of a new, functional alternative strategy and asking the patient to follow it up. The following example illustrates how empathic confrontation can be used to suggest to the patient that functional instead of dysfunctional behavior can be used to deal with a stressful interpersonal situation.

> Although I understand why you are so are upset about what Mark said, because it hurts you deep in your heart, and I understand that you now feel a strong inclination to physically hurt yourself, to show him what a bastard you think he is, I ask you not to do that because if you do, it will further complicate your relationship. He will get more angry, and you will become more afraid, and this escalation will strengthen your idea that other people are evil, and that there never will be someone for you to trust. In other words, by following your old strategy you will continue your problems. Instead, I ask you emphatically to try a new strategy, that is, to tell him that what he did was painful for you, and explain to him why it was painful for you, and ask him to stop it. In that way you don't hurt yourself; you remain in control of your behavior. This is a healthy way to deal with the problem. And, if he doesn't

stop, we will work on how you can react to that. I know this is difficult and even frightening for you to do, but I insist on it because it will help you to learn more healthy ways to deal with such problems.

CLINICAL APPLICATION OF THE INTERVENTION

Hierarchical Approach

In choosing which problem to address, it is wise to use a hierarchical approach. Table 17.1 offers an overview. Issues of life and death should always be given priority. Suicidal impulses and other dangerous behaviors are among them, including behaviors that threaten or endanger the lives of others, particularly dependent children. Next on the hierarchy are issues that threaten the therapeutic relationship. These include the premature wish of the patient to stop therapy, move to another city, not come to therapy, and start another therapy next to the current one; negative feelings of the patient toward the therapist and of the therapist toward the patient; coming late to sessions; using a cell phone during the sessions; and so on. The reason that issues that threaten the therapeutic relationship are so high on the hierarchy is that a good therapeutic relationship is a prerequisite for the other issues. Third, although not immediately life threatening, many self-damaging behaviors are so disruptive that there is no room to address underlying schemas. Self-injury, substance and medication abuse, not attending work, impulsive acts and decisions, not having adequate food and housing, and poorly controlled emotional outbursts are among the disruptive behaviors. Although it is useful to repeatedly address these behaviors, ask the patient to stop them, and work on alternatives and solutions, the therapist should not expect, and certainly not insist on, change early in treatment. The pathology of the patient can be so severe that the therapist has to bear it for a long time, which does not mean that it should not be placed repeatedly on the agenda. Last but not least, other issues, including schema work and trauma processing, should be addressed.

The hierarchy is not only an aid for deciding on agenda issues within a session but also for planning the therapy process as a whole. Therapists should be warned that it can be necessary to readdress issues 1–3 above when they are in a phase of therapy in which schema work is done. Addressing

TABLE 17.1. Hierarchy of Issues to Be Addressed

1. Life-threatening issues.
2. Therapeutic relationship.
3. Self-damaging issues.
4. Other problems, schema work, and trauma processing.

childhood traumas can, for instance, bring about life-threatening behavior, which should move into priority position, after which the focus can again be placed on trauma processing.

Handling Crises

Although there should always be a crisis facility, the therapist is the most important person in treating the crisis. As said, most crises are fueled by the patient's negative beliefs about experiencing intense emotions. The primary strategy to counter these beliefs is to take a calm, accepting, and soothing stance. Empathic listening to the patient, asking for feelings and interpretations, and validating the feelings are important. Often, self-punitive ideas and actions (in Young and colleagues' (2003) model: the punitive parent mode) play a dysfunctional role and it is important to actively inquire for these thoughts and to counter them (e.g., "That's not true, you are a good person," "It is absolutely okay to feel sad and angry when your husband leaves you," and "I'm happy that you tell me about your feelings").

Availability during a crisis can be helpful because an early intervention often prevents worsening, self-mutilation, drug abuse, or other maladaptive actions and reduces the need for hospitalization. Early or later in treatment it is possible to come to an agreement with the patient that he or she will not engage in dysfunctional behavior (like self-injury) before talking to the therapist. We have learned that in many cases empathic listening and talking to the patient on the phone dampens the crisis in 15–20 minutes. During treatment, the patient gradually internalizes this new attitude toward difficult feelings and can apply it to him- or herself, so that immediate help of others is less needed. The therapist can help with this transition by making an audiotape with soothing words spoken by the therapist, and by making flash cards the patient can use to recall soothing thoughts.

Starting too early to offer practical suggestions on how to handle the problem and the crisis is a common pitfall. This generally fuels the punitive beliefs ("So I did it wrong") and counteracts the creation of a healthy attitude toward experiencing emotions. Practical problems should be addressed when emotions are calmed down, and often the patient is then able to handle it for him- or herself. There are, however, circumstances when it is not productive to follow these guidelines. An example is when the patient is so intoxicated (alcohol, benzodiazepines, etc.) that talking to him or her makes little sense because he or she cannot control aggressive impulses. More medically oriented help is then indicated. Another example is when the patient engages in self-injury while talking to the therapist. The therapist should then set firm limits (e.g., "I want you to stop cutting yourself now, and then we will talk about your feelings, so put away that blade").

Limit Setting

Some behaviors are so unacceptable that they should be limited by the therapist. These include behaviors that cross the therapist's personal boundaries (e.g., stalking, threatening, or insulting the therapist). Unacceptable behaviors also include dangerous actions that threaten the patient's life or the continuation of therapy. Formal limit setting as outlined here should only be done when the therapist feels able to execute the last step: stopping therapy. If not ready for that step, the therapist should tolerate the behavior while continuing to confront the patient with it and working toward a change. In applying this technique, therapists should be firm about the limit, use their personal motives to explain it, and talk about the patient's behavior and not criticize the patient's character. Never assume that the patient should have known that the behavior was unacceptable for the therapist. The following example illustrates how limit setting can be used to address inappropriately calling the therapist.

> Yesterday you called me when you were in terrible emotional pain, as I asked you to do. But I learned that you were drunk and had taken a lot of benzos. Because you were intoxicated, I didn't think that I could talk to you in any reasonable way. It made no sense. So I want to ask you not to call me when you are already intoxicated. You are welcome to call me before you consider drinking so much and taking pills, so that I can really connect with you. Please call me before, not after, you do that.

The patient's behavior may persist, in which case, the therapist firmly repeats his or her limits:

> Two weeks ago I changed the conditions under which you could call me. I asked you not to call me when you are drunk and have used benzos. But last Wednesday you called me after taking pills and drinking a bottle of wine. I must say that I got a bit irritated when I found out that you were intoxicated. I don't like to talk to people who are drunk, and I don't want to start disliking you because you call me when you are intoxicated. So call me when you need me because you are in a crisis, but only when you are sober. Don't call me when you are intoxicated. Call me before you start to drink or take pills.

Table 17.2 summarizes the steps that should be taken in limit setting. As is clear from Table 17.2, consequences are only applied after a warning has been given, so that the patient has the chance to change his or her behavior. Furthermore, consequences should initially be light and, if possible, intrinsically related to the undesired behavior (e.g., a patient using too much of the therapist's time gets a shorter session next time). Limit setting can evoke strong anger, which can be dealt with according to the collaboration strategies outlined previously.

TABLE 17.2. Steps to Be Taken in Limit Setting

- Explain the rule; use personal motivation.
- Repeat the rule; show your feelings a little bit, repeat personal motivation.
- As above; add warning and announce consequence.
- As above; execute consequence.
- As above; announce stronger consequence.
- As above; execute stronger consequence.
- Announce a temporary break of therapy so that the patient can think it over.
- Execute temporary break of therapy so that the patient can decide whether he or she wants the present therapy with this limit.
- Announce the end of treatment.
- Stop treatment and refer the patient.

Note. Based on Young, Klosko, and Weishaar (2003, pp. 356–358).

Cognitive Techniques

Unraveling Underlying Schemas and Modes

Because patients with BPD have initially poor understanding of their own emotions, thoughts, and behaviors, an important part of treatment is devoted to help the patient understand them. Gaining clarity on which underlying schemas (or modes) play a role helps patients to reduce confusion and gain some control over their behavior. A daily diary of emotions, thoughts, and behaviors is useful in helping the patient to detect underlying schemas and modes. It is particularly useful to link unraveled underlying schemas (or modes) to the patient's history, so that the patient can see how the schema developed and what function it previously served.

As an example, Natasha (discussed in the beginning of this chapter) learned that she adapted a somewhat arrogant, challenging attitude, as if nobody could hurt her, when she felt uncertain and feared harm. This often triggered more hurtful behavior from others, which was the last thing she wanted. Natasha and her therapist found out that she had developed this attitude as a child to cope with her mother's threats and physical abuse. Showing her mother how she felt hurt or getting angry inevitably led to even more punishment, and adapting this attitude helped her, in a way, to maintain her self-worth and to punish her mother. This historical link made clear the protective function of her schema, and that it was adaptive when she was a child. Because it was triggered automatically when she became an adult, and she had been almost unaware of it until therapy, it took her a long time to understand how her own behavior led to more, rather than less, hurt in present situations. After that became clear, Natasha became interested in learning alternative ways to deal with situations that were threatening for her.

Tackling Dichotomous Thinking

Patients with BPD frequently think in dichotomous terms, fueling extreme emotions, polarizing conflicts, and prompting sudden, extreme, impulsive decisions. It is important to help them to become aware of this thinking style, its harmful implications, and teach them to evaluate situations in more nuanced ways. Structured exercises can be used to develop a more adaptive thinking style. One helpful method is to use a white board to illustrate the difference between black and white thinking and nuanced thinking. On the white board, the therapist compares putting an action or a person into one of two compartments (black or white), versus creating a visual analogue scale (VAS) of a horizontal line between two extremes. Thus, different people, actions, or character traits can be placed in the dichotomous system, or they can be placed along a continuum of the VAS. When multidimensional evaluations have to be made, it is wise to draw a separate VAS for each dimension.

Flash Cards

What has been achieved in a session is often difficult for patients with BPD to remember when they need it. If a schema has been really triggered, all their thinking and feeling seems to be determined by it, and they have great difficulty seeing other perspectives. Flash cards can be particularly useful as an aid to memory and to fight pathogenic schemas on the spot. Usually, on one side of the card the pathogenic reasoning and the activated schema (mode) are described, so that the patient can understand that his or her emotions are caused by the activation of that schema. On the other side, a healthy view is offered, together with a functional way to cope with the problems. Some patients always take flash cards with them as a sort of safety measure, not only because of the content but also because it makes them feel connected to the therapy and the therapist.

Experiential Techniques

Imagery Rescripting and Historical Role Play

A powerful technique to attain change in painful childhood memories on schema level is imagery rescripting. Detailed procedures are described elsewhere (Arntz, 2011; Arntz & Weertman, 1999). In most cases, a present negative feeling is taken as a memory bridge to a childhood memory, which the patient imagines with (if possible) the eyes closed. When the patient clearly imagines the childhood memory and affect is activated, the therapist (or another safe and strong person) should enter the scene and intervene. Patients with BPD are usually, at least in the beginning of treatment, not healthy and powerful enough to intervene themselves, so someone else can serve as the intervener. The intervener stops the maltreatment, creates safety for the child, and asks the child what he or she needs. Special attention should then be given to correction of negative interpretations and soothing of the child, during which imagined physical contact should be offered, as it is the most powerful way to convey comfort and love to a child. If the patient does not accept physical contact, it should not be forced in any way.

In the following example, Natasha imagines a threatening childhood memory with her mother.

NATASHA: I cannot do anything. I'm too afraid.

THERAPIST: I am joining you. Can you imagine me standing alongside you?

NATASHA: Yes, I can see you beside me.

THERAPIST: Good. I'm talking to little Natasha now . . . what is it what you need? Is there anything I can do?

NATASHA: (*Does not say anything, seems very afraid.*)

THERAPIST: Okay, listen to what I say to your mother then . . . Madam, you are Natasha's mother, aren't you? I have to tell you that you are doing terrible things to your daughter. Her bike was stolen, there was nothing she could do about that, and she is emotional about that. That is normal, everybody feels emotional when you lose something of importance. But you are humiliating her in front of the rest of the family because she is emotional. And what is even worse, you are accusing her that she caused the theft. You are saying that she has always been a bad girl, always causing problems, and that she is the cause of your misery. But that is not true, Natasha is a good girl. She should get sympathy and consolation from you because you are her mother and she is in pain. And if you are not able to give her what she needs, and what every other child needs, that is enough of a problem. But in any case you shouldn't accuse her because you have a problem in handling emotions and being a parent. So, stop accusing her and apologize for having done that!

Natasha, look at your mom now, what is she doing? What is she saying?

NATASHA: She looks a bit surprised . . . she is not used to being talked to like that . . . she does not know what to say . . . well, she says that I should be taught a lesson because I should have known beforehand that it would go wrong with what I did with the bike.

THERAPIST: Listen to me, madam. That's nonsense, Natasha didn't know that beforehand and she feels sad about losing her bike, and if you cannot comfort her, stop talking like this or leave the room. What is she doing now, Natasha?

NATASHA: She stops talking and just sits in her armchair.

THERAPIST: How does little Natasha feel now?

NATASHA: I'm afraid that she will punish me when you go away.

THERAPIST: Is there anything that I can do to help you? Ask me!

NATASHA: I want you to stay and care for me.

THERAPIST: That is okay, Natasha, I'll stay and take care of you . . . what do you need now?

NATASHA: That you not only take care of me but also of my sister.

THERAPIST: Should I send your mother away, or take you and your sister with me?

NATASHA: Take us with you.

THERAPIST: Okay, I take the two of you with me: imagine that you take your stuffed animals and everything else you want and that we leave the house together with your sister. We drive to my place. There we enter the house, and you take a seat. Do you want something to drink?

NATASHA: I'm feeling sad now. (*Starts to cry.*)

THERAPIST: That's okay, do you want me to comfort you? Let me take you in my arms . . . can you feel that?

NATASHA: (*Cries even harder.*)

Note that the therapist takes several roles, intervening and protecting the child, correcting dysfunctional ideas about guilt and badness, and comforting the child so that the experience can be emotionally processed. The therapist acts, in other words, as a good parent would have done. The purpose of the rescripting is not to distort or replace the reality of the patient's childhood (which was generally bad) but to correct dysfunctional beliefs, to provide corrective experiences, and to evoke feelings that were avoided or suppressed. Usually imagery with rescripting is highly confrontational, as the patient begins to realize what he or she has missed and how he or she was maltreated. This can lead to a period of mourning. The therapist should help the patient through this period, balancing the focus between here and now and the processing of childhood memories. Role plays of situations from childhood can be used instead of imagery (Arntz & van Genderen, 2009; Arntz & Weertman, 1999). However, some behaviors are awkward or unethical to practice in a role play (i.e., therapist taking child on his or her lap), and imagery may provide an easier and safer strategy.

Empty-Chair Techniques

Punitive caregivers, threatening persons in the present, or a punitive schema mode can be symbolically put on an empty chair, and the therapist and/or the patient can safely express feelings and opinions toward them. Often, it is wise that the therapist first models this technique, as patients might be too afraid to express themselves. As Natasha suffered frequently from her punitive schema mode, echoing her mother's verbal aggressiveness, the therapist repeatedly put this mode (i.e., her aggressive mother) on an empty chair, firmly contradicted her, told her to stop, and sent her away. It is helpful to make an audiotape that the patient can use at home. Later in treatment, the therapist helped Natasha to do this herself, and Natasha also started, with success, to do this at home, each time she was burdened by an activation of this mode.

Experiencing Emotions

Patients with BPD should learn to tolerate the experience of strong negative emotions, without acting out behaviors that serve to avoid or escape from the experience. Exposure techniques known from behavior therapy can be helpful, as are writing exercises, such as composing a letter to a former abuser (but not sending it) in which the patient expresses all of his or her feelings. Patients with BPD are especially afraid of experiencing anger, as they fear that they will lose control and become aggressive. As an intermediate stage, the therapist may model verbally expressing anger while banging on a cushion, asking the patient to join. This lowers the fear of anger. Later on, the patient can be asked to try to experience anger without engaging in any behavioral action. The patient then discovers that he or she can stand high levels of emotions without having to behaviorally express them and without losing control.

Behavioral Techniques

Role Plays

These techniques are useful for teaching interpersonal skills to patients, such as appropriate assertiveness and expressing feelings toward another person. The therapist usually models assertive expression first, as many patients with BPD are truly confused about how to execute an effective expression of feelings. Even when patients refuse to practice during a session, we have seen that the modeling is helpful to get them to begin appropriately expressing feelings and opinions outside the session.

Experimenting with New Behavior

A powerful way to reinforce new schemas and strategies is to ask the patient to behave according to them. Even when the patient reports that this new way of behaving feels strange (i.e., is not yet internalized), it is eventually helpful, so the therapist should continue to encourage the patient to try it out. This is an important part of the later phases of treatment. Later in treatment, Natasha started to show more uncertainty and emotional pain instead of putting on her tough attitude when she was uncertain or hurt inside, and she found out that this was more functional as it led most people to accept her. After she divorced her aggressive husband, she also tried out new ways of behaving during dating. She found out that other types of men, more caring and less threatening than her former partners, were consequently interested in her.

Pharmacological Interventions

Patients with BPD may experience very high levels of negative emotions while having little tolerance for affect. Consequently, they are often prescribed medication. Unfortunately, often when one prescription does not help, a new prescription is added, leading to exotic, unnecessary, and possible harmful polypharmacy (Gunderson, 2011; Lieb et al., 2004). Clinicians should also realize that there is no medication with proven efficacy for BPD or for the severity of BPD symptoms in general (Feurino & Silk, 2011; Lieb, Völlm, Rücker, Timmer, & Stoffers, 2010; NICE, 2009; Stoffers et al., 2010). Although some reviews concluded that specific medications can be used to reduce specific symptoms (Stoffers et al., 2010), others are more reluctant (NICE, 2009). There is little evidence that selective serotonin reuptake inhibitors (SSRIs) have any specific merits, not even for depression in BPD patients (Feurino & Silk, 2011; Lieb et al., 2010). Currently, mood stabilizers and atypical antipsychotics are believed to be the most effective for specific symptoms in BPD patients, though there is lack of robustness of findings and more trials are needed (Feurino & Silk, 2011; Lieb et al., 2010). In general, pharmacotherapy is considered as a possible adjunct to psychotherapy, not as a treatment of BPD in itself. Moreover, there are specific risks in prescribing medication in this population: paradoxical effects, abuse, dependency, and use for suicide attempts are among them. This is particularly true for benzodiazepines, which might be prescribed when patients are in a state of acute fear or suffer from sleep problems. Often, the fear is fueled by aggressive impulses that the patient feels unable to control. Use of benzodiazepines might lead to a reduction of fear of the expression of the impulses and lowered threshold for expression, similar to alcohol (see Cowdry & Gardner, 1988; Gardner & Cowdry, 1985, for empirical evidence). We have often observed the intensification of an emotional crisis, leading to self-injury and suicide attempts, after the use of benzodiazepines, especially when used in combination with alcohol. This "paradoxical" effect should be explained to the patient and the patient should be asked to stop the use of benzodiazepines and alcohol. A short use of antipsychotics or antihistaminics is often a safe alternative, when anxiety levels seem to become intolerable. Personal contact is often a better alternative. Long-term use of antipsychotics dampens many BPD symptoms but may make it impossible to address important feelings so is generally discouraged.

PROGRESS, LIFESPAN, AND TERMINATION CONSIDERATIONS

Because termination of treatment might be very frightening for the patient, it should be well prepared and discussed as part of the process of therapy. Feelings and negative beliefs about termination should be clarified. In addition, a list of remaining problems should be made and appropriate treatment strategies chosen. Gradually tapering off the frequency of sessions is recommended, so that the patient can find out how life is without the regular help of the therapist. Booster sessions may be especially helpful, to help the patient maintain functional strategies and prevent relapse into old schemas. Some therapists recommend an open end, in the sense that the patient can always come back for a few sessions when needed. Paradoxically, this possibility might lead to less relapse and health care use because it offers a safe base on which the patient can fall back. Because patients with BPD are generally not very healthy in their choice of partners, and treatment usually brings about enormous changes, subsequent relational problems can occur. A referral for marital therapy may be indicated, so that the couple can adapt to the new situation. However, many partners are so unhealthy that the patient decides to leave the relationship. The therapist can help the patient learn to choose healthier partners and thus prevent a relapse into old patterns. Some believe that former patients with BPD are, in the long run, best protected for relapse when in a good relationship with a caring partner.

Similarly, the patient should be encouraged to discover and develop his or her true interests and capacities. This might have implications for choice of study and work, as well as hobbies and friends. Creating a good and healthy context in the broadest sense should be high on the agenda in the final stage of therapy. There is a risk that the patient will want to terminate treatment too early, claiming that there are no longer problems, whereas the therapist knows that important issues were not addressed in treatment. When empathic confrontation with this detached strategy does not work, the best thing the therapist probably can do is offer that the patient can return for further treatment if the patient needs it.

BPD in Youth

There is no agreement as to whether BPD can be diagnosed in youth, given the rapid development and the rather common prevalence of some BPD features. Nevertheless, clinicians see youth with problems that can be classified as BPD and that need to be addressed in treatment. The approach described in this chapter can be used to treat these youth, though care should be taken that maltreatment and other forms of negative influences in the family (or other systems the patient depends on) stop. Otherwise it might be impossible to correct in say 2 hours a week what is reinforced in so many other hours during the week. Also, the patient might be afraid of being disloyal to parents, as this would create the risk of severe punishment or abandonment. Thus, parents should be corrected (sometimes they need treatment themselves) or patients should live in a more healthy context so that they don't need to depend any longer on those who put them back into dysfunctional patterns.

COMMON CHALLENGES AND CLINICIAN SELF-CARE

Treatment of patients with BPD is for most therapists challenging. Among the major risks are burnout, transgression of professional boundaries, and development of negative feelings toward the patient (countertransference). It is therefore important to have a safe peer supervision group of therapists who work with the same model and who can help one another. The peer supervision group should validate difficult feelings evoked by patients with BPD, support one another, and empathically confront one another with dysfunctional attitudes and actions of the therapists. Emotionally detached therapists who have difficulties in being open and personal are usually not a good match for patients with BPD, as these patients need more personal connection than usual. Therapists with high levels of unsatisfied personal needs might be at risk to transgress personal boundaries, as they might be seduced to use the patient to meet their needs. Recent piloting with the combination of group and individual schema therapy indicated that therapists like this format, as it offers both a shared responsibility between group and individual therapists, and offers possibilities to do intensive individual therapy while the patient also profits from experiences in the group.

CONCLUSION

The approach presented in this chapter is based on an integration of cognitive-, behavioral-, experiential-, and therapy-relationship techniques in the framework of a cognitive model. This approach helps therapists to adapt treatment to the needs of the patient, while at the same time maintaining focus. Empirical tests have yielded evidence that this approach is highly effective and has a high degree of acceptability for patients. In the future, the development of variants that lead to faster results are expected.

Dismantling studies, experimental tests of ingredients, and possibly the combination of group and individual formats will contribute to this.

ACKNOWLEDGMENTS

Thanks are due to Tim Beck, Christine Padesky, Jeffrey Young, Joan Farrell, and Ida Shaw for what they taught me during their workshops and during discussions I had with them. Colleagues, notably Hannie van Genderen and Gitta Jacob, as well as clients, helped to develop and validate the ideas and methods described in this chapter.

PART III

COMORBIDITY AND CLINICAL MANAGEMENT

CHAPTER 18

Symptomatic Comorbidity

Robert A. DiTomasso
Bradley Rosenfield

A high degree of comorbidity between personality and symptomatic disorders (formerly Axis I conditions; American Psychiatric Association, 2000) is well documented (Goodwin, Brook, & Cohen, 2005; Johnson, Cohen, Kasen, & Brook, 2005; Loranger, 1990). Lenzenweger, Lane, Loranger, and Kessler (2007) propose that personality disorders affect the precipitation, duration, and severity of comorbid symptomatic disorders. Personality disorders also negatively impact treatment outcome for a variety of symptomatic disorders (Reich & Green, 1991), most likely by adversely influencing the working alliance, aggravating pathology, and limiting the potential for self-reflection (Crits-Christoph & Barber, 2002). Personality pathology may also exert influence on symptomatic disorders as patients fail to appreciate the impact of their actions and emotions on others, as well as how their dysfunctional personality style contributes to their distress (Crits-Christoph & Barber, 2002). Crits-Christoph and Barber (2002) concluded that the effect of personality disorders on treatment outcome for symptomatic disorders is consistently negative, stressing the need for careful assessment of interpersonal problems, although these results are inconsistent (e.g., Mathew, Chamberlain, Szafranski, Smith, & Norton, 2013).

Personality disorders can predispose people to other disorders and complicate treatment (see Millon, 2011). Of the 11 personality disorders (American Psychiatric Association, 2013), the greatest risk for mood and anxiety disorders appears to be associated with borderline, avoidant, antisocial, dependent, obsessive-compulsive, and schizotypal (e.g., Alloy &

Abramson, 1999; Boyce & Mason, 1996; Grilo et al., 2010; Skodol et al., 1999; Smith, Grandin, Alloy, & Abramson, 2006). Below are 10 general considerations related to the co-occurrence of personality disorders and other specific conditions.

First, personality issues can threaten accurate assessment and case formulation. For example, patients with avoidant personality disorder are often unwilling to even think about relevant issues, which may block access to important information that should inform treatment for comorbid disorders. It is also important to avoid overdiagnosis when assessing personality disorders during symptomatic episodes to prevent spuriously inflating the prevalence of personality disorders (Hirschfeld et al., 1983). Conversely, underdiagnosis may occur by missing personality disorders while treating acute symptomatic disorders.

Second, specific symptomatic disorders may manifest quite differently in individuals with particular personality disorders. There is often a reciprocal interaction between conditions, with one exacerbating the other. Symptomatic disorders may magnify deficits associated with specific personality disorders by increasing overreliance on maladaptive coping strategies, whereas personality disorders predispose individuals to developing symptomatic disorders.

Third, personality disorders may interact with symptomatic disorders in ways that affect treatment. Yet, most manualized treatments for symptomatic disorders generally do not take personality disorders into consideration. Additionally, dysfunctional personality characteristics are egosyntonic, often impeding insight and interfering with motivation to change (Beck, Freeman, & Davis, 2004). The application of empirically based protocols often needs to be modified for patients with comorbid personality pathology.

Fourth, while the therapeutic relationship alone may not be sufficient to alter a symptomatic disorder, it is undoubtedly necessary to help patients engage in the therapy process and accept treatment recommendations. Informed flexibility and clinical innovation are critical to creating a therapeutic alliance and treating comorbid conditions that include personality disorders.

Fifth, an important issue is whether to divulge a personality disorder diagnosis to patients. Fusco and Freeman (2004) posit that patients have a right to know their diagnoses and to be educated about chronicity and the need for active commitment to increase the probability of symptom relief, unless such labeling would be countertherapeutic. According to Cory F. Newman (personal communication, June 17, 2013), it may be therapeutic to discuss personality strengths and problematic symptoms rather than labeling the patient with a personality "disorder." With genuine empathy, discussing specific symptoms and educating the patient that such problems are consistent with features of a specific "personality" may be advisable. If pressed for a diagnosis, however, Newman recommends asking patients if they would endorse relevant symptoms. If it is therapeutically appropriate, the therapist can inform the patient of the diagnosis. Then, it is helpful to explore the patient's cognitions regarding the diagnosis and to correct misconceptions. To consider personality disorders in a dichotomous fashion is itself a distortion, as no person is solely a personality disorder. All people have characteristics of various personality *types*, in some combinations and degrees. Nonetheless, an unwanted diagnosis can create cognitive dissonance and much needed motivation for change. The decision to disclose a personality disorder diagnosis to a patient who is symptomatic should be made in light of a good case conceptualization and the potential therapeutic benefit to the patient.

Sixth is the question of where to begin? Should one first address the symptomatic problem or the personality disorder? Freeman and Rock (2008) propose that symptomatic conditions should be the primary target, with some exceptions. Symptomatic conditions are generally the primary reason patients seek help so hope for their resolution can be a powerful motivator for treatment engagement and a bridge to establishing the working alliance. Moreover, symptomatic disorders are likely to yield more quickly to cognitive therapy than personality disorders and can establish patient hope and therapist credibility, while building patient skills that can be generalized to treat personality disorders. When the personality functioning is severely disrupted, as with borderline personality disorder, it may be best to target the personality difficulties first (Leichsenring, Leibing, Kruse, New, & Leweke, 2011) or at least clarify whether the borderline personality disorder is to be included in the symptomatic treatment plan (see Arntz, Chapter 17, this volume). Newman proposes that patients with co-occurring disorders often require parallel treatment for each specific disorder.

Seventh, when conceptualizing and planning treatment for co-occurring disorders, we must remain cognizant that we are treating individuals with complex presentations with much overlap among disorders. Eighth, the most efficient and enduring interventions are most likely to be those that target the underlying schema (and skills deficits) that form the common denominator among the individual's comorbid problems (K. Kuehlwein, personal communication, May 5, 2013). Ninth, plotting an effective treatment strategy should begin by identifying the patient's motivation and, then, modifying the maladaptive behaviors and cognitions that are the least rigid and most amenable to change (M. A. Layden, personal communication, August 5, 2013). Tenth, distinguishing co-occurring disorders can be challenging. All of the above is predicated upon a carefully conducted differential diagnosis.

In sum, comorbidity has important implications for assessment and treatment with regard to forming a therapeutic relationship, sharing diagnoses, eliciting motivation, and planning treatment. To effectively address the impact of personality pathology on symptomatic treatment, we must first accurately diagnose the patient's difficulty. Next, we must hypothesize how unique personality disorder features are likely to affect important facets of the cognitive-behavioral therapy (CBT) process. This allows us to plan strategies that may reduce predictable problems of resistance or unresponsiveness. In this manner, we can modify typical treatment plans to address unique aspects of personality disorder pathology that may undermine treatment. In the following sections, we consider the treatment implications for comorbidity of personality disorders with anxiety, mood, autism, and health spectrum disorders.

PERSONALITY DISORDERS AND ANXIETY DISORDERS

Anxiety disorders are common, costly, and debilitating (DiTomasso & Gosch, 2007), although highly responsive to CBT treatments (Tolin, 2010). Fear and avoidance appear to be a common pathway for the development of anxiety disorders and Cluster C personality disorders (Mathew et al., 2013). Mathew and colleagues (2013) propose a bidirectional model, whereby personality disorders impact the future development of anxiety disorders and early-onset anxiety disorders increase the risk for the development of personality disorders. However, the impact of personality disorders on co-occurring anxiety appears to be inconsistent (Mathew et al., 2013). Therefore, it seems that the effect of personality on anxiety disorders treatment may be idiosyncratic.

Anxiety appears to be most commonly manifested in patients with avoidant and dependent personalities (Millon, Millon, Meagher, Grossman, & Ramnath, 2004). In individuals diagnosed with an anxiety disorder, comorbidity for a personality disorder diagnosis is as follows: social phobia (22.9%), generalized anxiety disorder (21.4%), obsessive–compulsive disorder (15.6%), posttraumatic stress disorder (29.6%), and panic disorder (26.1%; McGlashan et al., 2000). Anxiety and borderline personality disorder are also frequently comorbid (Lenzenweger et al., 2007). These findings underscore that clinicians need to consider that approximately one-fourth of their patients who are anxious may need more than simply the typical empirically based protocol for a symptomatic disorder.

For example, early in treatment, a highly functioning patient who was borderline with dependent features and experiencing intense worriment and depression frequently called her therapist seeking reassurance. The therapist made a decision to be available for these crisis calls, gradually setting reasonable limits to 5-minute conversations and, then, decreasing their frequency and duration even further by having the patient agree to generate one (then two or three) possible solutions before calling the therapist. Such therapeutic maneuvers, based on valid case conceptualization, allow cognitive therapists to prepare the patient and increase receptivity for delivery of an empirically based protocol.

Personality disorders affect length of treatment and relapse rates (Ansell et al., 2011). Among patients with anxiety disorders, specific personality disorders are associated with higher rates of relapse (avoidant and schizotypal personality disorders in social phobia; borderline, obsessive–compulsive, and schizotypal personality disorders in general anxiety disorder; borderline and avoidant personality disorders in obsessive–compulsive disorder; schizotypal personality disorder in posttraumatic stress disorder [obsessive–compulsive personality disorder is protective]; borderline and avoidant personality disorders in panic disorder with agoraphobia; and obsessive–compulsive personality disorder in agoraphobia without panic) as well as increased treatment duration (avoidant personality disorder in social phobia). Personality disorders may also adversely impact outcomes. For example, exposure and ritual prevention for obsessive–compulsive disorder appears less effective with co-morbid obsessive–compulsive personality disorder (Pinto, Liebowitz, Foa, & Simpson, 2011), with greater obsessive–compulsive personality disorder severity predicting poorer outcome. However, only perfectionism predicted worse outcome. Leichsenring and colleagues (2011) have proposed that for patients with anxiety co-morbid for borderline personality disorder, it is more effective to treat the personality disorder as the primary target (Leichsenring et al., 2011); others argue that these pathological states are so not easily separated (Newman, Leahy, Beck, Reilly-Harrington, & Gyulai, 2002).

Based on comparisons of patients with specific anxiety disorders, *with and without complicating personality disorders*, Ansell and colleagues (2011) noted that when specific anxiety disorders are complicated by specific personality disorders, the result is higher levels of severity as well as an adverse impact on psychosocial functioning and prognosis, manifested by decreased remission, increased likelihood of developing a new episode, and greater length of episode as well as time spent in treatment. The most problematic personality disorders were schizotypal, obsessive–compulsive, and avoidant personality disorders. Chambless, Renneberg, Goldstein, and Gracely (1992) and Chambless, Renneberg, Gracely, Goldstein, and Fydrich (2000) found avoidant personality disorder was associated with poor clinical outcome when treating agoraphobia with exposure therapy as well as exposure therapy plus additional treatments. Minichiello, Baer, and Jenike (1987) reported poor outcome for the behavioral treatment of obsessive–compulsive disorder in patients with schizotypal personality disorder. The presence of personality disorder has also been associated with poor outcome for CBT treatment of social phobia (Turner, 1987) as well as panic disorder (Mennin & Heimberg, 2000), supporting the need for additional treatments. However, Kampman, Keijsers, Hoogduin, and Hendriks

(2008) and Steketee and Shapiro (1995) failed to find evidence for particular predictors of outcome for panic disorder.

A thorough assessment and case formulation are necessary to guide successful interventions. Some personality disorders are most likely to create interference with the treatment of specific anxiety disorders as in the following scenario.

John had severe social anxiety and avoidant personality disorder. The therapy relationship proved to be a significant source of threat for him. He offered limited information to his therapist and misinterpreted questions as criticisms. Fear of exposure to social situations precluded opportunities for *in vivo* exposure. His preoccupation about being criticized also prevented him from giving accurate feedback about the treatment process and from fully engaging in exposure exercises. Focusing on goals and framing therapy as a safe, noncritical, and supportive environment allowed John to gradually learn skills to manage increasing levels of perceived threat as he worked through an exposure hierarchy of feared stimuli. In the next section we examine comorbid personality disorders and mood disorders.

PERSONALITY DISORDERS AND MOOD SPECTRUM DISORDERS

Although the *Diagnostic and Statistical Manual of Mental Disorders* (DSM-5; American Psychiatric Association, 2013) documents the essential symptoms of major depressive disorder as depressed mood or anhedonia, it is the more cognitively based symptoms that appear to overlap with many personality disorder features, such as indecisiveness (in borderline personality disorder, dependent personality disorder, obsessive–compulsive personality disorder, avoidant personality disorder, histrionic personality disorder), worthlessness (in borderline personality disorder, antisocial personality disorder, avoidant personality disorder, dependent personality disorder, narcissistic personality disorder, obsessive–compulsive personality disorder, histrionic personality disorder), feelings of guilt (in borderline personality disorder, avoidant personality disorder, dependent personality disorder, obsessive–compulsive personality disorder), and suicidal ideation (in borderline personality disorder, histrionic personality disorder, antisocial personality disorder, narcissistic personality disorder, and others). Among individuals with depression, prevalence rates of comorbid personality disorders range from 28 to as much as 81% (Alnaes & Torgersen, 1988; Hirschfeld, 1999; Ilardi & Craighead, 1995).

Grilo and colleagues (2010) found that comorbid personality disorders with depression at baseline strongly predicted higher major depressive disorder relapse rates and shorter remissions. Patients with major depressive disorder with co-occurring borderline personality disorder, schizotypal personality disorder, and obsessive–compulsive personality disorder were particularly at risk. Borderline personality disorder, avoidant personality disorder, and dependent personality disorder have also been associated with the highest risk of depression (Boyce & Mason, 1996; Skodol et al., 1999). Skodol and colleagues (2011) determined that all personality disorders were associated with refractory major depressive disorder, although borderline personality disorder was the greatest predictor of major depressive disorder persistence.

Smith and colleagues (2006) determined that two maladaptive patterns of cognition, often found in personality disorders, predicted depression: cognitive risk (dysfunctional attitudes and negative attributional styles) and rumination. Cognitive risk correlated with symptoms of paranoid personality disorder, histrionic personality disorder, narcissistic personality disorder, avoidant personality disorder, dependent personality disorder, obsessive–compulsive personality disorder, and schizotypal personality disorder. Rumination was most highly related to borderline personality disorder and obsessive–compulsive personality disorder symptoms. Numerous prospective studies have determined that the interaction of life stressors and cognitive vulnerability predicted future depression (e.g., Hankin, Abramson, Miller, & Haeffel, 2004; Hankin, Abramson, & Siler, 2001; Lewinsohn, Joiner, & Rohde, 2001). Newman (2011) posits that chronic anger and severe avoidance, attendant to many personality disorders, also present unique obstacles to effective treatment.

Outcome studies clearly identify obstacles that impede the treatment of patients with depressive personality disorder, including lack of early symptom relief, negative treatment expectations, poor treatment engagement, a weak working alliance, failure to complete homework, low social support, anger, avoidance, rumination, and premature termination (Hollon & Beck, 2004; Newman, 2011; Persons, Burns, & Perloff, 1988; Schindler, Hiller, & Witthöft, 2013; Smith et al. 2006). Thus, overcoming those obstacles should be among the primary treatment goals.

Regarding specific comorbidities, the prevalence of borderline personality disorder among depressed samples ranges from 2 (Shea, Glass, Pilkonis, Watkins, & Docherty, 1987) to 24% (Pepper et al., 1995). In a borderline personality disorder sample, McGlashan and colleagues (2000) determined that almost 71% of patients also met criteria for major depressive disorder. So it may be fair to say that borderline personality disorder is somewhat common among patients who are depressed, while depression is highly prevalent among patients with borderline personality disorder. Improvement or exacerbation in either major depressive disorder or borderline personality disorder predicts similar changes in the other (Gunderson et al., 2004; Shea et al., 2004).

When comorbid with depression, borderline personality disorder symptoms, especially impulsivity and aggression, are associated with an increase in the severity and number of suicide attempts (Soloff, Lynch,

Kelly, Malone, & Mann, 2000). A startling 92% of inpatients with both disorders have attempted suicide at least once during their lifetimes, significantly more than those with either disorder alone (Friedman, Aronoff, Clarkin, Corn, & Hurt, 1983). Most alarming is that between 5 and 7% of those with borderline personality disorder complete suicide (Duberstein & Conwell, 1997). Yen and colleagues (2003) found that exacerbation of depressed mood, alcohol use, and/or substance use predicted a suicide attempt within the next month. Consequently, when treating comorbid borderline personality disorder and mood disorders, continual monitoring of suicidal ideation is necessary, especially when accompanied by chronic anger, worsening of mood, and substance use.

In a transnational study in 18 countries (Perugi et al., 2012), 14.5% of patients with borderline personality disorder also met criteria for bipolar disorder. Moreover, the comorbid group exhibited greater pathology than bipolar disorder alone as measured by earlier age of onset, mood instability, irritability, higher comorbidity with disorders of anxiety, eating, attention-deficit/hyperactivity disorder, mixed episodes, seasonal affective symptoms, substance use, psychosis, and suicide attempts. Notably, the group with borderline personality disorder–bipolar disorder had problems with antidepressant medication, including lower therapeutic response and antidepressant-induced irritability and lability.

According to DSM-5, differential diagnosis of borderline personality disorder and mood disorders can be difficult as extreme borderline personality disorder mood fluctuations can mimic both depressive and manic episodes (American Psychiatric Association, 2013). Evidence of distinct interepisode recovery supports a mood diagnosis, whereas persistent course and early onset are generally more indicative of borderline personality disorder. The diagnostic picture can get increasingly murky as bipolar episodes increase in frequency (American Psychiatric Association, 2013; Kramlinger & Post, 1996).

Once mood disorders are diagnosed, clinicians can provide early psychoeducation for both disorders by explaining the diathesis-stress model, with "brain chemistry" interacting with stress, which is influenced by subjective perception (Newman et al. 2002, p. 26), with genetic predisposition for both borderline personality disorder (Calati, Gressier, Balestri, & Serretti, 2013) and bipolar disorder (Belmaker, 2004). An early history of childhood abuse is common to both disorders (Trull, 2001; Weaver & Clum, 1993). Patients learn that high-risk, maladaptive behaviors in both disorders function as compensatory strategies in response to maladaptive beliefs that (1) "I can't tolerate negative feelings," (2) "My emotions are out of control and will go on forever," and (3) "Engaging in risky and self-injurious behavior provides temporary relief, and if there are negative consequences, I deserve it (or can handle it) anyway." Activation of these beliefs, attendant to both borderline personality disorder and mood disorders, produces wide fluctuations in affect. The resulting unstable behavior sabotages the patient's efforts and creates havoc in relationships. Resultant stress can trigger mood episodes (Bockian, 2006; Millon, 1999).

The most fundamental treatment goals for bipolar disorder include behavioral activation for depression and reducing activity during mania (Lam, Jones, & Hayward, 2010). Comorbid borderline personality disorder–bipolar disorder may be especially pernicious because the compensatory high-risk behaviors, cognitive deficits, and psychosocial stressors endemic to borderline personality disorder can trigger episodes of both depression and mania. Highly stimulating activity, sexual conquests, and even adaptive achievements (e.g., pay raise) that would be expected to ameliorate depression can actually trigger grandiosity and manic episodes (Johnson et al., 2005). Of course, mania and depression magnify borderline personality disorder personality traits.

During prodromes and hypomanic or manic episodes, behavioral interventions focus on maintaining behavioral routines, restraining unnecessary activity, reducing stimulation, and improving sleep and diet (Lam et al., 2010; Linehan, 1993). Treatment is especially difficult for the patient with borderline personality disorder with mood disorder, who has little tolerance for "boredom" (Linehan, 1993). Affect tolerance skills are useful for reducing the tendency to seek external modes of affect regulation such as drugs, unprotected sex, reckless driving, and self-mutilation (Layden, Newman, Freeman, & Morse, 1993; Linehan, 1993). Instead, Lam and colleagues (2010) recommend stimulus control to avoid people, places, and things associated with maladaptive behavior in favor of finding more adaptive alternative "safe thrills" (Lam et al., 2010, p. 210), such as moderate exercise, video games, and computer simulation of more risky behavior (martial arts, racing, mountain climbing). "Pleasurable non-task activities" (Lam et al., 2010, p. 197) are also recommended, including relaxation, quiet time with family or friends, hobbies, reading, religious activity, mindfulness, and gentle exercise such as walking.

Sleep deprivation is a red flag for the onset of mood episodes (e.g., Plante & Winkelman, 2008; Wirz-Justice & Van den Hoofdakker, 1999). Batterham, Glozier, and Christensen (2012) determined that sleep disturbance predicted major depressive disorder episodes at a 4-year follow-up. However, after controlling for ruminative style and neuroticism (frequent in borderline personality disorder), the impact of sleep disturbance was reduced to statistical insignificance. This illustrates the primacy of rumination and neuroticism as treatment targets in ameliorating insomnia and mood disorders. Baer and Sauer (2011) cite treatments specifically targeting rumination, including rumination-focused CBT (Watkins et al., 2007) and behavioral activation (Dimidjian et al., 2006), or mindfulness-based cognitive therapy (Segal, Williams, & Teasdale, 2002). These interventions are efficacious in treating anxiety and depression and clinical experience shows promise for treating borderline personality disorder–bipolar disorder. For insomnia, Perlis, Jungquist, Smith, and Posner (2005) offer a session-by-session CBT manual.

Finally, there is no evidence for purely psychosocial interventions for acute mania (Lam et al., 2010). The American Psychiatric Association guidelines and others recommend combined psychotherapy and pharmacotherapy (mood stabilizers, antipsychotics, anticonvulsants, and, more rarely, antidepressants) for the treatment of co-occurring mood disorders and borderline personality disorder (American Psychiatric Association, 2000, 2002; Kool, Dekker, Duijsens, de Jonghe, & Puite, 2003; Paris, 2005). Referral for psychiatric consultation is essential when comorbidity includes bipolar I disorder (see Rosenbluth, MacQueen, McIntyre, Beaulieu, & Schaffer, 2012, for a recent review).

In summary, comorbid mood disorders and borderline personality disorder can be treated with CBT to address dysfunctional cognitions, emotional dysregulation, and medication adherence; maintaining regular routines in the domains of sleep, exercise, social, and occupational activities; early prodrome detection; and couple or family concerns.

Avoidant personality disorder has a strong comorbid relationship with depressive disorders. Prevalence rates of comorbid avoidant personality disorder among individuals with depression range from 30.4 to (Pilkonis & Frank, 1988) to 6.9% (Zimmerman & Coryell, 1989). Among those with dysthymic disorder, avoidant personality disorder was found in 32 (Markowitz, Moran, Kocsis, & Frances, 1992) to 16% (Pepper et al., 1995). Conversely, in samples of participants with avoidant personality disorder, the prevalence rate of major depressive disorder was 81.5% (McGlashan et al., 2000).

The high comorbidity and similarity between avoidant personality disorder and major depressive disorder is understandable. DSM-5 diagnostic criteria for avoidant personality disorder sound like a near recapitulation of major depressive disorder symptoms and associated features (American Psychiatric Association, 2013). Patients who are depressed with avoidant personality disorder yearn for idealized, close relationships; however, all efforts in this direction are aborted for fear of rejection, stemming from chronic, pervasive, depressogenic core beliefs of being "unlovable," "disgusting," "worthless," "inadequate," or "stupid." They believe they cannot tolerate negative thoughts and emotions so they withdraw socially and feel intense loneliness, anxiety, and depression (Millon & Davis, 2000), perceiving their isolation and depression as evidence of personal defectiveness. A never-ending stream of self-criticism further maintains maladaptive schema and depression (Beck et al., 2004). These early maladaptive childhood schema (subjugation, abandonment, and emotional inhibition) largely mediate the relationship between retrospectively reported childhood experiences (family sociability and overprotective parenting) and adult avoidant personality disorder symptoms (Carr & Francis, 2010). Additionally, depression and anxiety magnify fearful and avoidant traits.

Early in the first treatment session, it is crucial to educate the patient who is depressed with avoidant personality disorder to the culture of disclosure as a normal part of cognitive therapy. Treatment can be framed as an exploration to find and then dismantle goal-interfering avoidance (Martell, Addis, & Jacobson, 2001). Cognitive and emotional avoidance often stem from beliefs that "If I don't think about problems, I don't have to do anything about them," "I can't handle emotions," and "They'll escalate out of control." But, avoidance is like coping with a small fire by hiding in the corner. It is best to deal with it immediately! A puff of air can extinguish a match and prevent greater harm. Furthermore, with the mantra "Avoidance is the enemy," it can be helpful to *get angry at avoidance*. Anger is an incompatible response to fear and depression and can spur action (Butler, 1975).

Behavioral activation is an excellent early intervention. Coffman, Martell, Dimidjian, Gallop, and Hollon (2007) determined that skills training and behavioral activation, targeting behavioral avoidance and inactivity in extreme nonresponders, was superior to more cognitive techniques. It is also useful to connect social behavior to improvements in mood via a mood log to demonstrate the positive effect of behavioral activation and to increase self-efficacy (Beck, Rush, Shaw, & Emery, 1979).

In session, patients' compensatory avoidance strategies may include silence, changing the topic, joking, and inattention. To address avoidance *in session* at times of silence and discomfort, it can be helpful to say "You look like you want to tell me something," rather than the more accurate "You look like you *don't* want to tell me something." It can also be useful to ask "Are you worried what I'll think?" (A. T. Beck, personal communication, June 18, 1996). Asking directly for both positive and corrective feedback in the session can open the door to assertive communication. Even when told everything is fine, therapists can ask "If there was something that I could improve on, how could you tell me?" Humor may help in this regard.

Hypersomnia and substance abuse may be extreme avoidance strategies that can exacerbate depression. Effective interventions include motivational interviewing, including goal setting, cost–benefit analysis of current situation and change, problem solving, and behavioral activation (Beck et al., 1979; Miller & Rollnick, 2013). With motivation established, CBT for substance abuse may be in order (Beck, Wright, Newman, & Liese, 1993).

In summary, CBT for avoidant personality disorder with depression should include techniques for undercutting core beliefs of unlovability, helplessness, and worthlessness that maintain depression, inhibition, and avoidance, while activating behavior and increasing self-efficacy, assertiveness, and tolerance of negative evaluation. Next, we consider antisocial personality disorder and depression.

Antisocial personality disorder alone is a negative predictor of treatment outcome. Many with antisocial personality disorder lack motivation and are mandated to treatment. Individuals with antisocial personality disorder often become depressed because they perceive that "They have been constrained in some way" (Bockian, 2006, p. 112) by authority or societal rules. While counterintuitive, it can be a mistake to attempt to precipitously assuage depression (e.g., Woody, McLellan, Luborsky, & O'Brien, 1985). Rather, an early treatment strategy is to explore presenting problems, thoughts, behaviors, and negative mood. Dysphoria can increase cognitive dissonance between current behavior and desirable goals—a powerful motivator for change (Miller & Rollnick, 2013). The next step is to relate dysphoria and life stressors to antisocial patterns. Subsequently, collaboratively set goals should be desirable, behavioral, and measurable (J. Beck, 1995; Miller & Rollnick, 2013). The focus on goals reduces "resistance" and the tendency to ruminate about the past while increasing hope and improving mood. Most patients endorse the metaphor that it is difficult to drive while looking in the rearview mirror. Instead, you have focus on where you want to go and then take action to get there.

After collaboratively developing willingness to change, the focus should shift to increasing self-efficacy, readiness for change, and behavioral activation with the patient's stated goals as a magnet for action. Rather than trying to inculcate a moral structure at this stage, therapy focuses on goal attainment. Patients with antisocial personality disorder generally perceive things in terms of their own self-interest rather than the good of others or society (Beck et al., 2004). When roadblocks to progress inevitably occur, identifying obstacles to change can be some of the most valuable experiences in therapy. These obstacles are often cognitive or practical in nature. Antisocial behavior is also framed as a barrier to goal attainment and ensuring a vicious depressogenic cycle.

Finally, anger and aggressive behavior can harm others and land patients with antisocial personality disorder in serious trouble, the consequences of which increase the risk of depression. Clinicians and patients can collaboratively create a written contract specifying clear boundaries and consequences in this regard. Clinicians can teach patients the difference between aggression versus assertiveness and effective communication (Alberti & Emmons, 2008; Burns, 1999) as a means of reaching immediate goals (e.g., quieting a noisy neighbors, etc.) and long-term goals (e.g., staying out of prison). Impulse control training might also be in order, especially in the case of reactive aggression (Cornell et al., 1996). Treatment for depression and antisocial personality disorder requires collaboration and mutual respect within the confines of specific boundaries.

PERSONALITY DISORDERS AND AUTISM SPECTRUM DISORDERS

Autism spectrum disorder has received comparatively little attention in the adult clinical literature. DSM-5 has subsumed Asperger's disorder and autism (American Psychiatric Association, 2000) under the now official diagnosis of autism spectrum disorder (American Psychiatric Association, 2013), conceptualizing autism spectrum disorder on three levels, rather than categories. Autism spectrum disorder is now included under the classification of "neurodevelopmental disorders."

There are similarities in the presentation between autism spectrum (Level 1) and schizoid personality disorder, obsessive–compulsive personality disorder, schizotypal personality disorder, and avoidant personality disorder. Communication deficits may arise earlier in childhood for autism spectrum disorder versus schizoid personality disorder and schizotypal personality disorder, although the previous DSM-IV-TR requirement of deficits before age 3 are now absent. Furthermore, patients with autism spectrum disorder can be quite avoidant.

The relationship between autism spectrum disorder and personality disorders remains unclear. Lugnegård, Hallerbäck, and Gillberg (2011) determined that, in a group of 54 young adults with Asperger's disorder, 26% also met criteria for schizoid personality disorder, 19% for obsessive–compulsive personality disorder, 13% for avoidant personality disorder, and 2% for schizotypal personality disorder. There were significant gender differences, with 65% of men versus only 32% of women with comorbid personality disorders. According to Lugnegård and colleagues, comorbidity between schizoid personality disorder and autism spectrum disorder may be accounted for by the overlap in symptom criteria. Criteria for obsessive–compulsive personality disorder also show substantial overlap such as rigidity, reduced interest in friends, and other restricted interests and behaviors. Avoidant symptoms may be compensatory strategies to elude the "elevated sensitivity to stressful environments because of visual and auditory perceptual difficulties" (Lugnegård et al., 2011, p. 6). Moreover, avoidance may arise from anxiety related to expectations of social ridicule and harassment.

The literature on CBT for autism spectrum disorder is a young but burgeoning science (Kincade & McBride, 2009). Results appear to support the efficacy of CBT in reducing anxiety, improving social cognition, and increasing social skills for high-functioning patients with autism spectrum disorder. Clinical experience militates for careful diagnosis of personality traits that can hinder treatment but also offer a path to effectively using personality disorder pathology in the service of improving function.

For example, Frank is a client who is anxious with high-functioning Level 1 autism spectrum disorder with narcissistic features who was failing miserably in college. Despite his keen intellect, he was not attending class, refused to participate in group projects, and was fearful of meeting with his professors. This pattern resulted from his unrelenting beliefs that he is perceived as "odd and different." Although he had a fantasy that someday he would become a computer tycoon, his academic performance was seriously undermining his prospects. Treatment was reframed as a means of assisting him in reaching his most desired goals. Tying these goals to specific behaviors (e.g., attending class) helped him to overcome the anxiety, change his behavior, and become more academically successful. To overcome his forgetfulness, daily appointments were saved as a screensaver on his smartphone, with accompanying alarms to prompt action. To surmount his social anxiety, the clinician requested a peer mentor from the college's Office for Students with Disabilities for social support and to model adaptive social behavior. Frank also benefited greatly by reading Segar's manual (1997), written by a young man with Asperger's disorder as a guide for navigating the social world.

PERSONALITY DISORDERS AND HEALTH SPECTRUM DISORDERS

Treatment of medical problems is often complicated by personality disorder traits. CBT therapists often interface with primary care physicians (PCPs) and other specialists in the treatment of patients who are comorbid (DiTomasso, Golden, & Morris, 2010). The literature reveals an increased incidence of problematic alcohol, cigarette, and drug use among individuals with personality disorders. A diagnosis of borderline, antisocial, and schizotypal personality predicted persistent substance problems (Hasin et al., 2011). Personality dysfunction is also associated with an increased risk for physical illness (Lahey, 2007). Borderline personality disorder is associated with a heightened risk for obesity and diabetes (Frankenburg & Zanarini, 2006). Patients diagnosed with schizoid personality disorder, avoidant personality disorder, and obsessive–compulsive personality disorder (Pietrzak, Wagner, & Petry, 2007) exhibit an increased risk for heart disease. Byrne, Cherniack, and Petry (2013) reported that patients with antisocial personality disorder have a fivefold increase in receipt of disability benefits related to substance abuse.

Patients with personality disorder also overutilize medical services. Patients with borderline personality disorder fill more prescriptions, visit their PCPs more frequently, and place more phone calls between appointments than those without borderline personality disorder (Ansell, Sanislow, McGlashan, & Grilo, 2007). Borderline personality disorder is associated with hypertension, hepatic disease, cardiovascular disease, gastrointestinal disease, arthritis, and venereal disease; individuals with borderline personality disorder with a history of suicide attempts had even higher rates of cardiovascular and venereal disease (El-Gabalawy, Katz, & Sareen, 2010).

Furthermore, individuals with borderline personality disorder show an increased frequency of changing PCPs, disrupting continuity and comprehensiveness of care, and preventing the formulation of a valid diagnosis and treatment plan (Sansone, Farukhi, & Wiederman, 2011). Feenstra and colleagues (2012) found that adolescents exhibiting personality pathology demonstrated a lower quality of life as well as high health care costs.

Personality disorders impact health in other ways, including nonadherence to medical advice and exposure to interpersonal aggression or physical abuse (Vickerman & Margolin, 2008; Whisman & Schonbrun, 2009). However, Pfohl, Barrash, True, and Alexander (1989) reported that personality disorder did not predict nonadherence in a sample of male patients who were hypertensive.

Individuals with personality disorders also often show poor coping with stressors and life transitions (Millon, Million, et al., 2004; Monroe, 2008) and frequently report that they experience more stressful life events than the average person, manifesting poorer functioning after such events. Finally, onset of new health problems can be particularly stressful for persons with personality disorders (Oltmanns & Balsis, 2011). All told, the unique characteristics of these patients may present marked challenges to the health care team working with them to maintain good health and reduce health risks.

Angstman and Rasmussen (2011) outlined challenges that patients with personality disorder present to health care providers. Patients in Cluster A may present significant problems in establishing relationships with physicians and nurse practitioners because of their mistrust and avoidance. Patients in Cluster B, such as borderlines, may present with anger problems, while narcissists may present with a sense of entitlement and being special, creating stress in the ongoing consultations. Patients who are Cluster C anxiety prone may have a tendency to overwhelm their care providers with irrelevant information, and can become quite demanding of the provider's time. Patients with obsessive–compulsive personality disorder exhibit perfectionism and significant overattention to details. Patients who are dependent may overattach to physicians and seek constant reassurance from them. Patients with borderline personality disorder are two times more likely to display disruptive behaviors (e.g., cursing and making threats) that undermine the physician–patient relationship (Sansone & Sansone, 2013), making them the most difficult, challenging, and demanding patents encountered by PCPs (Gross et al., 2002). These challenges include suicidal ideation, psychotic symptoms, psychiatric comorbidity, and decreased levels of emotional and physical health. Finally, Gross and colleagues (2002) report that personality disorders that are not recognized by PCPs probably contribute to poor physician–patient relationships.

In sum, the impact of personality disorders on the treatment of anxiety, depression, autism spectrum disorders, and health is fairly compelling.

Cognitive therapists would benefit from a standardized model for addressing personality disorder problems that complicate symptomatic treatment.

Proper assessment and diagnosis are essential for both personality and symptomatic disorders. In assessing and treating patients who are symptomatic with coexisting personality disorders, clinical experience and empirical studies offer the following clinical pearls: Avoid the risk of over- and underdiagnosis; chart where and how treatment interference from personality disorders is expected and adjust existing protocols accordingly; use distressing symptoms to motivate treatment engagement; consider the use of pharmacotherapy; focus on early symptom relief and positive treatment expectancies; educate patients about the benefits of homework on reducing dropout, fostering positive outcome, and improving mood; address the obstacles of chronic anger, rumination, and negative mood; teach problem-solving strategies to alleviate stress and reduce termination and relapse; and target underlying schemas that are common threads across disorders.

CONCLUSION

The comorbidity of symptomatic and personality disorders may complicate treatment, result in higher rates of relapse, exacerbate the symptomatic disorder, increase treatment duration, and yield poorer outcomes. Clinicians need to prudently tailor manualized treatments based on a thorough case conceptualization, recognizing that personality disorders may increase the likelihood that treatment will be extended.

Because outcome studies generally fail to incorporate case formulations that actually drive treatment in clinical practice, modifying treatment protocols for the presence of a personality disorder is often necessary. It is best to examine the specific characteristics of patients and to understand how their idiosyncratic cognitions relate to onset, maintenance, and relapse, and how to address these factors in treatment. Finally, it is important to remember that we do not treat disorders but, rather, individuals with their own unique patterns of cognition, emotion, and behavior. True to the cognitive model, the most efficient route to effective treatment appears to be identification and modification of maladaptive schema and skills deficits that underlie co-occurring disorders.

CHAPTER 19

Clinical Management
Working with Those Diagnosed with Personality Disorders

Gina M. Fusco

Caring for them can be difficult and frustrating.
—WARD (2004, p. 1505)

The treatment team sat in silence. Frustration escalated as they discussed the proposed discharge plan for Jonathan, a 37-year-old Caucasian male admitted to the psychiatric inpatient unit approximately 10 days ago. Jonathan was referred by the local emergency department after becoming highly aggressive secondary to a self-disclosed suicide attempt via an overdose of alcohol and medication. He fought with and insulted the police and medical staff, yelling that they were just "stupid workers" who didn't understand. After medical clearance determined that he would not require detoxification or admission into a medical facility, the emergency department recommended inpatient mental health services. He initially refused this recommendation, but continued to express suicidal ideation. With the "threat" looming of involuntary commitment, he agreed to be admitted. Once transferred, the inpatient multidisciplinary team worked closely with Jonathan. His psychosocial history revealed that alcohol abuse, argumentativeness, and "dramas" had "burned bridges' with his family, and therefore they refused to be involved with his care. Jonathan identified no other supports and no longer had insurance coverage due to losing his job, and he had recently been evicted from his apartment. Throughout his stay, Jonathan was argumentative and seemed to "hijack" all of the groups with dismissive and insulting statements, followed by abrupt withdrawal to his room. He gravitated toward the female staff, and at times made provocative statements. He vacillated between declaring to the staff that they were doing tremendous work in helping his symptoms to improve and angry hostile statements that the team had failed. He was antagonistic toward the direct care staff, but treated the clinical staff with a more respectful demeanor. This respectful nature quickly changed to complaints about the psychiatrist made to the social worker, and negative statements made to the nursing staff about the social worker. Tension, confusion, and a growing belief that their efforts were futile existed within the team. With mounting pressure to identify a discharge plan as he was no longer clearly meeting stringent inpatient criteria, the team pushed ahead to arrange his discharge. A particularly annoyed staff member stated, "When can we get him out of here—he's causing havoc in the milieu," while another member said, "I'm concerned about his suicidality and what he did," to which several responded that he had made the suicide attempt to garner sympathy and was "attention seeking" and "manipulating." The social worker in charge of creating discharge plans lamented that no outpatient providers would accept his referral given his lack of insurance coverage, and from her list of resources, there were 2-month waiting lists for community mental health centers, recovery houses, and group homes. She indicated she had no real plan at this point. Recognizing they were rushing the discharge by trying to piece things together, they requested a case consultation and review to ensure they were making sound clinical recommendations.

CLINICAL CHALLENGES AND COMMUNITY CONTEXT

The treatment team above is struggling to work as a cohesive group and identify an appropriate and effective discharge plan. Given the high rate of repeated suicide attempts and completed suicide for recently discharged patients within a week of inpatient care (Deisenhammer, Huber, Kemmler, Weiss, & Hinterhuber, 2007; Qin & Nordentoft, 2005), an increased risk of suicide during the transition from inpatient to outpatient care (Kleespies, Marshall, Pokrajac, & Amodio, 1994), and data concluding unplanned discharges from inpatient settings increase the risk of completed suicide (Burgess, Pirkis, Morton, & Croke, 2000), delaying Jonathan's discharge was a prudent and clinically sound decision.

The team experienced common issues related to working with a patient cohort presenting with high-risk symptoms and personality pathologies. Jonathan exhibited difficulty establishing and maintaining interpersonal relationships, isolation, limited social skills, inappropriate behaviors, aggression, and other challenging behaviors. Countertransference, lack of communication, and a pejorative stance pressured the team to produce a discharge plan and hindered further risk assessment. Interventions (or lack of) were not being driven by an objective clinical assessment, did not incorporate a strengths-based approach, and no postdischarge resources were identified. The clinical team's reactions exemplifies the need to consider Burgess and colleagues' (2000) findings that suboptimal clinician–patient relationships and inadequate risk assessment can be factors contributing to increasing risk of suicide postdischarge from inpatient settings. With limited training of the direct care staff combined with negative and differing views, a splintered frustrated team became ineffective in maintaining consistent treatment interventions and creating a therapeutic discharge plan to a vulnerable patient who required just that—a viable discharge plan.

With the rapidly changing landscape of health care delivery systems, clinicians are faced with the challenge of working with individuals who present with highly complex clinical problems along with limited resources and time frames. Clinicians are tasked not only to understand and conceptualize in a more thorough and robust way but to do so quickly and with greater efficiency, while also caring for and respecting the patient as a person. To further complicate treatment with this highly vulnerable population, social and therapeutic supports are often scarce or unavailable. As an example, Roggenbaum, Christy, and LeBlanc (2012) surveyed mental health professionals from four facilities that receive emergency commitments across the state of Florida. Nearly half of the respondents indicated that the availability of community mental health treatment was "less than adequate" (p. 741). With limited resources, many clinicians must advocate for individuals to access and secure ongoing traditional treatment services, and assist with meeting general human welfare needs such as housing, food, and health care.

Arguing from a public health perspective, Duberstein and Witte (2009) suggest that population-level initiatives such as public health campaigns may help to prevent morbidity and enhance wellness by creating an interconnected system of supports, providing an alternative to focusing only on the small group that tends to frequently use crisis and emergency services. The authors state, "Psychologists must work to actively construct a care delivery system that accommodates these at-risk individuals elsewhere" (p. 277), and "New treatments in novel venues are needed" (p. 263). As those with personality disorders tend to have higher use of emergency services among those presenting for inpatient admission (Hayward & Moran, 2007), a nontraditional care delivery system could provide important prevention initiatives, promote early intervention, and create an ongoing support network for those being discharged from crisis services, or who need support beyond traditional therapy. Recovery-oriented advocacy and grassroots groups such as National Alliance on Mental Illness (NAMI), provides a diverse resource network with supports beyond traditional approaches that include certified peer specialists, volunteers, education and support groups, and a sense of community in maintaining one's recovery (2013). Located throughout the country in state and local chapters, NAMI, and groups similar to NAMI, are easily accessible to patients (*www.nami. org*). Given that people with personality disorders struggle to establish and maintain lifelong relationships, accessing an interconnected network can be invaluable in maintaining stability and equilibrium.

Unique and creative programs to assist patients within the community are showing promise to maintain treatment gains. These programs include postdischarge contact with the patient that helps to establish an ongoing connection and support. The benefits of follow-up or aftercare contact are supported by the results of the Motto and Bostrom (2001) study, which demonstrated "caring letters" sent to those discharged after a suicide attempt significantly reduced the rate of subsequent attempts. Follow-up programs have included postcards, letters, phone calls, and use of modern technologies such as texting and e-mailing. Luxton, June, and Comtois (2013) conducted a literature review related to postdischarge follow-up and concluded that contacts appeared to reduce suicide and suicidal behavior. In practice, clinicians ideally need to have an active and evolving list of resources to access, and with patient permission, provide some follow-up support if possible, such as providing information about groups such as NAMI.

COMORBIDITY AND EARLY DETECTION

Early detection is important to adequate treatment, yet often a major challenge with personality disorders. Because of high comorbidity, those with personality disorders often present for clinical care due to symptoms of mood, anxiety, substance use, or trauma. High-risk behaviors such as self- or other injury suggest the presence of a personality disorder, but may be difficult to distinguish in the context of severe symptoms. Widiger and Samuel (2009) recommend an integrated general approach and strategy to the assessment of personality disorders that includes administering a self-report to alert to whether there is a presence of maladaptive personality traits, followed by a semistructured interview to assess and verify diagnostic symptoms consistent with identified self-report items. A comprehensive history in addition to information provided by family members or supports can further corroborate information (Widiger & Samuel, 2009). Krysinska, Heller, and De Leo (2006) note that personality disorders, especially Cluster B disorders comorbid with clinical disorders, have been linked to suicidal behaviors, attempts, and completed suicides. Lambert (2003) indicated that comorbidity between personality disorders and commonly co-occurring substance abuse and mood disorders increases the risk of completed suicide, in addition to a history of child sexual abuse and antisocial traits. In terms of childhood trauma, Johnson, Smailes, Cohen, Brown, and Bernstein (2000) concluded that adult mental health and personality disorders are associated with child sexual abuse, complex abuse, and early developmental trauma. As childhood abuse is often linked with Cluster B personality disorders (Allen, 2004), a trauma-informed lens is very helpful in assessing the impact of childhood trauma and developing schema. In sum, Cheng, Mann, and Chan (1997) demonstrated that the greatest risk of suicide is associated with the comorbidity of clinical disorders and personality disorders. Therefore, to ensure best practices in the provision of thorough patient care, a comprehensive assessment that includes review of safety risks, comorbid conditions and pathways to respective treatment, and a discharge and/or safety plan that is realistic and empowering with specific access to support are recommended.

Suicide risk is elevated when there is evidence of prior life-threatening suicide attempts (which may be the strongest predictor of completed suicide; Moscicki, 1997); high lethality (e.g., firearms); medical illness; recent discharge from an inpatient setting (Deisenhammer et al., 2007; Qin & Nordentoft, 2005); and self-harming command hallucinations (in forensic inpatients; Rogers, Watt, Gray, MacCulloch, & Gournay, 2002). A literature review by Sullivan and Bongar (2009) identify psychiatric conditions such as schizophrenia, and eating, mood, substance, obsessive–compulsive, and panic disorders; recent losses, stress, and life events; Caucasian male demographic (increases with age); adolescence; social isolation; and a family member who has completed suicide as additional suicide risk factors.

TREATMENT, THERAPIST VARIABLES, AND QUALITY OF CARE

Therapeutic outcomes for patients diagnosed with personality disorders were explored in a comprehensive research review conducted by the American Psychological Association's Division 12. Characteristics of patients and therapists, the therapeutic relationship, and techniques with suggested links to outcome for personality disorder treatments were summarized as unique to personality disorders, shared with other disorders, and generalized from other disorders to personality disorders. Specific to personality disorders, patient variables included the "willingness and ability to engage in treatment" (Critchfield & Benjamin, 2006, p. 664), and shared with other disorders, a history of positive attachment and coping style. Therapist-related variables unique to this population were comfort with long-term relationships, tolerance of feelings and the process, patience, open-mindedness, and specialized training related to those issues that can occur with specific personality disorder populations, such as management of high-risk behaviors and borderline personality disorder. A suggested link to outcomes was associated with the therapist stance of a relatively high activity level, availability and flexibility during crises, and maintaining the relationship with honesty regarding limits, a balanced focus regarding change, and ongoing supervision/consultation (Critchfield & Benjamin, 2006).

The complicated nature of the needs of this population require the clinician to be flexible, and also well prepared and trained in providing suicide and violence assessment. Mental health professionals regularly encounter or intervene with patients who are suicidal or are in crisis, yet may lack the requisite training to be fully effective. A survey conducted by Kleespies, Penk, and Forsyth (1993) of psychologists in training from 1985 to 1990 indicated that 97% of the respondents had encountered a patient who was suicidal during their training years. Practicing social workers reported a high rate of contact (87%) with patients who were suicidal (Feldman & Freedenthal, 2006), and 28.8% of practicing psychologists reported at least one patient suicide and identified the most widespread fear they experienced in practice was "a client would commit suicide" (Pope & Tabachink, 1993, p. 149). Despite these high numbers, Schmitz and colleagues (2012) state, "The lack of training available in the institutions that prepare mental health professionals has been documented for decades" (p. 294). In all settings therefore, clinicians can benefit from training in suicide, risk assessment, and management of high-risk behaviors that begin with new employee orientation and include ongoing maintenance of competency through review, in-service training, or continuing education.

Support to Treatment Teams Working in Higher Levels of Care

Working with patients diagnosed with personality disorders requires specialized training, consultation, and ongoing peer or supervisory supports. Clinical teams are challenged with increasing clinical and administrative demands, while continuing to provide treatment in a collaborative, consistent, and safe way. Training that equips staff with skills to increase effectiveness when working with patients, and to be aware of and manage their responses, can impact the delivery of treatment and assist in maintaining a coordinated and consistent approach. Specifically, Duff (2003, p. 28) suggests staff receive specialized "shop floor" skills to be part of a comprehensive training program that include (1) a specialized induction that reviews information about the actual setting in which they are working, the patient populations they care for, and associated problems with those populations such as self-harm; (2) mentorship; (3) personal development plans; (4) support and supervision teams; and (5) debriefing. In addition, self-awareness, information about personality disorders, and an understanding of systems associated with the relational difficulties that this population often exhibits can be helpful. System issues related to interpersonal functioning requires the staff to have a consistent, empathic, and supportive approach, and to learn to manage discrepant information between team members that may cause conflict, boundary challenges, and emotional reactions to difficult behaviors and volatility (Duff, 2003). Formal training packages that include evidence-based verbal and nonverbal deescalation programs provide standardized approaches to managing high-risk situations in a trauma-informed, culturally responsive, and systemized way. Kleespies and Dettmer (2000) suggest creating mentorship programs to assist staff to prepare cognitively and affectively to work with a high-risk population that engages in life-threatening behavior.

Several studies have demonstrated that clinicians may develop negative attitudes and stigma related to working with those diagnosed with personality disorders (Newton-Howes, Weaver, & Tyrer, 2008; Treloar & Lewis, 2008). Therefore, it is important to assess negative staff perception of the diagnostic label and pejorative terminology used to describe behaviors, and remediate this with training and education. With deprecating terms such as "manipulating" and "attention seeking" used to describe behavior, empathy wanes (Potter, 2006) and frustration can build. Staff can be encouraged to reframe negative perceptions of challenging patient behaviors as a maladaptive pattern of attempting to get needs met or resolve issues. Institutional policies also need to reflect competencies and related outcomes to guide staff in improving the quality of care. The Joint Commission Accreditation of Hospital Organization references a quality tool prepared for the U.S. Department Health and Human Services (Lewin Group, 2013), to describe a high-reliability organization as one that creates a systemic culture that sets safety as the priority, promotes openness, learning, transparency, and emphasis on quality initiatives.

Policy, procedures, assessment strategies, emergency activation systems for patient and staff safety (e.g., panic buttons), standardized approaches to manage a crisis situation, and ongoing quality review of protocol effectiveness contributes to creating a high standard for established practice. A process for accessing after-hours or emergency support can be communicated to the patient as part of the informed consent process. If the patient is in crisis, the clinician may need to adjust a standard session, respond to an emergent situation, or become a patient advocate in securing ongoing care. In respect to providing crisis and/or emergent intervention, Robertson (1988) defines the clinician's general obligation or "duty to care" as the legal and ethical duty to provide ordinary and reasonable care (as cited in Kleespies, Deleppo, Gallagher, & Niles, 1999).

Collaboration between Psychological and Medical Providers

Ideally, collaboration and coordination of care needs is consistent, proactive, and inclusive. Through the informed consent process, patients can provide authorization for release of protected health information. With patients who are personality disordered, it is especially useful to create clear expectations of communication among treatment and medical providers with the goal of supporting the patient's overall health and functioning. It is helpful for the clinician to be fully aware of any concurrent treatment (e.g., family, addiction therapy). Resistance to sharing of this information can be explored within a collaborative motivational interviewing approach supporting autonomy, while evoking commitment to change within the treatment process. Documented and consistent communication with the patient's medical providers including primary care physicians (PCPs) and treating psychiatrists is essential when there are issues of discrepant information, especially pertaining to medication compliance, harmful medication interactions such as those that result from substance abuse, and medical conditions.

MANAGING CLINICAL CHALLENGES

Crisis Presentation

Patients with personality disorders may have a long history of maladaptive coping strategies leading to self- or other harm, self-medication, unhealthy relationships, difficulty in social and vocational arenas, and frequent overwhelming intrapersonal distress. When stressed, patients typically present with discomfort, dysfunction, dyscontrol, disorganization, and inability to resolve the difficulty through internal or external resources. A compromised problem-solving ability creates vulnerability to being overwhelmed or unable to cope (Fusco & Freeman, 2007b). For some, "Being in crisis is a way of life" (Freeman & Fusco, 2000, p. 28), and they may experience life as a series of the crisis du jour. Intense emotional states and related crises can create the expectation that life is unpredictable, and certainly out of their control.

Within the cognitive-behavioral model, emotions have a powerful and determining role in the overall scheme of personality organization (see A. Beck, Chapter 2, this volume). During a crisis, intense and powerful emotions activate compelling schema that through a distorted perceptual filter create maladaptive behaviors and coping strategies. Highlighting emotionality and its role in high-risk behaviors, Yen and colleagues (2009) demonstrated that within a predominately personality-disordered sample, the personality trait of negative affectivity (negative temperament/emotionality) was a more robust predictor of suicide attempts than traits of disinhibition or impulsivity. The profound influence of emotions on problem solving and cognitive processing, where the emotional priority overriding the cognitive system is likely related to seeking pleasure or avoiding pain, need to be considered when attempting intervention. Consistent with this view, Kleespies and Richmond (2009) stress the role of emotions in crisis, and suggest that the major tasks of conducting an emergency interview is to (1) contain the patient's emotional turmoil, (2) define the problem(s), (3) estimate the risk to self or others, and (4) provide treatment that is appropriate to the presenting or identified problem. Throughout assessment, the clinician can use verbal limits, active listening, and frame questions that help to contain emotional turmoil. If the patient presents disorganized or losing emotional control, brief closed-ended questions that the patient can focus on help to distract and calm. For example, "I'm going to ask you some questions . . I want you to focus on just the questions I'm asking, okay? Let's start with how did you get here?" Kleespies and Richmond (2009) suggest that multiple short interviews with breaks can also help to defuse and calm the patient.

Crisis Versus Emergency

Crisis intervention, depending on the nature of the situation, can be an evaluation to determine level-of-care (LOC) requirements such as those conducted within a psychiatric emergency room or emergency department, conducting an assessment of an already engaged patient who presents in crisis, or a series of brief therapy sessions designed to assist the patient in returning to a previous level of functioning. Ascertaining the safety of the patient, both to him or herself and to others is imperative in any crisis intervention. This aspect of crisis intervention involves an in-depth evaluation and requires rapid development of the therapeutic relationship.

Within crisis intervention literature, there is often a demarcation between crisis services and emergency interventions. Specifically, Kleespies and colleagues (1999) define a crisis as "a serious disruption of a person's baseline level of functioning such that his or her usual coping mechanisms are inadequate to restore equilibrium" (p. 454), is emotionally significant, and can result in a positive or negative outcome. Callahan (2009) states that crisis intervention includes the providing of a response within 24–48 hours, therapy to develop or reestablish equilibrium, and resolution within 4–6 weeks. In comparison, Kleespies and colleagues define an emergency, "when an individual reaches a state of mind in which there is imminent risk that he or she will do something (or fail to do something) that will result in serious harm or death to self or others unless there is some immediate intervention" (p. 454). Callahan states in response to an emergency situation that the clinician must provide an immediate response to the imminent risk, manage the intervention to prevent harm, and resolve the threat of immediate risk within a single encounter. Thus, clinical skills for crisis and emergency management include ascertaining imminent risk, having knowledge about how to access emergency services, working with responding medical personnel, ensuring the safety of themselves and others during the process, and referring or providing crisis stabilization within an appropriate time frame.

In considering the crisis intervention process, Roberts (2000, 2005) has suggested a seven-stage process for conducting an intervention. The stages include the following: (1) assess lethality and safety needs, (2) make psychological contact and rapidly establish rapport, (3) examine the dimension of the problem in order to define it, (4) encourage feelings, (5) explore past coping attempts, (6) formulate an action plan, and (7) follow up. If imminent risk is determined at Step 1, then steps for handling the crisis as an emergency need to be taken.

Suicide Risk Management

First and foremost, the patient's safety is paramount. Schneider and colleagues (2008) state that the treatment of personality disorders is an essential component in reducing rates of completed suicides. Personality disorders are associated with suicide risk (Chioqueta & Stiles, 2004) with estimates derived from psychological autopsies of those who committed suicide indicating 30–40% met criteria for a personality disorder (Duberstein & Conwell, 1997). Although recent studies indicate tremendous variation, which may be in part due to geographical differences, the median rates of personality disorders in postmortem samples is 32% (Duberstein & Witte, 2009). Specifically, borderline and Cluster B (Chioqueta & Stiles, 2004; Pompili, Giraldi, Ruberto, & Tatarelli, 2005), personality disorder diagnosis in more than one cluster and males in Cluster C (Schneider et al., 2006), schizoid, and avoidant (Duberstein & Conwell, 1997) personalities have demonstrated higher rates of suicidality, with dependent and paranoid personalities showing increased risk as concluded in a data review conducted by Duberstein and Witte (2009). A thorough review of suicide and harm assessment procedure and strategies is beyond the scope of this chapter. However, Schmitz and colleagues (2012) refers to Quinnett's definition that defines the competence and capacity to conduct a suicide assessment to include the following:

> A one-to-one assessment/intervention interview between a suicidal respondent in a telephonic or face-to-face setting in which the distressed person is thoroughly interviewed regarding current suicidal desire/ideation, capability, intent, reasons for dying, reasons for living, and especially suicide attempt plans, past attempts and protective factors. The interview leads to a risk stratification decision, risk mitigation intervention and a collaborative risk management/safety plan, inclusive of documentation of the assessment and interventions made and/or recommended. (p. 294)

At minimum, Sullivan and Bongar (2009) suggest that a thorough diagnostic assessment include the following: psychiatric disorders; suicide accelerants such as hopelessness, psychological pain, recent losses, substance abuse, firearm access, and insomnia. Additional factors to assess include potential for harm, trauma history, change in mental status, and potential situations that may involve abuse of children and the elderly, and interpersonal violence. Direct inquires about suicidal ideation, behaviors, risk, and protective factors are included in the interview. As a means to determine suicide risk, clinicians rely primarily on the clinical interview and observation. However, psychological testing can assist in further identifying risk of self-harm. No one scale or test can delineate risk, and all means to assess risk should be utilized. Commonly used psychological tests include the Minnesota Multiphasic Personality Inventory–2 (MMPI-2; Butcher et al., 2001), and the recent addition to the Rorschach comprehension system (Exner, 2003) that includes the Suicide Constellation (S-CON) among the special indexes (as cited in Sullivan & Bongar, 2009). Suicide assessment measures including the Beck Depression Inventory–II (Beck, Steer, & Brown, 1996), which assesses level of depression and has two items that directly address suicidality, and the Beck Hopelessness Scale (Beck & Steer, 1993b), which assesses future-oriented thinking, motivation, and expectations, are commonly used and have been determined as reliable and valid instruments. It is important to note that some patients tend to disclose more information in self-report instruments rather than verbally to a clinician (Kaplan, Asnis, Sanderson, & Keswani, 1994), and frequently discrepancies between patient and clinician assessment of risk exist (Bewick, McBride, & Barkham, 2006).

A thorough interview, which may or may not include psychological testing, provides an overall estimation of risk and is utilized (often with psychiatric assessment) to determine LOC, or disposition. The LOC may include a referral for an outpatient psychiatric evaluation, substance abuse or specialized assessment or treatment, more frequent contacts with the treating clinician (intensive outpatient), partial hospitalization, inpatient hospitalization, or immediate transfer to a medical facility for medical clearance if a suicide attempt is suspected, and/or assessment to rule out any medical issues. White (2010) states that medical clearance indicates that although the patient may be in crisis, a medical illness is not considered present; a medical illness may be present but is not thought to be the cause of the current behavioral symptoms; or it is thought that the medical illness no longer requires medical treatment. Clarification of medical clearance is essential to promote an appropriate transfer and handoff of care, ensuring that the patient's psychological, as well as medical needs, are met. It is vital to ensure that clinicians do not disregard medical evaluation or clearance, as many major medical illnesses can mimic many psychological symptoms (White, 2010).

The clinician must remain observant of verbal and nonverbal communication at all times when working with a patient who may be suicidal. Suicide experts suggest clinician "gut feelings" as a warning sign of suicide potential should not be ignored, but rather safely explored with thorough assessment and follow-up (Tartakavosky, 2011). If the patient has called the clinician or scheduled an urgent or emergent session indicating suicidal ideation, clarify if an attempt has already been made (remaining aware of the patient's breathing, slurring, voice changes, etc.). If the patient has taken self-harming action, the amounts of medications used to overdose or depth of cuts are confirmed only through the medical clearance process (many patients may underestimate amounts or potential for harm). As family members may have motives for nondisclosure of seriousness, denial, or belief that they can handle the patient or situation, clinical judgment must be exercised if family members are involved. If a situation requires contacting emergency services, the clinician should inform responding personnel of any safety risks, including patient ownership of firearms, or any high-risk symptomology such as suicidality, paranoia, and homicidality. Advising emergency department medical staff of the pending arrival of the patient with any known information including medications, medical problems, nature and method of suicide plan or attempt, and a brief synopsis can be helpful. Other information can include contact information of the patient's psychiatrist and PCP. Members of the patient's treatment team (psychiatrist, PCP), considering consents, should be contacted, and if applicable, the patient's insurance company (Fusco & Freeman, 2007b).

Voluntary and Involuntary Hospitalization

Inpatient admission may be necessary if a patient demonstrates he or she is at risk for self- or other harm, or exhibits an inability to care for him- or herself. Depending on the setting, and the insurance carrier, a psychiatric face-to-face evaluation may be needed to determine medical necessity and payment authorization for admission. Best practices include knowing what programs and facilities are available in the community, and how to access psychiatric emergency services. Mobile crisis services can provide intervention within the community, but may lack psychiatric intervention or assessment. During the process of the assessment, if the patient requires an admission but is refusing or unable to consent to being admitted, an involuntary commitment may be necessary to ensure the safety of the patient and others. The commitment process requires clear documentation of specific behaviors, verbal statements, and observations detailed in the patient record. All states have civil statutes that provide for the involuntary hospitalization of those who may be mentally ill, a danger to self, or to others (Kaufman & Way, 2010). However, the statutes and regulations vary including time-frame differences (Tebaldi, 2012). It is essential that the clinician is informed and trained as to how to petition, access, or initiate this process within his or her region. If safe to do so, all avenues of possible clinical or medical alternative care should be pursued as the commitment process deprives one of liberty, and may be stigmatizing (Kaufman & Way,

2010). Ethically, clinical providers have to balance the need for patient and others' safety and well-being, with the idea of self-determination (Sehiralti & Er, 2012). McGarvey, Leon-Verdin, Wancheck, and Bonnie (2013) suggest that investment into creating a continuum of intensive community services may reduce the need for involuntary interventions, as emergency service clinicians employed by community service boards throughout Virginia indicated that 27% of committed patients could have been served in a voluntary residential, short-term crisis stabilization had it been available.

Tarasoff and Duty to Warn/Protect

In the landmark case *Tarasoff v. Regents of the University of California* in 1974, the duty to warn (DTW) ruling set the precedence that mental health professionals must warn third parties of danger disclosed by patients during psychotherapeutic treatment (Edwards, 2013). In a subsequent ruling in 1976, the court modified and replaced that responsibility with a broader duty to protect, an obligation for mental health professionals to utilize reasonable care to protect an intended victim (as cited in Pabian, Welfel, & Beebe, 2009). The *Tarasoff* case was the first to address outpatient clinicians and their duty to protect the public in a way that might compel them to breach confidentiality in providing information to an outside party. In subsequent years, all states have in some way addressed the law, but vary in their requirements in enacting the duty including the following: the requirement of a specific DTW an intended victim of a specific threat of bodily harm, a broader duty to protect from harm, permission to (but not require) breach of confidentiality, or for some states, an absence of a requirement. The *Tarasoff* case highlighted the importance for the clinician to have specific knowledge relating to the understanding of a fiduciary relationship, prediction of dangerousness, foreseeability, identifiable victim(s), reasonable care, and the duty statutes (Simone & Fulero, 2005). Pabian and colleagues (2009) demonstrated in a survey of psychologists from four states that 76% were misinformed about their specific state laws with many believing they had the legal obligation of DTW, and were not aware that other protective actions were permitted. To meet the legal standards, clinicians must understand the law specific to the state in which they practice regarding informed consent requirements, what triggers the DTW or protect (Pabian et al., 2009), and how that duty can be discharged under the provisions of the law, including the option to use clinical discretion.

Violence Assessment

There is empirical evidence to support a linkage between personality disorders and violent behavior (Gilbert & Daffern, 2011). Those with antisocial and borderline personalities, and those who were violent before admission were more likely to be violent postdischarge from an inpatient setting than those without personality disorders (Tardiff, Marzuk, Leon, & Portera, 1997). Ranked second to schizophrenia, those with personality disorders were the majority of assailants toward psychologists working in various settings who responded in a national survey (Guy, Brown, & Poelstra, 1990). For their own safety and the safety of others, it is important for clinicians to have some level of competence in detecting or estimating the risk of patient violence toward others. The prediction of violence however, is a complex and controversial issue effecting patient care and public policies. Specific assessment tools have produced inconsistent results, although they have profound impact on treatment intervention, current practices, and the implementation of community policies in various settings such as no-tolerance rules in schools (Yang, Wong, & Coid, 2010). Risk assessment tools identify variables that are most frequently associated with an outcome of violence, providing the clinician with a list of risk factors that when indicated denote through a quantifiable rating, an estimation of risk (Doyle & Logan, 2012). McNeil (2009) provides a comprehensive overview of current acute risk assessment tools utilized to screen and assess for violence risk. In comparison to solely utilizing a tool for assessment, the structured professional judgment (SPJ) approach to estimating risk attempts to "bridge the gap" between unstructured clinical interviews and actuarial approaches in risk assessment (Kropp, 2008, p. 207). The SPJ approach involves formal steps incorporating empirically identified risk factors with an individualized assessment that generates risk management strategies and summary of judgment. For example, a clinician may use a formal assessment tool that incorporates variables associated with risk, and gather further information on the presence of risk factors (history, current, context, and protective) and individualized risk formulation and scenarios to develop targeted risk management strategies and summary recommendations (Doyle & Logan, 2012).

When working with those who may be at risk to become violent, the safety of all involved is critical. This includes the patient, clinician, other patients, and the public. For all settings, safety protocols need to be part of standardized trainings, practiced with drills, and assessed in a quality review process. The physical setting should be carefully considered in any type of service, including crisis-oriented programs or centers. This includes the types and placement of furniture (e.g., anchored, secured, sharp edges), access to egress, areas not easily viewed or observed due to layout (corners), staffing patterns that provide support when needed, objects that can be used as weapons or projectiles, safety risks (e.g., ligature), and sound levels that invariably can activate or further patient escalation. Waiting area design and flow of service provided to patients should consider potential agitating elements such as the often used television turned to what may be triggering television shows (e.g., crime dramas, news, talk shows), unclear or confusing process of registration, reading material, music, temperature, overcrowding, loud or piercing alarms related to calling codes or announcements, access to refreshment (e.g., water fountain, snacks), little privacy or confining spaces, limited cultural responsiveness, insensitive search for contraband or requests for clothing removal, poorly fitting gowns or scrubs, and a lack of empathy for those patients struggling with rules related to smoking.

Kleespies and colleagues (1999) note clinician response to increasing aggression will vary in response to the setting. Training of clinicians should include safety issues such as choice of clothing and grooming (e.g., neckties, scarves, necklaces), and basic skills related to setting verbal limits (clarifying what is acceptable behavior, neutral/positive tone), proximity, and nonverbal (e.g., avoiding intense eye contact) responses. Clinician awareness of increasing agitation, frustration, and verbal and nonverbal signals of increased tension such as clenching, pacing, elevated or voice changes, grimacing, and so on can alert the need for support or intervention that may include recommending a higher LOC, initiating an involuntary commitment, warning an intended victim, escaping for self-protection, contacting the police, ambulance, or if in an inpatient setting, initiating a code or show of force, or more restrictive measures including therapeutic holds or restraints (Kleespies et al., 1999).

McNeil, Binder, and Greenfield (1988) indicate that when conducting a violence assessment, patient history of violent behavior is consistently shown to be the best predictor of future violent behavior, and conclude that those who were violent in the community are more likely to be violent in a hospital. LOC and decisions related to risk involve the assessment of the imminence of aggression, the nature (types of abuse), how often it occurs, level of aggression, and the attempt to predict occurrence (Kropp, 2008), keeping in mind specific state-mandated reporting of child abuse and/or elder abuse and other required reporting statutes. An informative assessment may include the following: queries about any stated intention or desire to harm or veiled threats toward others; recent aggressive behavior; past harm to others; frequency of aggression; patterns and/or triggers related to aggression; psychiatric symptoms associated with aggression (e.g., hallucinations, mood changes); context of past aggression; planned versus impulsive aggression; attitude toward past aggression; violent threats or fantasies; specific threats (related to DTW laws); and extent of planning harm, means, and preparation to fulfill fantasy or threat (McNeil, 2009). Additional queries optimally include thorough assessment of legal history including past and current protection from abuse orders (restraining orders); incarceration; current involvement with legal system (e.g., probation or parole); prior psychiatric treatment (voluntary and involuntary); and thorough assessment of weapon access and ownership including firearms, knives, and so on. Clinical judgment in conducting such interviews is paramount with consideration of settings and available support, particularly in more isolated outpatient settings, with pacing as needed to maintain rapport and moderate any risk of aggravating the potentially violent patient in a way that could increase imminent risk to the clinician or others. McNeil, Weaver, and Hall (2007) suggest that specific queries into the availability of firearms should be part of a standard screening process "in contexts in which patients are undergoing behavioral emergencies and therefore tend to be at elevated risk of impulsive suicidal or violent behavior—for example, inpatient units and emergency departments" (p. 552) versus querying on an as-needed basis, as higher reports of firearm ownership were reported when routinely assessed. The mental status examination can identify acute symptoms such as paranoia, hostility, excitement, hallucinations, and disorganization that can indicate increasing risk of imminent violence (McNeil, 2009).

Relationship Crises and Intimate Partner Violence

For those with personality disorders, the struggle to establish and maintain relationships creates the inevitable crises related to interpersonal functioning. The activation of relationship-oriented powerful schema, such as abandonment, rejection, isolation, hostility, and worthlessness, can exacerbate and overwhelm an already compromised coping system. Depending on the intensity and compelling nature of the schema, crises can erupt from either the realistic appraisal or inaccurate perception of relationship turmoil. Through a collaborative process, the exploration, examination, and challenge of automatic thoughts and assumptions can create a more balanced and realistic appraisal. The building of coping strategies to manage reactions to conflict, disruption, or stability of relationships is a necessary component in treatment planning. Social skills and communication building can help to create a more adaptive and positive interaction style, with behavioral experiments creating the opportunity for an "adaptive spiral" of functioning (Yalom, 1995, p. 43).

Comprehensive assessment of intimate partner violence (IPV) is essential. Dutton (2006) notes that recent studies have identified that among partner-abusing men, rates of those with personality disorders were six times higher than those within the general population (as cited in Ross & Babcock, 2009). Batterer typologies that are anchored in personality pathologies include borderline/dysphoric, low-level antisocial, generally violent/antisocial, and family-only violence (Holtzworth-Munroe, Meehan, Herron, Rehman, & Stuart, 2000). Eckhardt, Holtzworth-Munroe, Norlander, Sibley, and Cahill (2008) demonstrated that specific typologies are linked to batterer intervention program completion (borderline/dysphoric and generally violent/antisocial showing high levels of dropout), and associated resistance and low readiness to change with recidivism and rearrest. Dutton (2006, cited in Ross & Babcock, 2009) further notes that symptom patterns of those with personality disorders are related to the types of abuse batterers exhibit. For example, the patient with borderline personality disorder who struggles with dysregulation may be at risk to exhibit IPV when mood instability or schema is activated related to abandonment. For couples engaging in treatment, motivational interviewing strategies have been found to reduce physical aggression and harmful alcohol use in a study of 50 college dating couples between the ages of 18 and 25 who had reported at least one incident of male to female aggression (Woodin & O'Leary, 2010). Safety plans with identified resources such as a women's shelter should be readily available for those who decide to vacate their home and be in a protective setting.

Safety Plans

For those who have demonstrated high-risk behaviors or are living in high-risk situations, establishing a safety plan, accessing supports, and patient empowerment is essential as often those with personality disorders demonstrate "the lack of ability to organize and plan their activities" (Morana & Camara, 2006, p. 541). Information to prompt the patient can be organized in an individualized written safety plan for crisis situations that denotes identified triggers, positive coping strategies, emergency services information, supports with specific phone numbers or contact information, and follow-up appointment date and time. The identification and provision of access to local support networks—both formal and informal—friends, family, spiritual affiliations, employee assistance programs (EAPs), employees, support groups, 12-step groups, sponsors, hotlines, recovery-oriented groups, and peer groups or services can help to support the patient between sessions and postdischarge. Family and support resources can be invaluable in challenging held beliefs, related worthlessness, isolation, reinforcing safety plans, and other issues. The use of no-harm contracts (NHCs) remains controversial in its effectiveness in reducing or preventing suicidal or harming behavior. Hyldahl and Richardson (2011) suggest careful consideration if an NHC is used and for the clinician to "Remember that contracting is just one piece of an ongoing risk assessment and treatment process" (p. 125).

Insurance

With emphasis on short lengths of stay or treatment, many insurance carriers do not authorize payment for treatment for an individual with a primary diagnosis of a personality disorder, likely due to the chronic nature of the condition. There may also be a negative perception and attitude regarding efficacy of treatment (American Psychological Association, 2004). Higher levels of care are generally approved for authorization of payment by the insurance company if the patient exhibits behaviors that are creating imminent risk such as self- or other harm, inability to care for him- or herself, and/or substance use that requires treatment within a structured setting. Clear documentation within the patient record can help substantiate medical necessity of continued treatment focused on the specific behaviors that led to the need for treatment, and consistent communication between medical and treatment providers (e.g., formal treatment teams with a specific agenda targeting treatment goals). Clinicians may need to assist their financial departments to create protocols to help patients without insurance gain access and maintain their coverage by assisting patients to complete the required documentation. Insurance carriers often have specialty teams such as intensive case managers and prevention programs to assist the patient.

CLINICIAN SELF-CARE AND RESILIENCE

The ability to empathize, the very attribute that makes a clinician exceptional in what he or she does, can also create distress (Kleespies & Dettmer, 2000). A regimen of clinician self-care and attentiveness to personal limits is essential. Patients with personality disorders often present with a complicated case conceptualization that can include high-risk behaviors and variable treatment compliance (Gudjonsson & Main, 2008), which can prove to be taxing and challenging. For the clinician, exposure to life-threatening behavior can create stress, relationship issues, vicarious traumatization, and clinical disorders. Surveys have indicated that psychologists are at risk for mental health problems, including depression (Kleespies et al., 2011), and therefore must exercise great care in ensuring that they are aware of becoming overwhelmed; have social, peer support and/or supervision; and a realistic schedule. A prevention focus that is highlighted during training years and in current practice can strengthen and create resiliency to the rigors of clinical practice. Making self-care a priority and viewing it as integral to well-being can include maintaining health, nutrition, use of relaxation strategies such as meditation, and an overall balance of work life and personal time. With electronic technology allowing 24/7 access, it is often difficult for a clinician to experience true downtime. Personal time that includes scheduled time off and creating consistent practice coverage, perhaps shared with colleagues, can be helpful to avoid fatigue and ensure the clinician is well rested. Formal colleague assistance programs introduce preventative initiatives such as frequent self-assessments, and a confidential platform to seek support (Kleespies et al., 2011). Ongoing awareness and support by one's colleagues and the organizations that employ clinicians can promote clinician health and well-being, ultimately benefiting the patients they serve.

Revisiting the Case of Jonathan and the Treatment Team

Having recognized the need for formal procedures within the institution to promote quality practice and support to clinical staff, the hospital had created a case review process for all team participants and several nonteam professional members as objective consultants. The multidisciplinary group accessed and initiated the supportive and open process and reviewed Jonathan's history, case formulation, and treatment plan, and discussed how well the team worked together in providing treatment. Clinically, the team discussed how Jonathan's personality style and patterns of coping tended to influence his reactions and attempts to manage significant stressors. Treatment goals were subsequently added to build specific adaptive coping and problem-solving skills related to his many recent life challenges, including losing his apartment. Because he often alienated others with dismissive and provocative statements, Jonathan's treatment plan was expanded to include specific groups for social interaction skills. To build cohesion, the team was encouraged to discuss their frustrations and suggestions to improve the team's process. Frustrations included the lack of pertinent clinical information that could help guide treatment decisions, and their feelings of inadequacy and incompetency in managing challenging behaviors. To meet this need, a referral for psychological testing that included a substance abuse screen was generated. Thereafter, protocols were refined to make referrals for in-house psychological testing easier and quicker. An ongoing training was organized for all staff related to the management of challenging behaviors, use of pejorative terms and how they impact team perception and reactions to patients, maintaining boundaries, and how to use debriefing after an incident of aggression or occurrence of a restrictive intervention, such as a therapeutic hold. Social work staff were provided access to linkage databases from affiliated hospitals that listed discharge resources, support and advocacy groups, and other specialty supports. Empowered with an enhanced and clarified understanding of Jonathan's needs and risks, the team recommended that Jonathan remain in the hospital for an additional week. After an assessed indication of low risk of self-harm and access to additional community resources, he was successfully discharged with a comprehensive safety plan that included intensive outpatient services and admission to a halfway house that provided structure and a supportive milieu, with additional supports from local recovery-oriented and advocacy groups.

CHAPTER 20

Synthesis and Prospects for the Future

Denise D. Davis
Arthur Freeman

The concept of personality disorders is continuously evolving. Successive editions of the American Psychiatric Association's *Diagnostic and Statistical Manual of Mental Disorders* have marked significant changes in the theoretical view, range of problems, definitions, and terminology used to denote personality disorders. New disorders are identified as others are eliminated. For example, the inadequate personality (301.82) and the asthenic personality (301.7) in DSM-II disappeared in DSM-III. Narcissistic personality disorder (301.81) emerged for the first time in DSM-III. Passive–aggressive personality disorder was declassified from a formal disorder to a provisional diagnosis in DSM-IV, and then dropped to a personality trait in DSM-5. Depressive personality was a provisional diagnosis in DSM-IV, and then also "downgraded" to a personality trait in DSM-5. However, it is still possible to diagnose these clinically relevant conditions under the category "other specified personality disorder" (301.89). Other terms have changed across the history of diagnosis. For example, the emotionally unstable personality (51.0) in DSM-I became the hysterical personality (301.5) in DSM-II, and histrionic personality disorder (301.5) in DSM-III through DSM-5. Low face validity and high levels of overlap in meaning for several of the personality disorders has been an ongoing concern (Blashfield & Breen, 1989). Nevertheless, the distinctive cognitive profiles can be mapped out, and work is progressing in valid measurement of specific cognitive factors that distinguish among the different personality disorders (Fournier, DeRubeis, & Beck, 2011).

Ongoing confusion is compounded as clinicians increasingly navigate between the DSM-5 system and the *International Classification of Diseases* (ICD; World Health Organization) criteria for personality disorders. It is important that diagnostic categories offer a valid and useful conceptual framework to support effective clinical interventions and continuity in clinical research.

ASSESSMENT

Effective treatment hinges on ongoing assessment, monitoring of cognitive processes, and case conceptualization. One overarching objective in assessment is to ensure that enduring traits are differentiated from more transient states attributable to circumstances or symptomatic disorders, and that maladaptive implications are tested for cultural biases. The cognitive therapist most likely integrates multiple sources of data, including diagnostic interviews, review of collateral data, behavioral observations, self-report inventories, and ongoing discussion. Idiographic details of the patient's operative beliefs can be pinpointed with specifically designed instruments such as the Personality Belief Questionnaire (Beck & Beck, 1995a, Beck & Beck, 1995b) or the Schema Questionnaire (Young, 2006), and relative dimensions of personality features can be profiled.

CLINICAL GUIDELINES

As the preceding chapters show, considerable progress has been made in applying cognitive therapy in the treatment of personality disorders. However, the practitioner faces the challenge of treating a complex disorder without having a reliable, validated treatment protocol. Furthermore, to a large extent the treatment of each of the personality disorders has been considered in isolation. However, individuals seeking treatment rarely fall neatly into a single diagnostic category. When individuals with personality disorders seek treatment, they may present features of several personality disorders without fully meeting diagnostic criteria for any single one, or they may qualify for more than one personality disorder diagnosis. Characteristics of one personality disorder may either attenuate or magnify characteristics of another disorder, further altering the pattern of clinical signs. In addition, individuals typically have comorbid symptomatic disorders as well, so it may take some time to sort out the stable and pervasive features that maintain the patient's distress over time.

It is not simple to provide effective treatment in the complex situations encountered in clinical practice. Fortunately, therapists do not have to start from scratch in figuring out how to approach treatment with patients who have personality disorders. Reviews of the empirical and clinical literature noted in this volume have provided the basis for general guidelines for cognitive therapy with patients whose personality functioning results in significant functional impairment or subjective distress. These applied guidelines are summarized as follows:

1. *Interventions are most effective when based on an individualized conceptualization of the patient's problems.* Patients with personality disorders have complex, ingrained, and hypertrophied problems that coexist with transient or situation difficulties. The therapist is often faced with choosing among many possible targets for intervention and a variety of possible intervention techniques. Not only does this present a situation in which treatment can easily become confused and disorganized if the therapist does not have a rational treatment plan, but the interventions that seem appropriate after a superficial examination of the patient can easily prove ineffective or counterproductive. Turkat and his colleagues (especially Turkat & Maisto, 1985) have demonstrated the value of developing an individualized conceptualization based on a detailed evaluation and testing the validity of that conceptualization through collecting additional data and through observing the effects of clinical interventions.

The conceptualizations presented in this volume can provide a starting framework. Nevertheless, it is important to base interventions on an individualized conceptualization rather than presuming that the "standard" conceptualization will fit every patient with a particular diagnosis. Although developing an understanding of a complex patient is challenging, cognitive therapy can be a self-correcting process because the conceptualization is refined over the course of treatment. When the therapist begins conceptualization on the basis of an initial evaluation, and seeks corroboration from the patient before proceeding, the effects of these efforts will provide valuable feedback. The "litmus test" for any conceptualization is whether it explains past behavior, accounts for present behavior, and predicts future behavior. If the interventions work as expected, this shows that the conceptualization is accurate enough for the time being. If the interventions prove ineffective or produce unexpected results, this shows that the conceptualization is insufficient or only partially correct. Furthermore, examination of the thoughts and feelings evoked by the interventions may provide valuable data for refining the conceptualization and the treatment plan.

2. *It is important for therapist and patient to work collaboratively toward specifying an agreement on treatment goals.* With patients as complex as those with personality disorders, clear, consistent goals for therapy are necessary to avoid skipping from problem to problem without making lasting progress. However, it is important for these goals to be mutually agreed on to minimize the noncollaboration and power struggles that can

impede treatment of patients with personality disorders. It can be difficult to develop shared goals for treatment when patients present numerous vague complaints and, at the same time, may be unwilling to modify behaviors that the therapist sees as particularly problematic. The time and effort spent developing mutually acceptable goals can be a good investment. It is likely to maximize the patient's motivation for change, minimize resistance, and make it easier to maintain a consistent focus to treatment. A general strategy for developing goals can be found in asking patients what it means to them to get "better," and articulating what this might look like in functional, real-life circumstances. The therapist often needs to help patients build and maintain investment in pursuing these goals through discussions about change that draw out their ambivalence and allow them to formulate the reasons to pursue change. This may require the therapist to moderate his or her own goal orientation, and to use skills such as motivational interviewing to avoid provoking the patient's resistance and instead facilitate his or her successful resolution of ambivalence.

3. *It is important to focus more than the usual amount of attention on the therapist–patient relationship.* A good therapeutic relationship is as necessary for effective intervention in cognitive therapy as in any other approach to therapy. Behavioral and cognitive-behavioral therapists are generally accustomed to being able to establish a straightforward collaborative relationship at the outset of therapy and then to proceed without paying much attention to the interpersonal aspects of therapy. However, when working with patients who have personality disorders, therapy often is not this straightforward. The dysfunctional schemas, beliefs, and assumptions that bias patients' perceptions of others also bias their perception of the therapist, and the dysfunctional interpersonal behaviors manifest in relationships outside therapy are likely to be manifested in the therapist–patient relationship as well. Attachment patterns that are evident across the patient's lifespan can often be identified in how the patient regards therapy and the therapist, as he or she may relate in anxious, ambivalent, disorganized, or detached ways. Interpersonal difficulties manifested in the therapist–patient relationship can disrupt therapy if they are not addressed effectively. However, these difficulties also provide the therapist with an opportunity to do *in vivo* observation and intervention rather than having to rely on the patient's report of interpersonal problems occurring between sessions (Freeman, Pretzer, Fleming, & Simon, 1990; Mays, 1985; Padesky, 1986).

One issue in the therapist–patient relationship that is more pronounced and central to the treatment process among individuals with personality disorder is the phenomenon traditionally termed "transference." This term refers to times when the patient manifests an extreme or persistent misperception of the therapist based on the patient's previous experience in significant relationships, rather than on the therapist's behavior. This phenomenon can be understood in cognitive terms as resulting from the individual overgeneralizing the beliefs and expectancies he or she acquired in significant relationships. Individuals with personality disorders are typically vigilant for any sign that their fears may be realized and are prone to react quite intensely when the therapist's behavior appears to confirm their anticipations. When these strongly emotional reactions occur, it is important for the therapist to recognize the impact of the patient's biased view of others, to quickly develop an understanding of what the patient is thinking, and to directly but sensitively address these misconceptions within the therapy. Although these reactions can be quite problematic, they also provide opportunities to identify beliefs, expectations, and interpersonal strategies that play an important role in the patient's problems. This also is an opportunity for the therapist to respond to the patient in ways that disconfirm the patient's dysfunctional beliefs and expectancies, and to help the patient understand the workings of the cognitive model and how it can provide a means of breaking out of problematic relationship patterns. The techniques of empathic interpersonal feedback and limited or partial reparenting are especially relevant to this process.

4. *Consider beginning with interventions that do not require extensive self-disclosure, especially with highly anxious or fearful patients who view others with mistrust.* Many patients with personality disorders are initially uncomfortable with self-disclosure in psychotherapy. They may not trust the therapist, may be uncomfortable with even mild levels of intimacy, may fear rejection, and so on. It is sometimes necessary to begin treatment with interventions that require extensive discussion of the patient's thoughts and feelings, but often treatment can begin with behavioral interventions that gradually introduce self-disclosure. Starting with small recommendations for concrete actions that give the patient something specific to do allows time for the patient to become more comfortable with therapy and for the therapist to gain the patient's trust and explore the reasons for discomfort with self-disclosure.

5. *Interventions that increase the patient's sense of self-efficacy often reduce the intensity of symptoms and facilitate other interventions.* The intensity of the emotional and behavioral responses manifested by individuals with personality disorders is often exacerbated by the individual's doubts regarding his or her ability to cope. This doubt regarding one's ability to cope effectively not only intensifies emotional responses to the situation but also predisposes the individual to drastic responses. When it is possible to increase the individual's confidence that he or she will be able to handle problem situations as they arise, this often lowers the patient's level of anxiety, moderates his or her symptoms, enables him or her to react more deliberately, and makes it easier to implement other interventions. The individual's sense of self-efficacy, his or her confidence that he

or she can deal effectively with specific situations when they arise, can be increased by correcting any exaggerations of the demands of the situation or minimization of the individual's capabilities, adding new coping skills, or through a combination of the two (Freeman et al., 1990; Pretzer, Beck, & Newman, 1989). Increasing the patient's self-efficacy early in treatment also conveys the therapist's confidence in the patient as a capable person, and instills a sense of encouragement from others that may be lacking.

6. *Do not rely primarily on verbal interventions.* The more severe a patient's problems are, the more important it is to use behavioral interventions to accomplish cognitive as well as behavioral change (Freeman et al., 1990). Experiential tools such as role playing within the session and a hierarchy of "behavioral experiments" between sessions provides an opportunity for desensitization to occur, helps the patient to gain confidence, and can be quite effective in challenging unrealistic beliefs and expectations. When it is necessary to rely on purely verbal interventions, concrete, real-life examples often are more effective than abstract, philosophical discussions. Other experiential methods including mindfulness practices, imagery, schema dialogues, and affective awareness training are important in creating a sufficiently intense therapeutic experience.

7. *Try to identify and address the patient's fears before implementing changes.* Patients with personality disorders often have strong, unexpressed fears embedded in their beliefs and assumptions that give rise to a global fear that something bad might happen if they change. Attempts to induce the patient to simply go ahead without addressing these fears are often unsuccessful (Mays, 1985). If the therapist makes a practice of discussing the patient's expectations and concerns before each change is attempted, it is likely to reduce the patient's level of anxiety regarding therapy and to improve compliance. General goals can be subdivided into much smaller subcomponents to make change more manageable, so it is easier to see how good things might happen. For example, the patient with a broad goal of being more assertive might work on a subcomponent of handling low-level provocation from a difficult coworker in a more proactive way.

8. *Help the patient deal adaptively with aversive emotions.* Patients with personality disorders often experience very intense aversive emotional reactions in specific situations. These intense reactions can be a significant problem in their own right. More importantly, the individual's attempts to avoid experiencing these emotions, his or her attempts to escape the emotions, and his or her cognitive and behavioral response to the emotions often play an important role in the patient's problems. Many individuals with personality disorders were raised in emotionally distorted or invalidating environments, and have little or no experience to draw upon for tolerating and managing aversive emotions, much less discerning how to effectively recover from them. This lack of coping skills perpetuates fears

about the consequences of experiencing the emotions and fears about the meaning of having these emotions in the first place. When this is the case, it can be important to work systematically to increase the patient's ability to tolerate intense affect and cope effectively with it (Farrell & Shaw, 1994). Patients often appreciate the therapist's use of empathic confrontation, where the therapist validates the emotion and then points out the risks of acting on these emotions in maladaptive ways (internalizing or externalizing), and then explains more functional options and encourages the patient to use the latter approach.

9. *Help patients cope with aversive emotions that can be elicited by therapeutic interventions.* In addition to the intense emotions patients experience in day-to-day life, therapy itself can elicit strong emotions. When therapy involves facing one's fears about self and others, making life changes, risking self-disclosure, addressing painful memories, and so on, it can provoke a range of emotional responses. It is important for the therapist to recognize painful emotions provoked by therapy and to be understanding and sympathetic, guiding the patient toward newly developing coping skills. Otherwise, there is a risk that these emotions will drive the patient from therapy. If the therapist makes a habit of obtaining feedback from the patient on a regular basis and watches for nonverbal signs of emotional reactions during the therapy session, it usually is not difficult to recognize problematic emotional reactions. When these reactions occur, it is important for the therapist to develop an understanding of the patient's thoughts and feelings and to help the patient understand his or her own reactions. It is important to pace therapy so that the benefits of therapy outweigh the drawbacks and to make sure that the patient recognizes this.

10. *Anticipate problems with completion of assignments.* Many factors contribute to a high rate of assignment default among patients with personality disorders. In addition to the complexities in the therapist–patient relationship and the fears regarding change discussed earlier, the dysfunctional behaviors of individuals with personality disorders are strongly ingrained and often are reinforced by aspects of the patient's environment. However, rather than simply being an impediment to progress, episodes of default can provide an opportunity to look more closely at active schemas and modes. The most important response may be a collaborative one that asks the patient to speculate on the obstacles and assess for interfering issues. A plan to pinpoint the thoughts that occur at the times when the patient thinks of acting on the therapy assignment but decides not to often reveals the most significant impediments that need to be considered. It may be that the assignment is too complex, not focused on a goal that is relevant to the patient, or wasn't developed in an optimally collaborative way.

11. *Do not presume that the patient exists in a reasonable environment.* Some behaviors, such as assertion, are so frequently adaptive that

it is easy to assume they are always a good idea. However, patients with personality disorders are often the product of seriously atypical families and often live in atypical environments. When implementing changes, it is important to assess the likely responses of significant others in the patient's environment rather than presuming that others will respond in a reasonable way. Often it is useful to have the patient initially experiment with new behaviors in low-risk situations. This arouses less anxiety and provides the patient with a chance to polish his or her skills before facing more challenging situations. Validations from the therapist that the patient's environment may be atypical and particularly challenging can significantly contribute to the patient's persistence and sense of self-efficacy. Receiving feedback that the patient's circumstances might be hard for anyone helps the patient to develop a more refined concept of what is normal and what isn't, which aids his or her skill in fact-based thinking.

12. *Be prepared to allocate time for reviewing a developmental narrative.* Seldom do we see personality disorders without some significant developmental antecedents of a social nature, whether from an invalidating and critical childhood environment; a cold and demanding one; an unstable, chaotic, or emotionally unpredictable one; or other traumatic events of significant impact, especially interpersonal trauma. Exploring these historical experiences as potential contributing factors can help the patient to build a conceptualization of schema modes as constructed over time, and increases his or her self-understanding for how his or her beliefs and behaviors made sense at some point in time. The goal of this developmental narrative is not to locate and blame caretakers, but rather to understand how and why painful conclusions that shaped the patient's beliefs developed in the first place. It can be explained that stored memories have become part of the biased information processing that causes a problem to be maintained, and that can be altered with therapy. The timing and intensity of developmental review will depend on the patient. As noted, patients with a mistrusting stance toward others may need more time to become comfortable with self-disclosure and prefer focusing on action steps early on. Others may be comfortable enough with self-disclosure but need help in approaching the strong emotions that this exploration may provoke. These reflections may be covered briefly during assessment, and then further explored at several later points, in brief bits or in extended narrative recall. Whatever the pace, the purpose is to assess how these important experiences either support or contradict the working theory about the patient's problematic beliefs and assumptions, and how they might be understood or modified to facilitate change.

13. *Limit setting is often an essential part of the overall treatment program.* Setting firm, reasonable limits and enforcing them consistently serves several purposes in treating patients with personality disorders.

First, consistency helps patients to organize their lives in more adaptive ways and protects them from behavioral excesses that cause problems for them and others. Second, it provides an opportunity for the therapist to model a reasoned approach to problem solving. Third, it provides a safe structure for maintaining a long-term and possible stormy therapeutic relationship. Finally, appropriate limits minimize the risk that the therapist will feel taken advantage of and become resentful, or that the therapy will become derailed in some way.

It might seem a good thing for the therapist to be generous and extend him- or herself in attempting to help a patient who is in great distress, but such "generosity" can easily backfire. Special treatment that seems acceptable in the short run can become galling when demands for special treatment persist month after month. If the therapist allows a situation to develop that causes him or her to feel resentful, a major impediment to effective treatment has also developed. It is particularly important not to inadvertently reinforce dysfunctional behavior by responding in ways that reward the patient for impaired limits, entitlement expectations, or manipulation of attention.

14. *Attend to your own emotional reactions during the course of therapy.* Interactions with patients who are personality disordered elicit many emotional reactions from the therapist, ranging from empathic feelings of depression to strong anger, discouragement, fear, or sexual attraction. It is important for the therapist to be aware of these many possible responses so that they can be used as a source of potentially useful data. Therapists may benefit from using cognitive techniques (such as the dysfunctional thought record; Beck, Rush, Shaw, & Emery, 1979), reviewing their case conceptualization, and/or seeking consultation with an objective colleague. Emotions within the therapist should be considered an expected response that can inform the process of therapy, and should not be considered mistakes or errors per se. Attempts to avoid or suppress emotional responses may increase the risk of mismanaging the therapeutic interaction.

Emotional responses do not occur randomly. An unusually strong emotional response on the therapist's part is often a reaction to some aspect of the patient's behavior, although there may well be other more salient determinants, such as the therapist's history or professional issues. Because a therapist may respond emotionally to a pattern in the patient's behavior long before it has been recognized intellectually, accurate interpretation of one's own responses can speed recognition of these patterns.

Careful thought is needed regarding whether to disclose these reactions to the patient and how to manage any disclosure therapeutically. On the one hand, patients with personality disorders may react strongly to therapist self-disclosure, easily misinterpreting this information. On the other hand, if the therapist does not disclose an emotional reaction that

is apparent to the patient from nonverbal cues or that the patient antici-
pates on the basis of experiences in other relationships, it can easily lead
to misunderstandings or distrust. This decision is best considered within
a thoughtful context of the case conceptualization, the patient's current
issues, the state of the therapeutic rapport, and the therapist's level of
arousal and ability to cope. The use of empathic interpersonal feedback is
an important skill, and essential to effective intervention with certain personality disorders such as narcissism, where the manipulation of others is
a central aspect of the psychopathology. This feedback is always delivered
in a warm and supportive way, but makes use of the therapist's reactions to
maladaptive behavior when it occurs in session. Providing feedback on the
spot, when the mode is active, creates an emotionally arousing experience
that improves the chance of having an impact.

15. *Be realistic regarding the length of therapy, goals for therapy, and
standards for therapist self-evaluation.* Many therapists using behavioral
and cognitive-behavioral approaches are accustomed to accomplishing substantial results relatively quickly. One can easily become frustrated and
angry with the "resistant" patient when therapy proceeds slowly, or become
self-critical and discouraged when the interactions become complicated or
highly emotionally charged. When treatment is only partially successful or
unsuccessful, it is important to remember that many factors influence outcome, and therapist competence is only one of those factors. When therapy
proceeds slowly, it is important neither to give up prematurely nor to perseverate with an unsuccessful approach. Behavioral and cognitive-behavioral
interventions can accomplish substantial, lasting changes in some patients
with personality disorders, but more modest results are achieved in other
cases, and little is accomplished in others, at least in the immediate term.

CONCLUSION

The past two decades have marked rapid growth in mapping specific cognitive features of personality disorders and refining a range of technology
for cognitive intervention. Perhaps the newest frontier for future work, in
addition to further establishing clinical efficacy of the cognitive treatment
of personality disorders, may be in articulating the common pathways of
development and process of change in disorders of personality. As we move
well into the future, we have even more hope that personality conditions,
once widely considered refractory to therapeutic interventions, will be
found to be modifiable in the same way as affective and anxiety disorders.

References

Abi-Dargham, A., Kegeles, L. S., Zea-Ponce, Y., Mawlawi, O., Martinez, D., Mitropoulou, V., et al. (2004). Striatal amphetamine-induced dopamine release in patients with schizotypal personality disorder studied with single photon emission computed tomography and [123I] iodobenzamide. *Biological Psychiatry, 55*(10), 1001–1006.

Abramson, L. Y., Metalsky, G. I., & Alloy, L. B. (1989). Hopelessness depression: A theory-based subtype of depression. *Psychological Review, 96*, 358–372.

Ackerman, R. A., Witt, E. A., Donnellan, M. B., Trzesniewski, K. H., Robins, R. W., Kashy, D. A. (2011). What does the narcissistic personality inventory really measure? *Assessment, 18*(1), 67–87.

Adams, P. (1973). *Obsessive children: A sociopsychiatric study.* New York: Brunner/Mazel.

Adeponle, A. B., Thombs, B. D., Groleau, D., Jarvis, E., & Kirmayer, L. J. (2012). Using the cultural formulation to resolve uncertainty in diagnoses of psychosis among ethnoculturally diverse patients. *Psychiatric Services, 63*(2), 147–153.

Adshead, G., & Sarkar, J. (2012). The nature of personality disorder. *Advances in Psychiatric Treatment, 18*, 162–172.

Aggarwal, N. K., Nicasio, A. V., DeSilva, R., Boiler, M., & Lewis-Fernández, R. (2013). Barriers to implementing the DSM-5 Cultural Formulation Interview: A qualitative study. *Culture, Medicine, and Psychiatry, 37*(3), 505–533.

Akiskal, H. P. (1983). Dysthymic disorder: Psychopathology of proposed depressive subtypes. *American Journal of Psychiatry, 140*, 11–20.

Alarcón, R. D., Becker, A. E., Lewis-Fernández, R., Like, R. C., Desai, P., Foulks, E., et al. (2009). Issues for DSM-V: The role of culture in psychiatric diagnosis. *Journal of Nervous and Mental Disease, 197*(8), 559–560.

Alarcón, R. D., & Foulks, E. F. (1995a). Personality disorders and culture: Contemporary clinical views (Part A). *Cultural Diversity and Mental Health, 1*(1), 3–17.

Alarcón, R. D., & Foulks, E. F. (1995b). Personality disorders and culture: Contemporary clinical views (Part B). *Cultural Diversity and Mental Health, 1*(2), 79–91.

Alberti, R. E., & Emmons, M. L. (2008). *Your perfect right: Assertiveness and equality in your life and relationships* (9th ed.). Atascadero, CA: Impact.

Alden, L. (1989). Short-term structured treatment for avoidant personality disorder. *Journal of Consulting and Clinical Psycholology, 57*, 756–764.

Allen, J. (2004). *Traumatic relationships and serious mental disorders.* Chichester, UK: Wiley.

Alloy, L. B., & Abramson, L. Y. (1999). The Temple–Wisconsin Cognitive Vulnerability to

Depression (CVD) Project: Conceptual background, design, and methods. *Journal of Cognitive Psychotherapy: An International Quarterly, 13*, 227–262.

Alnaes, R., & Torgersen, S. (1988). The relationship between DSM-III symptom disorders (Axis I) and personality disorders (Axis II) in an outpatient population. *Acta Psychiatrica Scandinavica, 78*, 485–492.

Alnaes, R., & Torgerson, S. (1991). Personality and personality disorders among patients with various affective disorders. *Journal of Personality Disorders, 5*(2), 107–121.

American Psychiatric Association. (1952). *Diagnostic and statistical manual of mental disorders* (1st ed.). Washington, DC: Author.

American Psychiatric Association. (1968). *Diagnostic and statistical manual of mental disorders* (2nd ed.). Washington, DC: Author.

American Psychiatric Association. (1980). *Diagnostic and statistical manual of mental disorders* (3rd ed.). Washington, DC: Author.

American Psychiatric Association. (1987). *Diagnostic and statistical manual of mental disorders* (3rd ed., rev.). Washington, DC: Author.

American Psychiatric Association. (1989). Passive–aggressive personality disorder. In *Treatments of psychiatric disorders: A task force report of the American Psychiatric Association* (pp. 2783–2789). Washington, DC: Author.

American Psychiatric Association. (1994). *Diagnostic and statistical manual of mental disorders* (4th ed.). Washington, DC: Author.

American Psychiatric Association. (2000). *Diagnostic and statistical manual of mental disorders* (4th ed., text rev.). Washington, DC: Author.

American Psychiatric Association. (2002). *Guideline for the treatment of patients with bipolar disorder* (2nd ed.). Washington, DC: Author.

American Psychiatric Association. (2013). *Diagnostic and statistical manual of mental disorders* (5th ed.). Arlington, VA: Author.

American Psychological Association. (2002). *Ethical principles of psychologists and code of conduct*. Washington, DC: Author.

American Psychological Association. (2004). Axis II gets short shrift. *American Psychological Association Monitor, 35*(3). Retrieved from *www.apa.org/monitor/mar04/axis.aspx*.

Amrod, J., & Hayes, S. C. (2014). ACT for the incarcerated. In R. C. Tafrate & D. Mitchell (Eds.), *Forensic CBT: A handbook for clinical practice* (pp. 43–65). Chichester, UK: Wiley.

Andrews, D. A., & Bonta, J. (1995). *The Level of Service Inventory—Revised*. Toronto, Ontario, Canada: Multi-Health Systems.

Andrews, D. A., & Bonta, J. (2010). *The psychology of criminal conduct* (5th ed.). New Providence, NJ: LexisNexis Bender.

Andrews, D. A., Bonta, J., & Hoge, R. D. (1990). Classification for effective rehabilitation: Rediscovering psychology. *Criminal Justice and Behavior, 17*, 19–52.

Andrews, D. A., Bonta, J., & Wormith, J. S. (2006). The recent past and near future of risk and/or need assessment. *Crime and Delinquency, 52*, 7–27.

Andrews, D. A., & Dowden, C. (2005). Managing correctional treatment for reduced recidivism: A meta-analytic review of program integrity. *Legal and Criminological Psychology, 10*, 173–187.

Andrews, D. A., Zinger, I., Hoge, R. D., Bonta, J., Gendreau, P., & Cullen, F. T. (1990). Does correctional treatment work?: A clinically relevant and psychologically informed meta-analysis. *Criminology, 28*, 369–404.

Angstman, K. B., & Rasmussen, N. H. (2011). Personality disorders: Review and clinical application in daily practice. *American Family Physician, 84*, 1253–1260.

Ansell, E. B., Pinto, A., Edelen, M. O., Markowitz, J. C., Sanislow, C. A., Yen, S., et al. (2011). The association of personality disorders with the prospective 7-year course of anxiety disorders. *Psychological Medicine, 41*, 1019–1028.

Ansell, E. B., Sanislow, C. A., McGlashan, T. H., & Grilo, C. M. (2007). Psychosocial impairment and treatment utilization by patients with borderline personality disorder, other personality disorders, mood and anxiety disorders, and a healthy comparison group. *Comprehensive Psychiatry, 48,* 329–336.

APA Presidential Task Force on Evidence-Based Practice. (2006). Evidence-based practice in psychology. *American Psychologist, 61*(4), 271–285.

Arnevik, E., Wilberg, T., Urnes, Ø., Johansen, M., Monsen, J. T., & Karterud, S. (2010). Psychotherapy for personality disorders: 18 months' follow-up of the Ullevål Personality Project. *Journal of Personality Disorders, 24*(2), 188–203.

Arntz, A. (1994). Treatment of borderline personality disorder: A challenge for cognitive-behavioural therapy. *Behaviour Research and Therapy, 32,* 419–430.

Arntz, A. (2011). Imagery rescripting for personality disorders. *Cognitive and Behavioral Practice, 18,* 466–481.

Arntz, A. (2014). Treatment of comorbid anxiety disorders and personality disorders. In P. M. G. Emmelkamp & T. Ehring (Eds.), *Handbook of anxiety disorders: Theory, research and practice.* Hoboken, NJ: Wiley-Blackwell.

Arntz, A., Bernstein, D., Gielen, D., van Nieuwenhuyzen, M., Penders, K., Haslam, N., et al. (2009). Taxometric evidence for the dimensional structure of Cluster-C, paranoid, and borderline personality disorders. *Journal of Personality Disorders, 23*(6), 606–628.

Arntz, A., Dietzel, R., & Dreessen, L. (1999). Assumptions in borderline personality disorder: Specificity, stability, and relationship with etiological factors. *Behaviour Research and Therapy, 37,* 545–557.

Arntz, A., Dreessen, L., Schouten, E., & Weertman, A. (2004). Beliefs in personality disorders: A test with the Personality Disorder Belief Questionnaire. *Behaviour Research and Therapy, 42,* 1215–1225.

Arntz, A., & van Genderen, H. (2009). *Schema therapy for borderline personality disorder.* Chichester, UK: Wiley.

Arntz, A., & Weertman, A. (1999). Treatment of childhood memories: Theory and practice. *Behaviour Research and Therapy, 37,* 715–740.

Ascoli, M., Lee, T., Warfa, N., Mairura, J., Persaud, A., & Bhui, K. (2011). Race, culture, ethnicity and personality disorder: Group care position paper. *World Cultural Psychiatry Research Review, 6*(1), 52–60.

Baer, R. A., & Sauer, S. E. (2011). Relationships between depressive rumination, anger rumination, and borderline personality features. *Personality Disorders: Theory, Research, and Treatment, 2,* 142–150.

Bagby, R. M. (2013). Introduction to special issue on the Personality Inventory for DSM-5 (PID-5). *Assessment, 20*(3), 267–268.

Bagby, R. M., Costa, J. P. T., Widiger, T. A., Ryder, A. G., & Marshall, M. (2005). DSM-IV personality disorders and the five-factor model of personality: A multi-method examination of domain- and facet-level predictions [Special issue]. *European Journal of Personality. Personality and Personality Disorders, 19*(4), 307–324.

Bagby, R. M., Watson, C., & Ryder, A. G. (2012). Depressive personality disorder. In T. A. Widiger (Ed.), *The Oxford handbook of personality disorders* (pp. 628–647). Oxford, UK: Oxford University Press.

Bagby, R. M., Watson, C., & Ryder, A. G. (2013). Depressive personality disorder and the five-factor model. In T. A. Widiger, & P. T. Costa (Eds.), *Personality disorders and the five-factor model of personality* (pp. 179–192). Washington, DC: American Psychological Association.

Ball, S. A., Maccarelli, L. M., LaPaglia, D. M., & Ostrowski, M. J. (2011). Randomized trial of dual-focused versus single-focused individual therapy for personality disorders and substance dependence. *Journal of Nervous and Mental Disease, 199*(5), 319.

Bamelis, L. L. M., Evers, S. M. A. A., & Arntz, A. (2012). Design of a multicentered randomized controlled trial on the clinical and cost effectiveness of schema therapy for personality disorders. *BMC Public Health, 24,* 12–75.

Bamelis, L. L. M., Evers, S. M. A. A., Spinhoven, P., & Arntz, A. (2014). Results of a multicenter randomized controlled trial of the clinical effectiveness of schema therapy for personality disorders. *American Journal of Psychiatry, 171*(3), 305–322.

Bandelow, B., Schmahl, C., Falkai, P., & Wedekind, D. (2010). Borderline personality disorder: A dysregulation of the endogenous opioid system? *Psychological Review, 117*(2), 623.

Barber, J. P., & Muenz, L. R. (1996). The role of avoidance and obsessiveness in matching patients to cognitive and interpersonal psychotherapy: Empirical findings from the Treatment for Depression Collaborative Research Program. *Journal of Consulting and Clinical Psychology, 64*(5), 951–958.

Barlow, D. H. (2004). Psychological treatments. *American Psychologist, 59*(9), 869–878.

Baron, J. (2000). *Thinking and deciding.* Cambridge, UK: Cambridge University Press.

Bartlett, F. C. (1932). *Remembering.* New York: Columbia University Press.

Bartlett, F. C. (1958). *Thinking: An experimental and social study.* New York: Basic Books.

Bateman, A. W., & Tyrer, P. (2004). Psychological treatment for personality disorder. *Advances in Psychiatric Treatment, 10*, 378–388.

Batterham, P. J., Glozier, N., & Christensen, H. (2012). Sleep disturbance, personality and the onset of depression and anxiety: Prospective cohort study. *Australian and New Zealand Journal of Psychiatry, 46*, 1089–1098.

Baumeister, R. (2001, April). Violent pride. *Scientific American, 284*(4), 96–101.

Baumeister, R., Bushman, B., & Campbell, W. K. (2000). Self-esteem, narcissism, and aggression: Does violence result from low self-esteem or from threatened egotism? *Current Directions in Psychological Science, 9*, 26–29.

Baumeister, R., Smart, L., & Boden, J. (1996). Relation of threatened egotism to violence and aggression: The dark side of high self-esteem. *Psychological Review, 103*, 5–33.

Bebbington, P. E., McBride, O., Steel, C., Kuipers, E., Radovanovic, M., Brugha, T., et al. (2013). The structure of paranoia in the general population. *British Journal of Psychiatry, 202*, 419–427.

Beck, A. (1991). *Beck Scale for Suicide Ideation.* San Antonio, TX: Psychological Corporation.

Beck, A., Freeman, A., & Davis, D. B. (2004). *Cognitive therapy of personality disorders* (2nd ed.). New York: Guilford Press.

Beck, A. T. (1963). Thinking and depression: I. Idiosyncratic content and cognitive distortions. *Archives of General Psychiatry, 9*, 324–344.

Beck, A. T. (1964). Thinking and depression: II. Theory and therapy. *Archives of General Psychiatry, 10*, 561–571.

Beck, A. T. (1967). *Depression: Clinical, experimental and theoretical aspects.* New York: Harper & Row. (Republished as *Depression: Causes and treatment.* Philadelphia: University of Pennsylvania Press, 1972)

Beck, A. T. (1976). *Cognitive therapy and the emotional disorders.* New York: International Universities Press.

Beck, A. T. (1983). Cognitive therapy of depression: New perspectives. In P. J. Clayton & J. E. Barrett (Eds.), *Treatment of depression: Old controversies and new approaches.* New York: Raven Press.

Beck, A. T. (1987). Cognitive models of depression. *Journal of Cognitive Psychotherapy: An International Quarterly, 1*, 5–37.

Beck, A. T. (1988a). *Beck Hopelessness Scale.* San Antonio, TX: Psychological Corporation.

Beck, A. T. (1988b). *Love is never enough.* New York: Harper & Row.

Beck, A. T. (1996). Beyond belief: A theory of modes, personality, and psychopathology. In P. Salkovskis (Ed.), *Frontiers of cognitive therapy* (pp. 1–25). New York: Guilford Press.

Beck, A. T., & Beck, J. S. (1991). *The Personality Belief Questionnaire.* Unpublished instrument, Beck Institute for Cognitive Therapy and Research, Bala Cynwyd, PA.

Beck, A. T., & Beck, J. S. (1995a). *PBQ-PBD.* Unpublished instrument, Beck Institute for Cognitive Therapy and Research, Bala Cynwyd, PA.

Beck, A. T., & Beck, J. S. (1995b). *PBQ-SF*. Unpublished instrument, Beck Institute for Cognitive Therapy and Research, Bala Cynwyd, PA.

Beck, A. T., Butler, A. C., Brown, G. K., Dahlsgaard, K. K., Newman, C. F., & Beck, J. S. (2001). Dysfunctional beliefs discriminate personality disorders. *Behaviour Research and Therapy, 39*, 1213–1225.

Beck, A. T., & Emery, G. (with Greenberg, R. L.). (1985). *Anxiety disorders and phobias: A cognitive perspective.* New York: Basic Books.

Beck, A. T., Freeman, A., & Associates. (1990). *Cognitive therapy of personality disorders.* New York: Guilford Press.

Beck, A. T., & Haigh, E. (2014). Advances in cognitive theory and therapy: The generic cognitive model. *Annual Review of Clinical Psychology, 10*, 1–24.

Beck, A. T., Rush, A. J., Shaw, B. F., & Emery, G. (1979). *Cognitive therapy of depression.* New York: Guilford Press.

Beck, A. T., & Steer, R. A. (1993a). *Beck Anxiety Inventory Manual.* San Antonio, TX: Psychological Corporation.

Beck, A. T., & Steer, R. A. (1993b). *Manual for Beck Hopelessness Inventory.* San Antonio, TX: Psychological Corporation.

Beck, A. T., Steer, R., & Brown, G. (1996). *Manual for the Beck Depression Inventory–II.* San Antonio, TX: Psychological Corporation.

Beck, A. T., Wright, F., Newman, C., & Liese, B. (1993) *Cognitive therapy of substance abuse.* New York: Guilford Press.

Beck, J. S. (1995). *Cognitive therapy: Basics and beyond.* New York: Guilford Press.

Beck, J. S. (2005). *Cognitive therapy for challenging problems: What to do when the basics don't work.* New York: Guilford Press.

Beck, J. S. (2006). *Cognitive therapy worksheet packet* (rev. ed.). Bala Cynwyd, PA: Beck Institute for Cognitive Behavior Therapy.

Beck, J. S. (2011). *Cognitive behavior therapy: Basics and beyond* (2nd ed.). New York: Guilford Press.

Beesdo, K., Lau, J. Y., Guyer, A. E., McClure-Tone, E. B., Monk, C. S., Nelson, E. E., et al. (2009). Common and distinct amygdala-function perturbations in depressed vs. anxious adolescents. *Archives of General Psychiatry, 66*(3), 275–285.

Behary, W. (2012). Schema therapy for narcissism. In M. van Vreeswijk, J. Broersen, & M. Nadort (Eds.), *The Wiley-Blackwell handbook of schema therapy: Theory, research and practice* (pp. 81–90). Malden, MA: Wiley-Blackwell.

Behary, W., & Dieckmann, E. (2011). Schema therapy for narcissism: The art of empathic confrontation, limit-setting, and leverage. In W. K. Campbell & J. D. Miller (Eds.), *The handbook of narcissism and narcissistic personality disorder: Theoretical approaches, empirical findings, and treatments* (pp. 445–456). Hoboken, NJ: Wiley.

Behary, W., & Dieckmann, E. (2013). Schema therapy for pathological narcissism: The art of adaptive re-parenting. In J. S. Ogrodniczuk (Ed.), *Understanding and treating pathological narcissism* (pp. 285–300). Washington, DC: American Psychological Association.

Behary, W. T. (2013). *Disarming the narcissist: Surviving and thriving with the self-absorbed* (2nd ed.). Oakland, CA: New Harbinger.

Bellino, S., Rinaldi, C., Bozzatello, P., & Bogetto, F. (2011). Pharmacotherapy of borderline personality disorder: A systematic review. *Current Medicinal Chemistry, 18*(22), 3322–3329.

Belmaker, R. H. (2004). Bipolar disorder. *New England Journal of Medicine, 351*, 476–486.

Bender, D. S., Skodol, A. E., Dyck, I. R., Markowitz, J. C., Shea, M. T., Yen, S., et al. (2007). Ethnicity and mental health treatment utilization by patients with personality disorders. *Journal of Consulting and Clinical Psychology, 75*(6), 992–999.

Benjamin, L. (1993). *Interpersonal diagnosis and treatment of personality disorders.* New York: Guilford Press.

444 *References*

Benjamin, L. (2003). *Interpersonal diagnosis and treatment of personality disorders* (2nd ed.). New York: Guilford Press.

Benjamin, L., & Cushing, G. (2004). An interpersonal family-oriented approach to personality disorder. In M. M. MacFarlane (Ed.), *Family treatment of personality disorders advances in clinical practice* (pp. 41–69). New York: Haworth Clinical Practice Press.

Bergman, S. M., Fearrington, M. E., Davenport, S. W., & Bergman, J. Z. (2011). Millennials, narcissism, and social networking: What narcissists do on social networking sites and why. *Personality and Individual Differences, 50*(5), 706–711.

Bernal, G., Jiménez-Chafey, M. I., & Domenech Rodríguez, M. M. (2009). Cultural adaptation of treatments: A resource for considering culture in evidence-based practice. *Professional Psychology: Research and Practice, 40*(4), 361–368.

Bernstein, D. P. (2005). Cognitive therapy for clients with personality disorders and comorbid Axis I psychopathology. In J. Reich (Ed.), *Personality disorders: Current research and treatments* (pp. 154–159). New York: Routledge.

Bernstein, D. P., Arntz, A., & de Vos, M. E. (2007). Schema-focused therapy in forensic settings: Theoretical model and recommendations for best clinical practice. *International Journal of Forensic Mental Health, 6,* 169–183.

Bernstein, D. P., & Useda, J. D. (2007). Paranoid personality disorder. In W. O'Donohue, K. A. Fowler, & S. O. Lilenfeld (Eds.), *Personality disorders: Toward the DSM-V* (pp. 41–62). Thousand Oaks, CA: Sage.

Berridge, K. C. (2007). The debate over dopamine's role in reward: The case for incentive salience. *Psychopharmacology, 191*(3), 391–431.

Betancourt, H., & Lopez, S. R. (1993). The study of culture, ethnicity, and race in American psychology. *American Psychologist, 48*(6), 629–637.

Bewick, B. M., McBride, J., & Barkham, M. (2006). When clients and practitioners have differing views of risk: Benchmarks for improving assessment and practice. *Counseling and Psychotherapy Research, 6*(1), 50–59.

Bhar, S. S., Beck, A. T., & Butler, A. C. (2012). Beliefs and personality disorders: An overview of the Personality Beliefs Questionnaire. *Journal of Clinical Psychology, 68*(1), 88–100.

Bhugra D., & de Silva, P. (2007). Sexual dysfunctions across cultures. In K. Bhui (Ed.), *Textbook of cultural psychiatry* (pp. 364–378). Cambridge, UK: Cambridge University Press.

Black, D. W., Monahan, P., Wesner, R., Gabel, J., & Bowers, W. (1996). The effect of fluvoxamine, cognitive therapy, and placebo on abnormal personality traits in 44 patients with panic disorder. *Journal of Personality Disorders, 10*(2), 185–194.

Blackford, J. U., Buckholtz, J. W., Avery, S. N., & Zald, D. H. (2010). A unique role for the human amygdala in novelty detection. *NeuroImage, 50*(3), 1188–1193.

Blashfield, R. K., & Breen, M. J. (1989). Face validity of the DSM-III-R personality disorders. *American Journal of Psychiatry, 146,* 1575–1579.

Blum, N., John, D., Pfohl, B., Stuart, S., McCormick, B., Allen, J., et al. (2008). Systems training for emotional predictability and problem solving (STEPPS) for outpatients with borderline personality disorder: A randomized controlled trial and 1-year follow-up. *American Journal of Psychiatry, 165*(4), 468–478.

Bockian, N. R. (2006). Depression in borderline personality disorder. In N. R. Bockian (Ed.), *Personality-guided therapy for depression* (pp. 135–167). Washington, DC: American Psychological Association.

Bornstein, R. (1992). The dependent personality: Developmental, social, and clinical perspectives. *Psychological Bulletin, 112*(1), 3–23.

Bornstein, R. (2005). The dependent individual: Diagnosis, assessment, and treatment. *Professional Psychology: Research and Practice, 36*(1), 82–89.

Bornstein, R. (2012a). From dysfunction to adaptation: An interactionist model of dependency. *Annual Review of Clinical Psychology, 8*(1), 291–316.

Bornstein, R. (2012b). Illuminating a neglected clinical issue: Societal costs of interpersonal dependency and dependent personality disorder. *Journal of Clinical Psychology, 68*(7), 766–781.

Bornstein, R., Riggs, J., Hill, E., & Calabrese, C. (1996). Activity, passivity, self-denigration, and self-promotion: Toward an interactionist model of interpersonal dependency. *Journal of Personality, 64*(3), 637–673.

Bornstein, R. F. (1998). Reconceptualizing personality disorder diagnosis in the DSM-V: The discriminant validity challenge. *Clinical Psychology: Science and Practice, 5*(3), 333–343.

Bornstein, R. F. (2001). A meta-analysis of the dependency-eating disorders relationship: Strength, specificity, and temporal stability. *Journal of Psychopathology and Behavioral Assessment, 23,* 151–162.

Bornstein, R. F. (2011). Reconceptualizing personality pathology in DSM-5: Limitations in evidence for eliminating dependent personality disorder and other DSM-IV syndromes. *Journal of Personality Disorders, 25*(2), 235–247.

Bourgeois, J. A., & Hall, M. J. (1993). An examination of narcissistic personality traits as seen in a military population. *Military Medicine, 158,* 170–174.

Bowlby, J. (1969). *Attachment and loss: Vol. 1. Attachment.* New York: Basic Books.

Boyce, P., & Mason, C. (1996). An overview of depression-prone personality traits and the role of interpersonal sensitivity. *Australian and New Zealand Journal of Psychiatry, 30,* 90–103.

Bradley, R., Shedler, J., & Westen, D. (2006). Is the appendix a useful appendage?: An empirical examination of depressive, passive–aggressive (negativistic), sadistic, and self-defeating personality disorders. *Journal of Personality Disorders, 20*(5), 524–540.

Brennan, K., & Shaver, P. (1998). Attachment styles and personality disorders: Their comnnections to each other and to parental divorce, parental death, and perceptions of parental caregiving. *Journal of Personality, 66,* 835–878.

Bricker, D., Young, J. E., & Flanagan, C. (1993). Schema-focused cognitive therapy: A comprehensive framework for characterological problems. In K. Kuehlwein & H. Rosen (Eds.), *Cognitive therapies in action: Evolving innovative practice* (pp. 88–125). San Francisco: Jossey-Bass.

Brown, G. K., Newman, C. F., Charlesworth, S., Crits-Cristoph, P., & Beck, A. T. (2004). An open clinical trial of cognitive therapy for borderline personality disorder. *Journal of Personality Disorders, 18*(3), 257–271.

Buckholtz, J. W., Treadway, M. T., Cowan, R. L., Woodward, N. D., Benning, S. D., Li, R., et al. (2010). Mesolimbic dopamine reward system hypersensitivity in individuals with psychopathic traits. *Nature Neuroscience, 13*(4), 419–421.

Buckholtz, J. W., Treadway, M. T., Cowan, R. L., Woodward, N. D., Li, R., Ansari, M. S., et al. (2010). Dopaminergic network differences in human impulsivity. *Science, 329*(5991), 532.

Bukh, J. D., Bock, C., Vinberg, M., Gether, U., & Kessing, L. V. (2010). Clinical utility of Standardised Assessment of Personality—Abbreviated Scale (SAPAS) among patients with first episode depression. *Journal of Affective Disorders, 127*(1), 199–202.

Burgess, P., Pirkis, J., Morton, J., & Croke, E. (2000). Lessons from a comprehensive clinical audit of users of psychiatric services who committed suicide. *Psychiatric Services, 51*(12), 1555–1560.

Burns, D. D. (1999). *10 days to self-esteem.* New York: HarperCollins.

Bushman, B., & Baumeister, R. (1998). Threatened egotism, narcissism, self-esteem, and direct and displaced aggression: Does self-love or self-hate lead to violence? *Journal of Personality and Social Psychology, 75,* 219–229.

Buss, A. H. (1987). Personality: Primitive heritage and human distinctiveness. In J. Aronoff, A. I. Robin, & R. A. Zucker (Eds.), *The emergence of personality* (pp. 13–48). New York: Springer.

Butcher, J. N., Graham, J. R., Ben-Porath, Y. S., Tellegen, Y. S., Dahlstrom, W. G., & Kaemmer, B. (2001). *Minnesota Multiphasic Personality Inventory–2: Manual for administration and scoring* (rev. ed.). Minneapolis: University of Minnesota Press.

Butler, A. C., Beck, A. T., & Cohen, L. H. (2007). The Personality Belief Questionnaire—Short Form: Development and preliminary findings. *Cognitive Therapy and Research, 31,* 357–370.

Butler, A. C., Brown, G. K., Beck, A. T., & Grisham, J. R. (2002). Assessment of dysfunctional beliefs in borderline personality disorder. *Behaviour Research and Therapy, 40*(1), 1231–1240.

Butler, R. N. (1975). *Why survive?: Being old in America.* New York: Harper & Row.

Byrne, S. A., Cherniack, M. G., & Petry, N. M. (2013). Antisocial personality disorder is associated with receipt of physical disability benefits in substance abuse treatment patients. *Drug and Alcohol Dependence, 132*(1–2), 373–377.

Calati, R., Gressier, F., Balestri, M., & Serretti, A. (2013). Genetic modulation of borderline personality disorder: Systematic review and meta-analysis. *Journal of Psychiatric Research, 47,* 1275–1287.

Callahan, J. (2009). Emergency intervention and crisis intervention. In P. M. Kleespies (Ed.), *Behavioral emergencies: An evidence-based resource for evaluating and managing risk of suicide, violence, and victimization* (pp. 13–32). Washington, DC: American Psychological Association.

Carcione, A., Nicolo, G., Pedone, R., Popolo, R., Conti, L., Fiore, D., et al. (2011). Metacognitive mastery dysfunctions in personality disorder psychotherapy. *Psychiatry Research, 190,* 60–71.

Carlson, J., Melton, K., & Snow, K. (2004). Family treatment of passive–aggressive (negativistic) personality disorder. In M. M. MacFarlane (Ed.), *Family treatment of personality disorders advances in clinical practice* (pp. 241–272). New York: Haworth Clinical Practice Press.

Carr, S. N., & Francis, A. P. (2010). Do early maladaptive schemas mediate the relationship between childhood experiences and avoidant personality disorder features?: A preliminary investigation in a non-clinical sample. *Cognitive Therapy and Research, 34,* 343–358.

Carroll, A. (2009). Are you looking at me?: Understanding and managing paranoid personality disorder. *Advances in Psychiatric Treatment, 15,* 40–48.

Chadwick, P. (2006). *Person-based cognitive therapy for distressing psychosis.* Chichester, UK: Wiley.

Chamberlain, J., & Huprich, S. K. (2011). The Depressive Personality Disorder Inventory and current depressive symptoms: Implications for the assessment of depressive personality. *Journal of Personality Disorders, 25,* 668–680.

Chambless, D. L., & Hollon, S. D. (1998). Defining empirically supported therapies. *Journal of Consulting and Clinical Psychology, 66*(1), 7–18.

Chambless, D. L., Renneberg, D., Goldstein, A., & Gracely, E. J. (1992). MCMI-diagnosed personality disorders among agoraphobic outpatients: Prevalence and relationship to severity and treatment outcome. *Journal of Anxiety Disorders, 6,* 193–211.

Chambless, D. L., Renneberg, D., Gracely, E. J., Goldstein, A. J., & Fydrich, T. (2000). Axis I and II comorbidity in agoraphobia: Prediction of psychotherapy outcome in a clinical setting. *Psychotherapy Research, 10,* 279–295.

Cheng, A. T. A., Mann, A. H., & Chan, K. A. (1997). Personality disorder and suicide: A case-control study. *British Journal of Psychiatry, 170*(5), 441–446.

Chioqueta, A., & Stiles, T. C. (2004). Assessing suicide risk in Cluster C personality disorders. *Crisis, 25*(3), 128–133.

Clark, D. A., & Beck, A. T. (with Alford, B. A.). (1999). *Scientific foundations of cognitive theory and therapy of depression.* New York: Wiley.

Clark, L. A. (1992). Resolving taxonomic issues in personality disorders: The value of large-scale analyses of symptom data. *Journal of Personality Disorders, 6*(4), 360–376.

Clark, L. A. (2005a). *SNAP Schedule for Nonadaptive and Adaptive Personality: Manual for administration, scoring, and interpretation.* Minneapolis: University of Minnesota Press.

Clark, L. A. (2005b). Stability and change in personality pathology: Revelations of three longitudinal studies [Special issue]. *Journal of Personality Disorders: Longitudinal Studies, 19*(5), 524–532.

Clark, L. A. (2005c). Temperament as a unifying basis for personality and psychopathology. *Journal of Abnormal Psychology. Special Issue: Toward a Dimensionally Based Taxonomy of Psychopathology, 114*(4), 505–521.

Clark, L. A., & Livesley, W. J. (2002). Two approaches to identifying the dimensions of personality disorder: Convergence on the five-factor model. In P. T. Costa, Jr. & T. A. Widiger (Eds.), *Personality disorders and the five-factor model of personality* (2nd ed., pp. 161–176). Washington, DC: American Psychological Association.

Clark, L. A., Livesley, W. J., & Morey, L. (1997). Personality disorder assessment: The challenge of construct validity. *Journal of Personality Disorders, 11*(3), 205–231.

Clark, L. A., Vorhies, L., & McEwen, J. L. (2002). Personality disorder symptomatology from the five-factor model perspective. In P. T. Costa, Jr. & T. A. Widiger (Eds.), *Personality disorders and the five-factor model of personality* (2nd ed., pp. 125–147). Washington, DC: American Psychological Association.

Clarke, S., Thomas, P., & James, K. (2013). Cognitive analytic therapy for personality disorder: Randomised controlled trial. *British Journal of Psychiatry, 202*(2), 129–134.

Clifford, C. A., Murray, R. M., & Fulker, D. W. (1984). Genetic and environmental influences on obsessional traits and symptoms. *Psychological Medicine, 14*(4), 791–800.

Cloninger, C. R. (1986). A unified biosocial theory of personality and its role in the development of anxiety states. *Psychiatrics Development, 4*(3), 167–226.

Coffman, S., Martell, C. R., Dimidjian, S., Gallop, R., & Hollon, S. D. (2007). Extreme nonresponse in cognitive therapy: Can behavioral activation succeed where cognitive therapy fails? *Journal of Consulting and Clinical Psychology, 75*, 531–541.

Cohen, P., Chen, H., Crawford, T. N., Brook, J. S., & Gordon, K. (2007). Personality disorders in early adolescence and the development of later substance use disorders in the general population. *Drug and Alcohol Dependence, 88*, S71–S84.

Collins, N., & Read, S. (1990). Adult attachment, working models, and relationship quality in dating couples. *Journal of Personality and Social Psychology, 58*, 644–663.

Colvin, C. R., Block, J., & Funder, D. C. (1995). Overly positive self-evaluations and personality: Negative implications for mental health. *Journal of Personality and Social Psychology, 68*, 1152–1162.

Constantino, M. J., Arnkoff, D. B., Glass, C. R., Ametrano, R. M., & Smith, J. Z. (2011). Expectations. *Journal of Clinical Psychology: In Session, 67*, 184–192.

Corbisiero, J. R., & Reznikoff, M. (1991). The relationship between personality type and style of alcohol use. *Journal of Clinical Psychology, 47*(2), 291–298.

Cornell, D. G., Warren, J., Hawk, G., Stafford, E., Oram, G., & Pine, D. (1996). Psychopathy in instrumental and reactive violent offenders. *Journal of Consulting and Clinical Psychology, 64*(4), 783–790.

Costa, P. T., & McCrae, R. R. (1992). *Revised NEO Personality Inventory (NEO-PI-R) and NEO Five-Factor Inventory (NEO-FFI) professional manual.* Odessa, FL: Psychological Assesssment Resources.

Costa, P. T., & McCrae, R. R. (2010). *NEO inventories: NEO Personality Inventory-3 (NEO-PI-3).* Lutz, FL: Psychological Assessment Resources.

Costa, P. T., Patriciu, N. S., & McCrae, R. R. (2005). Lessons from longitudinal studies for new approaches to the DSM-V [Special issue]: The FFM and FFT. *Journal of Personality Disorders: Longitudinal Studies, 19*(5), 533–539.

Cottraux, J., Druon Note, I. D., Boutitie, F., Milliery, M., Genouihlac, V., Nan Yao, S., et al. (2009). Cognitive therapy versus Rogerian supportive therapy in borderline personality disorder: Two-year follow-up of a controlled pilot study. *Psychotherapy and Psychosomatics, 78*, 307–316.

Cowdry, R. W., & Gardner, D. (1988). Pharmacotherapy of borderline personality disorder: Alprazolam, carmabazepine, trifluoperazine and tranylcypromine. *Archives of General Psychiatry, 45*, 111–119.

Craig, A. D. (2002). How do you feel?: Interoception: The sense of the physiological condition of the body. *Nature Reviews Neuroscience, 3*(8), 655–666.

Craig, A. D. (2009). How do you feel—now?: The anterior insula and human awareness. *Nature Reviews Neuroscience, 10*(1), 59–70.

Cremers, H. R., Demenescu, L. R., Aleman, A., Renken, R., van Tol, M.-J., van der Wee, N. J., et al. (2010). Neuroticism modulates amygdala–prefrontal connectivity in response to negative emotional facial expressions. *NeuroImage, 49*(1), 963–970.

Critchfield, K. L., & Benjamin, L. (2006). Principles for psychosocial treatment of personality disorder: Summary of the APA Division 12 Task Force/NASPR review. *Journal of Clinical Psychology, 62*(6), 661–674.

Crits-Christoph, P., & Barber, J. (2002). Psychological treatment for personality disorders. In P. Nathan & J. Gorman (Eds.), *A guide to treatments that work* (2nd ed., pp. 611–624). New York: Oxford University Press.

Cumyn, L., French, L., & Hechtman, L. (2009). Comorbidity in adults with attention-deficit hyperactivity disorder. *Canadian Journal of Psychiatry, 54*(10), 673–683.

Czajkowski, N., Kendler, K. S., Jacobson, K. C, Tambs, K., Roysamb, E., & Reichborn-Kjennerud, T. (2008). Passive–aggressive (negativistic) personality disorder: A population-based twin study. *Journal of Personality Disorders, 22*(1), 109–122.

Damasio, A. (2005). *Descartes' error: Emotion, reason, and the human brain.* New York: Penguin.

Dattilio, F. M., & Padesky, C. A. (1990). *Cognitive therapy with couples.* Sarasota, FL: Professional Resource Exchange.

David, D. (2003). Rational emotive behavior therapy (REBT): The view of a cognitive psychologist. In W. Dryden (Ed.), *Theoretical developments in REBT.* London: Brunner/Routledge.

David, D. (in press). Rational emotive behavior therapy. In R. L. Cautin & S. O. Lilienfeld (Eds.), *Encyclopedia of clinical psychology.* Hoboken, NJ: Wiley-Blackwell.

David, D., & DiGiuseppe, R. (2010). Social and cultural aspects of rational and irrational beliefs: A brief reconceptualisation. In D. David, S. J. Lynn, & A. Ellis (Eds.), *Rational and irrational beliefs: Research, theory, and clinical practice* (pp. 130–159). New York: Oxford University Press.

David, D., Lynn, S., & Ellis. A. (Eds.). (2010). *Rational and irrational beliefs. Implications for research, theory, and practice* (pp. 49–62). New York: Oxford University Press.

David, D., Matu, S., & David, O. A. (2013). New directions in virtual reality-based therapy for anxiety disorders. *International Journal of Cognitive Therapy, 6*, 114–137.

David, D., & Montgomery, G. H. (2011). The scientific status of psychotherapies: A new evaluative framework for evidence-based psychosocial interventions. *Clinical Psychology: Science and Practice, 18*, 89–99.

David, D., & Szentagotai, A. (2006). Cognition in cognitive behavior psychotherapies. *Clinical Psychology Review, 26*, 284–298.

Davidson, K., Norrie, J., Tyrer, P., Gumley, A., Tata, P., Murray, H., et al. (2006). The effectiveness of cognitive behavior therapy for borderline personality disorder: Results from the borderline personality disorder study of cognitive therapy (BOSCOT) trial. *Journal of Personality Disorders, 20*, 450–465.

Davidson, K. M., Tyrer, P., Norrie, J., Palmer, S. J., & Tyrer, H. (2010). Cognitive therapy

v. usual treatment for borderline personality disorder: Prospective 6-year follow-up. *British Journal of Psychiatry, 197*(6), 456–462.

Davidson, R. J., Pizzagalli, D., Nitschke, J. B., & Putnam, K. (2002). Depression: Perspectives from affective neuroscience. *Annual Review of Psychology, 53*, 545–574.

Davies, E., & Burdett, J. (2004). Preventing schizophrenia. Creating the conditions for saner societies. In J. Read, L. R. Mosher, & R. P. Bentall (Eds.), *Models of madness: Psychological, social and biological approaches to schizophrenia* (pp. 271–282). Hove, UK: Brunner-Routledge.

Davins-Pujols, M., Perez-Testor, C., Salamero-Baro, M., & Castillo-Garayoa, J. (2012). Personality profiles in abused women receiving psychotherapy according to the existence of childhood abuse. *Journal of Family Violence, 27*(2), 87–96.

Davis, D. (2008). *Terminating psychotherapy: A professional guide to ending on a positive note.* Hoboken, NJ: Wiley.

Davis, D., & Younggren, J. (2009). Ethical competence in psychotherapy termination. *Professional Psychology: Research and Practice, 40*(6), 572–578.

Davis, M., Ressler, K., Rothbaum, B. O., & Richardson, R. (2006). Effects of D-cycloserine on extinction: Translation from preclinical to clinical work. *Biological Psychiatry, 60*(4), 369–375.

Davison, S. E. (2002). Principles of managing patients with personality disorder. *Advances in Psychiatric Treatment, 8*, 1–9.

Deisenhammer, E. A., Humber, M., Kemmler, G., Weiss, E. M., & Hinterhuber, H. (2007). Psychiatric hospitalizations during the last 12 months before suicide. *General Hospital Psychiatry, 29*, 63–65.

Depue, R. A., & Collins, P. F. (1999). Neurobiology of the structure of personality: Dopamine, facilitation of incentive motivation, and extraversion. *Behavioral and Brain Sciences, 22*(3), 491–517; discussion 518-469.

DeRubeis, R. J., Siegle, G. J., & Hollon, S. D. (2008). Cognitive therapy versus medication for depression: Treatment outcomes and neural mechanisms. *Nature Reviews Neuroscience, 9*(10), 788–796.

Dickhaut, V., & Arntz, A. (2014). Combined group and individual schema therapy for borderline personality disorder: A pilot study. *Journal of Behavior Therapy and Experimental Psychiatry, 45*(2), 242–251.

DiGiuseppe, R. (1996). The nature of irrational and rational beliefs: Progress in rational emotive behavior theory. *Journal of Rational-Emotive and Cognitive-Behavior Therapy, 4*, 5–28.

DiGiuseppe, R., Doyle, K., Dryden, W., & Backx, W. (2013). *A practitioner's guide to rational-emotive therapy* (3rd ed.). New York: Oxford University Press.

DiGiuseppe, R., Leaf, R., Exner, T., & Robin, M. W. (1988, September). *The development of a measure of rational/irrational thinking.* Paper presented at the World Congress of Behavior Therapy, Edinburgh, UK.

Dimaggio, G., Attina, G., Popolo, R., & Salvatore, G. (2012). Complex case personality disorders with over-regulation of emotions and poor self-reflectivity: The case of a man with avoidant and not otherwise specified personality disorder and social phobia treated with metacognitive interpersonal therapy. *Personality and Mental Health, 6*, 156–162.

Dimaggio, G., Carcione, A., Salvatore, G., Nicolo, G., Sisto, A., & Semerari, A. (2011). Progressively promoting metacognition in a case of obsessive–compulsive personality disorder treated with metacognitive interpersonal therapy. *Psychology and Psychotherapy: Theory, Research and Practice, 84*, 70–83.

Dimeff, L., & Linehan, M. M. (2001). Dialectical behavior therapy in a nutshell. *California Psychologist, 34*, 10–13.

Dimidjian, S., Hollon, S. D., Dobson, K. S., Schmaling, K. B., Kohlenberg, R. J., Addis, M.

E., et al. (2006). Randomized trial of behavioral activation, cognitive therapy, and antidepressant medication in the acute treatment of adults with major depression. *Journal of Consulting and Clinical Psychology, 74*, 658–670.

Disner, S. G., Beevers, C. G., Haigh, E. A., & Beck, A. T. (2011). Neural mechanisms of the cognitive model of depression. *Nature Reviews Neuroscience, 12*(8), 467–477.

Disney, K. L. (2013). Dependent personality disorder: A critical review. *Clinical Psychology Review, 33*(8), 1184–1196.

DiTomasso, R. A., Golden, B. A., & Morris, H. J. (Eds.). (2010). *Handbook of cognitive behavioral approaches in primary care*. New York: Springer.

DiTomasso, R. A., & Gosch, E. A. (2007). *Anxiety disorders: A practitioner's guide to comparative treatments*. New York: Springer.

Dixon-Gordon, K. L., Turner, B. J., & Chapman, A. L. (2011). Psychotherapy for personality disorders. *International Review of Psychiatry, 23*(3), 282–302.

Doyle, M., & Logan, C. (2012). Operationalizing the assessment and management of violence risk in the short-term. *Behavioral Sciences and the Law, 30*, 406–419.

Dreessen, L., & Arntz, A. (1995). *The Personality Disorder Beliefs Questionnaire (short version)*. Maastricht, The Netherlands: Author.

Duberstein, P. R., & Conwell, Y. (1997). Personality disorders and completed suicide: A methodological and conceptual review. *Clinical Psychology: Science and Practice, 4*(4), 359–376.

Duberstein, P. R., & Witte, T. (2009). Suicide risk in personality disorders: An argument for a public health perspective. In P. M. Kleespies (Ed.), *Behavioral emergencies: An evidence-based resource for evaluating and managing risk of suicide, violence, and victimization* (pp. 257–286). Washington, DC: American Psychological Association.

Duff, A. (2003). Managing personality disorders: Making positive connections. *Nursing Management, 10*(6), 27–30.

Duman, R. S., & Aghajanian, G. K. (2012). Synaptic dysfunction in depression: Potential therapeutic targets. *Science, 338*(6103), 68–72.

Dutton, D. G. (2006). *Rethinking domestic violence*. Vancouver: University of British Columbia Press.

Dutton, D. G., & Hart, S. D. (1992). Risk markers for family violence in a federally incarcerated population. *International Journal of Law and Psychiatry, 15*, 101–112.

Eckhardt, C., Holtzworth-Munroe, A., Norlander, B., Sibley, A., & Cahill, M. (2008). Readiness to change, partner violence subtypes, and treatment outcomes among men in treatment for partner assault. *Violence and Victims, 23*(4), 446–475.

Edens, J. F., Marcus, D. K., Lilienfeld, S. O., & Poythress, N. G., Jr. (2006). Psychopathic, not psychopath: Taxometric evidence for the dimensional structure of psychopathy. *Journal of Abnormal Psychology, 115*(1), 131–144.

Edwards, G. (2013). Tarasoff, duty to warn laws, and suicide. *International Review of Law and Economics, 34*, 1–8.

Eisely, L. (1961). *Darwin's century*. Garden City, NY: Doubleday/Anchor.

Ekselius, L., Tillfors, M., Furmark, T., & Fredrikson, M. (2001). Personality disorders in the general population: DSM-IV and ICD-10 defined prevalence as related to sociodemographic profile. *Personality and Individual Differences, 30*, 311–320.

El-Gabalawy, R., Katz, L. Y., & Sareen, J. (2010). Comorbidity and associated severity of borderline personality disorder and physical health conditions in a nationally representative sample. *Psychosomatic Medicine, 72*, 641–647.

Ellis, A. (1957). Rational psychotherapy and individual psychology. *Journal of Individual Psychology, 13*, 38–44.

Ellis, A. (1962). *Reason and emotion in psychotherapy*. New York: Stuart.

Ellis, A. (1994). *Reason and emotion in psychotherapy* (rev. ed.). Secaucus, NJ: Birch Lane. (Original work published 1962)

Ellis, A. (2003). Similarities and differences between rational emotive behavior therapy and cognitive therapy. *Journal of Cognitive Psychotherapy: An International Quarterly,* 17, 225–240.

Emmelkamp, P. M. G., Benner, A., Kuipers, A., Feiertag, G. A., Koster, H. C., & van Apeldoorn, F. J. (2006). Comparison of brief dynamic and cognitive–behavioural therapies in avoidant personality disorder. *British Journal of Psychiatry, 189,* 60–64.

Etkin, A., & Schatzberg, A. F. (2011). Common abnormalities and disorder-specific compensation during implicit regulation of emotional processing in generalized anxiety and major depressive disorders. *American Journal of Psychiatry, 168*(9), 968–978.

Evans, K., Tyrer, P., Catalan, J., Schmidt, U., Davidson, K., Dent, J., et al. (1999). Manual-assisted cognitive behavior therapy (MACT): A randomized controlled trial of a brief intervention with bibliotherapy in the treatment of recurrent deliberate self-harm. *Psychological Medicine, 29,* 19–25.

Evershed, S. (2011). Treatment of personality disorder: Skills-based therapies. *Advances in Psychiatric Treatment, 17,* 206–213.

Exner, J. E. (2003). *The Rorschach: A comprehensive system: Vol. I. Basic foundations* (4th ed.). New York: Wiley.

Fagin, L. (2004). Management of personality disorders in acute care settings: Part 2. Less common personality disorders. *Advances in Psychiatric Treatment, 10,* 100–106.

Falicov, C. J. (1995). Training to think culturally: A multidimensional comparative framework. *Family Process, 34*(4), 373–388.

Farmer, R. F., & Chapman, A. L. (2002). Evaluation of DSM-IV personality disorder criteria as assessed by the structured clinical interview for DSM-IV personality disorders. *Comprehensive Psychiatry, 43*(4), 285–300.

Farrell, J. M., & Shaw, I. A. (1994). Emotion awareness training: A prerequisite to effective cognitive-behavioral treatment of borderline personality disorder. *Cognitive and Behavioral Practice, 1,* 71–91.

Farrell, J. M., Shaw, I. A., & Webber, A. A. (2009). A schema-focused approach to group psychotherapy for outpatients with borderline personality disorder: A randomized controlled trial. *Behavior Therapy and Experimental Psychiatry, 40,* 317–328.

Feenstra, D. J., Hutsebaut, J., Laurenssen, E. M. P., Verheul, R., Busschbach, J. J. V., & Soeteman, D. I. (2012). The burden of disease among adolescents with personality pathology: Quality of life and costs. *Journal of Personality Disorders, 26,* 593–604.

Feldman, B. N., & Freedenthal, S. (2006). Social work education in suicide intervention and prevention: An unmet need? *Suicide and Life-Threatening Behavior, 36*(4), 467–480.

First, M., Gibbon, M., Spitzer, R., Williams, J., & Benjamin, L. (1997). *Structured Clinical Interview for DSM-IV Axis II Personality Disorders (SCID-II).* Washington, DC: American Psychiatric Press.

First, M. B., Bell, C. C., Cuthbert, B. N., Krystal, J. H., Malison, R., Offord, D. R., et al. (2002). Personality disorders and relational disorders: A research agenda for addressing crucial gaps in DSM. In D. J. Kupfer (Ed.), *A research agenda for DSM-V* (pp. 123–200). Washington, DC: American Psychiatric Press.

First, M. B., Spitzer, R. L., Gibbon, M., & Williams, J. B. W. (1995). The Structured Clinical Interview for DSM-III-R Personality Disorders (SCID-II): Part I. Description. *Journal of Personality Disorders, 9,* 83–91.

Fossati, A., Beauchaine, T. P., Grazioli, F., Carretta, I., Cortinovis, F., & Maffei, C. (2005). A latent structure analysis of diagnostic and statistical manual of mental disorders: Fourth edition. Narcissistic personality disorder criteria. *Comprehensive Psychiatry, 46*(5), 361–367.

Fossati, A., Maffei, C., Bagnato, M., Donati, D., Donini, M., Fiorelli, M., & Norella, L. (2000). A psychometric study of DSM-IV passive–aggressive (negativistic) personality disorder criteria. *Journal of Personality Disorders, 14*(1), 72–83.

Fournier, J. C., DeRubeis, R. J., & Beck, A. T. (2011). Dysfunctional cognitions in personality pathology: The structure and validity of the Personality Belief Questionnaire. *Psychological Medicine, 42*(4), 1–11.

Frankenburg, F., & Zanarini, M. (2006). Personality disorders and medical comorbidity. *Current Opinions in Psychiatry, 19,* 428–431.

Freeman, A. (2002). *Cognitive-behavioral therapy for severe personality disorders.* In S. G. Hofmann & M. C. Thompson (Eds.), *Treating chronic and severe mental disorders* (pp. 382–402). New York: Guilford Press.

Freeman, A., & Dolan, M. (2001). Revisiting Prochaska and DiClemente's stages of change theory: An expansion and specification to aid in treatment planning and outcome evaluation. *Cognitive and Behavioral Practice, 8*(3), 224–234.

Freeman, A., Felgoise, S., & Davis, D. (2008). *Clinical psychology: Integrating science and practice.* Hoboken, NJ: Wiley.

Freeman, A., & Fusco, G. (2000). Treating high-arousal patients: Differentiating between patients in crisis and crisis-prone patients. In F. M. Dattilio & A. Freeman (Eds.), *Cognitive-behavioral strategies in crisis intervention* (2nd ed., pp. 27–58). New York: Guilford Press.

Freeman, A., & Leaf, R. (1989). Cognitive therapy applied to personality disorders. In A. Freeman, K. Simon, L. Beutler, & H. Arkowitz (Eds.), *Comprehensive handbook of cognitive therapy* (pp. 403–433). New York: Plenum Press.

Freeman, A., Pretzer, J., Fleming, B., & Simon, K. M. (1990). *Clinical applications of cognitive therapy.* New York: Plenum Press.

Freeman, A., Pretzer, J., Fleming, B., & Simon, K. M. (2004). *Clinical applications of cognitive therapy* (2nd ed.). New York: Springer.

Freeman, A., & Rock, G. E. (2008). Personality disorders. In M. A. Whisman (Ed.), *Adapting cognitive therapy for depression: Managing complexity and comorbidity* (pp. 255–279). New York: Guilford Press.

Friedman, R. C., Aronoff, M. S., Clarkin, J. F., Corn, R., & Hurt, S. W. (1983). History of suicidal behavior in depressed borderline inpatients. *American Journal of Psychiatry, 140,* 1023–1026.

Fuller, J. R., DiGiuseppe, R., O'Leary, S., Fountain, T., & Lang, C. (2010). An open trial of a comprehensive anger treatment program on an outpatient sample. *Behavioural and Cognitive Psychotherapy, 38*(4), 485.

Furnham, A., & Trickey, G. (2011). Sex differences in the dark side traits. *Personality and Individual Differences, 50,* 517–522.

Fusco, G. M., & Freeman, A. (2004). *Borderline personality disorder: A patient's guide to taking control.* New York: Norton.

Fusco, G. M., & Freeman, A. (2007a). Negativistic personality disorder in children and adolescents. In A. Freeman & M. A. Reinecke (Eds.), *Personality disorders in children and adolescents* (pp. 639–679). Hoboken, NJ: Wiley.

Fusco, G. M., & Freeman, A. (2007b). Treating high-arousal patients: Differentiating between patients in crisis and crisis-prone patients. In F. M. Dattilio & A. Freeman (Eds.), *Cognitive-behavioral strategies in crisis intervention* (3rd ed., pp. 122–150). New York: Guilford Press.

Gardner, D. L., & Cowdry, R. W. (1985). Alprazolam-induced dyscontrol in borderline personality disorder. *American Journal of Psychiatry, 142,* 98–100.

Germer, C. K., Siegel, R. D., & Fulton, P. R. (2013). *Mindfulness and psychotherapy* (2nd ed). New York: Guilford Press.

Gibbon, S., Duggan, C., Stoffers, J., Huband, N., Völlm, B. A., Ferriter, M., et al. (2010). Psychological interventions for antisocial personality disorder. *Cochrane Database of Systematic Reviews,* Article No. CD007668.

Giesen-Bloo, J., van Dyck, R., Spinhoven, P., van Tilburg, W., Dirksen, C., van Asselt, T., et al. (2006). Outpatient psychotherapy for borderline personality disorder, randomized trial of schema-focused therapy vs transference-focused psychotherapy. *Archives of General Psychiatry, 63*, 649–658.

Gilbert, F., & Daffern, M. (2011). Illuminating the relationship between personality disorder and violence: Contributions of the general aggression model. *Psychology of Violence, 1*(3), 230–244.

Gilbert, P. (1989). *Human nature and suffering.* Hillsdale, NJ: Erlbaum.

Gilbert, P. (2009). *The compassionate mind: A new approach to life's challenges.* Oakland, CA: New Harbinger.

Gilbert, P. (2010). *Compassion focused therapy: Distinctive features.* New York: Routledge.

Gilbert, P., McEwan, K., Mitra, R., Franks, L., Richter, A., & Rockliff, H. (2008). Feeling safe and content: A specific affect regulation system?: Relationship to depression, anxiety, stress, and self-criticism. *Journal of Positive Psychology, 3*, 182–191.

Gilson, M. L. (1983). Depression as measured by perceptual bias in binocular rivalry. *Dissertation Abstracts International, 44*(8B), 2555. (University Microfilms No. AAD83–27351)

Glynn, L. H., & Moyers, T. B. (2010). Chasing change talk: The clinician's role in evoking client language about change. *Journal of Substance Abuse Treatment, 39*, 65–70.

Goodwin, R. D., Brook, J. S., & Cohen, P. (2005). Panic attacks and the risk of personality disorders. *Psychological Medicine, 35*, 227–235.

Gore, W. L., & Widiger, T. A. (2013). The DSM-5 dimensional trait model and five-factor models of general personality. *Journal of Abnormal Psychology, 122*(3), 816–821.

Grace, A. A., & Bunney, B. S. (1984). The control of firing pattern in nigral dopamine neurons: Burst firing. *Journal of Neuroscience, 4*(11), 2877–2890.

Grant, B. F., Stinson, F. S., Dawson, D. A., Chou, S. P., Ruan, W. J., & Pickering, R. P. (2004). Co-occurrence of 12-month alcohol and drug use disorders and personality disorders in the United States: Results from the National Epidemiologic Survey on Alcohol and Related Conditions. *Archives of General Psychiatry, 61*(4), 361–368.

Gratz, K., & Gunderson, J. (2006). Preliminary data on acceptance-based emotion regulation group intervention for deliberate self-harm among women with borderline personality disorder. *Behavior Therapy, 37*, 25–35.

Gray, J. A. (1987). *The neuropsychology of anxiety: An enquiry into the functions of the septo-hippocampal system.* New York: Oxford Univerisity Press.

Grecucci, A., Giorgetta, C., Brambilla, P., Zuanon, S., Perini, L., Balestrieri, M., et al. (2013). Anxious ultimatums: How anxiety disorders affect socioeconomic behaviour. *Cognition and Emotion, 27*(2), 230–244.

Grecucci, A., Giorgetta, C., Van't Wout, M., Bonini, N., & Sanfey, A. G. (2013). Reappraising the ultimatum: An fMRI study of emotion regulation and decision making. *Cerebral Cortex, 23*(2), 399–410.

Greenberger, D., & Padesky, C. A. (1995). *Mind over mood: Change how you feel by changing the way you think.* New York: Guilford Press.

Gresham, F. M., MacMillan, D. L., Bocian, K. M., Ward, S. L., & Forness, S. R. (1998). Comorbidity of hyperactivity–impulsivity–inattention and conduct problems: Risk factors in social, affective, and academic domains. *Journal of Abnormal Child Psychology, 26*, 393–406.

Grilo, C. M., McGlashan, T. H., Morey, L. C., Gunderson, J. G., Skodol, A. E., Shea, M. T., et al. (2001). Internal consistency, intercriterion overlap and diagnostic efficiency of criteria sets for DSM-IV schizotypal, borderline, avoidant and obsessive–compulsive personality disorders. *Acta Psychiatrica Scandinavica, 104*(4), 264–272.

Grilo, C. M., Stout, R. L., Markowitz, J. C., Sanislow, C. A., Ansell, E. B., Skodol, A. E., et al. (2010). Personality disorders predict relapse after remission from an episode of major depressive disorder: A 6-year prospective study. *Journal of Clinical Psychiatry, 71*, 1629–1635.

Gross, R., Olfson, M., Gameroff, M., Shea, S., Feder, A., Fuentes, M., et al. (2002). Borderline personality disorder in primary care. *Archives of Internal Medicine, 162*, 53–60.

Gudjonsson, G. H., & Main, N. (2008). How are personality disorders related to compliance? *Journal of Forensic Psychiatry and Psychology, 19*(2), 180–190.

Gunderson, J. G. (1996). The borderline patient's intolerance of aloneness: Insecure attachments and therapist availability. *American Journal of Psychiatry, 153*, 752–758.

Gunderson, J. G. (2010). Commentary on "Personality traits and the classification of mental disorders: Toward a more complete integration in DSM-5 and an empirical model of psychopathology." *Personality Disorders: Theory, Research, and Treatment, 1*(2), 119–122.

Gunderson, J. G. (2011). Clinical practice: Borderline personality disorder. *New England Journal of Medicine, 364*, 2037–2042.

Gunderson, J. G., Morey, L. C., Stout, R. L., Skodol, A. E., Shea, M. T., McGlashan, T. H, et al. (2004). Major depressive disorder and borderline personality disorder revisited: Longitudinal interactions. *Journal of Clinical Psychiatry, 65*, 1049–1056.

Gunderson, J. G., Phillips, K. A., Triebwasser, J., & Hirschfeld, R. M. A. (1994). The Diagnostic Interview for Depressive Personality. *American Journal of Psychiatry, 151*, 1300–1304.

Gunderson, J. G., Stout, R. L., McGlashan, T. H., Shea, M. T., Morey, L. C., Grilo, C. M., et al. (2011). Ten-year course of borderline personality disorder psychopathology and function from the Collaborative Longitudinal Personality Disorders Study. *Archives of General Psychiatry, 68*, 827–837.

Gutierrez, F., Vall, G., Peri, J. M., Bailles, E., Ferraz, L., Garriz, M., et al. (2012). Personality disorder features through the life course. *Journal of Personality Disorders, 26*(5), 763–774.

Guy, J., Brown, C., & Poelstra, P. (1990). Who gets attacked?: A national survey of patient violence directed at psychologists in clinical practice. *Professional Psychology: Research and Practice, 21*, 493–495.

Guzzo, L., Cadeau, N. D., Hogg, S. M., & Brown, G. (2012, June). *Mental health, criminogenic needs, and recidivism: An in depth look into the relationship between mental health and recidivism.* Paper presented at the 73rd annual convention of Canadian Psychological Association, Halifax, Nova Scotia.

Haaland, A. T., Vogel, P. A., Launes, G., Haaland, V. Ø., Hansen, B., Solem, S., et al. (2011). The role of early maladaptive schemas in predicting exposure and response prevention outcome for obsessive–compulsive disorder. *Behaviour Research and Therapy, 49*(11), 781–788.

Haas, B. W., Omura, K., Constable, R. T., & Canli, T. (2007). Emotional conflict and neuroticism: Personality-dependent activation in the amygdala and subgenual anterior cingulate. *Behavioral Neuroscience, 121*(2), 249.

Hadjipavlou, G., & Ogrodniczuk, J. S. (2010). Promising psychotherapies for personality disorders. *Canadian Journal of Psychiatry, 55*(4), 202–210.

Hamilton, J. P., Etkin, A., Furman, D. J., Lemus, M. G., Johnson, R. F., & Gotlib, I. H. (2012). Functional neuroimaging of major depressive disorder: A meta-analysis and new integration of base line activation and neural response data. *American Journal of Psychiatry, 169*(7), 693–703.

Hankin, B. L., Abramson, L. Y., Miller, N., & Haeffel, G. J. (2004) Cognitive vulnerability–stress theories of depression: Examining affective specificity in the prediction of depression versus anxiety in three prospective studies. *Cognitive Therapy and Research, 28*, 309–345.

Hankin, B. L., Abramson, L. Y., & Siler, M. (2001). A prospective test of the hopelessness theory of depression in adolescents. *Cognitive Therapy and Research, 25*, 607–625.

Hardy, G. E., Barkham, M., Shapiro, D. A., Stiles, W. B., Rees, A., & Reynolds, S. (1995). Impact of Cluster C personality disorders on outcomes of contrasting brief psychotherapies for depression. *Journal of Consulting and Clinical Psychology, 63*(6), 997–1004.

Hare, R. D. (1996). Psychopathy: A clinical construct whose time has come. *Criminal Justice and Behavior, 23*, 25–54.

Hare, R. D. (2003). *The Hare Psychopathy Checklist—Revised manual* (2nd ed.). Toronto, Ontario, Canada: Multi-Health Systems.

Hare, R. D., & Neumann, C. S. (2008). Psychopathy as a clinical and empirical construct. *Annual Review of Clinical Psychology, 4*, 217–246.

Harper, R. G. (2004). Personality disorders not otherwise specified. In T. Millon (Ed.), *Personality guided therapy in behavioral medicine* (pp. 277–318). Washington, DC: American Psychological Association.

Harris, D., & Batki, S. L. (2000). Stimulant psychosis: Symptom profile and acute clinical course. *American Journal on Addictions, 9*(1), 28–37.

Harris, G. T., Rice, M. E., & Quinsey, V. L. (1994). Psychopathy as a taxon: Evidence that psychopaths are a discrete class. *Journal of Consulting and Clinical Psychology, 62*(2), 387–397.

Hasin, D., Fenton, M. C., Skodol, A., Krueger, R., Keyes, K., Geier, T., et al. (2011). Personality disorders and the three-year course of alcohol, drug, and nicotine use disorders. *Archives of General Psychiatry, 68*, 1158–1167.

Hathaway, W., & Tan, E. (2009). Religiously oriented mindfulness-based cognitive therapy. *Journal of Clinical Psychology: In Session, 65*(2), 158–171.

Hawke, L. D., Provencher, M. D., & Arntz, A. (2011). Early maladaptive schemas in the risk for bipolar spectrum disorders. *Journal of Affective Disorders, 133*(3), 428–436.

Hayes, S. C., & Strosahl, K. D. (2004). *A practical guide to acceptance and commitment therapy.* New York: Springer.

Hayes, S. C., Strosahl, K. D., & Wilson, K. G. (Eds.). (2011). *Acceptance and commitment therapy: The process and practice of mindful change.* New York: Guilford Press.

Hayward, M., & Moran, P. (2007). Personality disorder and pathways to inpatient psychiatric care. *Social Psychiatry and Psychiatric Epidemiology, 42*, 502–506.

Hazlett, E. A., Zhang, J., New, A. S., Zelmanova, Y., Goldstein, K. E., Haznedar, M. M., et al. (2012). Potentiated amygdala response to repeated emotional pictures in borderline personality disorder. *Biological Psychiatry, 72*(6), 448–456.

Heisel, M. J., Links, P. S., Conn, D., van Reekum, R., & Flett, G. L. (2007). Narcissistic personality and vulnerability to late-life suicidality. *American Journal of Geriatric Psychiatry, 15*, 734–741.

Hend, S., Baker, J., & Williamson, D. (1991). Family environment characteristics and dependent personality disorder. *Journal of Personality Disorders, 5*, 256–263.

Hesse, M., & Moran, P. (2010). Screening for personality disorder with the Standardised Assessment of Personality: Abbreviated Scale (SAPAS): Further evidence of concurrent validity. *BMC Psychiatry, 10*(1), 10.

Hill, A. B. (1976). Methodological problems in the use of factor analysis: A critical review of the experimental evidence for the anal character. *British Journal of Medical Psychology, 49*, 145–159.

Hinton, D. E., Rivera, E. I., Hofmann, S. G., Barlow, D. H., & Otto, M. W. (2012). Adapting CBT for traumatized refugees and ethnic minority patients: Examples from culturally-adapted CBT (CA-CBT). *Transcultural Psychiatry, 49*(2), 340–365.

Hirschfeld, R. M. A. (1999). Personality disorders and depression: Comorbidity. *Depression and Anxiety, 10*, 142–146.

Hirschfeld, R. M. A., Klerman, G. L., Clayton, P. J., Keller, M. B., McDonald-Scott, P., & Larkin, B. H. (1983). Assessing personality: Effects of the depressive state on trait measurement. *American Journal of Psychiatry, 140*, 695–699.

Hofmann, S. G. (2007). Enhancing exposure-based therapy from a translational research perspective. *Behaviour Research and Therapy, 45*(9), 1987–2001.

Hofmann, S. G., Glombiewski, J., Asnaani, A., & Sawyer, A. T. (2011). Mindfulness and acceptance: The perspective of cognitive therapy. In J. D. Herbert & E. M. Forman (Eds.), *Acceptance and mindfulness in cognitive behavior therapy: Understanding and applying the new therapies* (pp. 267–290). Hoboken, NJ: Wiley.

Hofmann, S. G., Meuret, A. E., Smits, J. A., Simon, N. M., Pollack, M. H., Eisenmenger, K., et al. (2006). Augmentation of exposure therapy with D-cycloserine for social anxiety disorder. *Archives of General Psychiatry, 63*(3), 298–304.

Hofmann, S. G., Pollack, M. H., & Otto, M. W. (2006). Augmentation treatment of psychotherapy for anxiety disorders with D-cycloserine. *CNS Drug Reviews, 12*(3–4), 208–217.

Hogan, R. (1987). Personality psychology: Back to basics. In J. Aronoff, A. I. Robin, & R. A. Zucker (Eds.), *The emergence of personality* (pp. 141–188). New York: Springer.

Hogan, R., Johnson, J., & Briggs, S. (Eds.). (1997). *Handbook of personality psychology.* New York: Academic Press.

Hollandsworth, J., & Cooley, M. (1978). Provoking anger and gaining compliance with assertive versus aggressive responses. *Behavior Therapy, 9*(4), 640–646.

Hollon, S. D., & Beck, A. T. (2004). Cognitive and cognitive behavioral therapies. In M. J. Lambert (Ed.), *Bergin and Garfield's handbook of psychotherapy and behavior change* (5th ed., pp. 447–492). New York: Wiley.

Hollon, S. D., & Kendall, P. C. (1980). Cognitive self-statements in depression: Development of an Automatic Thoughts Questionnaire. *Cognitive Therapy and Research, 4*, 383–395.

Holtzworth-Munroe, A., Meehan, J. C., Herron, K., Rehman, U., & Stuart, G. L. (2000). Testing the Holtzworth-Munroe and Stuart (1994) batterer typology. *Journal of Consulting and Clinical Psychology, 68*, 1000–1019.

Hopwood, C. J., Morey, L. C., Markowitz, J. C., Pinto, A., Skodol, A. E., Gunderson, J.G., et al. (2009). The construct validity of passive–aggressive personality disorder. *Psychiatry: Interpersonal and Biological Processes, 72*(3), 256–267.

Hopwood, C. J., Schade, N., Krueger, R. F., Wright, A. G., & Markon, K. E. (2013). Connecting DSM-5 personality traits and pathological beliefs: Toward a unifying model. *Journal of Psychopathology and Behavioral Assessment, 35*(2), 1–11.

Howes, O. D., Bose, S. K., Turkheimer, F., Valli, I., Egerton, A., Valmaggia, L. R., et al. (2011). Dopamine synthesis capacity prior to the subsequent onset of psychosis: An [18F]-DOPA PET imaging study. *American Journal of Psychiatry, 168*(12), 1311.

Huprich, S. K. (2004). Convergent and discriminant validity of three measures of depressive personality disorder. *Journal of Personality Assessment, 8*, 321–328.

Huprich, S. K. (2005). Differentiating avoidant and depressive personality disorders. *Journal of Personality Disorders, 19*, 659–673.

Huprich, S. K. (2009). What should become of depressive personality disorder in DSM-V? *Harvard Review of Psychiatry, 17*, 41–59.

Huprich, S. K. (2012). Considering the evidence and making the most empirically informed decision about depressive personality disorder in DSM-5. *Personality Disorders: Theory, Research and Treatment, 3*, 470–482.

Huprich, S. K., Margrett, J., Barthelemy, K. J., & Fine, M. A. (1996). The Depressive Personality Disorders Inventory: An initial examination of its psychometric properties. *Journal of Clinical Psychology, 52*, 153–159.

Huttlinger, K. W. (2013). People of Appalachian heritage. In L. D. Purnell (Ed.), *Transcultural health care: A culturally competent approach* (4th ed., pp. 137–158). Philadelphia: Davis.

Hyldahl, R. S., & Richardson, B. (2011). Key considerations using no-harm contracts with clients who self-injure. *Journal of Counseling and Development, 89*, 121–127.

Hyler, S. E., & Rieder, R. O. (1987). *PDQ-R: Personality Diagnostic Questionnaire—Revised.* New York: New York State Psychiatric Institute.

Ilardi, S., & Craighead, W. E. (1995). Personality pathology and response to somatic treatments for major depression: A critical review. *Depression, 2,* 200–217.

Iwamasa, G. Y., Larrabee, A. L., & Merritt, R. D. (2000). Are personality disorder criteria ethnically biased?: A card-sort analysis. *Cultural Diversity and Ethnic Minority Psychology, 6*(3), 284–296.

Jacobs, G. A., & Arntz, A. (2013). Schema therapy for personality disorders—a review. *International Journal of Cognitive Therapy, 6,* 171–185.

John, O. P., Robinson, R. W., & Pervin, L. A. (Eds.). (2010). *Handbook of personality: Theory and research.* New York: Guilford Press.

Johnson, J., Smailes, E., Cohen, P., Brown, J., & Bernstein, D. (2000). Associations between four types of childhood neglect and personality disorder symptoms during adolescence and early adulthood: Findings of a community-based longitudinal study. *Journal of Personality Disorders, 14*(2), 171–187.

Johnson, J. G., Cohen, P., Chen, H., Kasen, S., & Brook, J. S. (2006). Parenting behaviors associated with risk for offspring personality disorder during adulthood. *Archives of General Psychiatry, 63,* 579–587.

Johnson, J. G., Cohen, P., Kasen, S., & Brook, J. S. (2005). Personality disorder traits associated with risk for unipolar depression during middle adulthood. *Psychiatry Research, 136,* 113–121.

Johnson, J. G., Cohen, P., Kasen, S., & Brook, J. S. (2006). Personality disorders evident by early adulthood and risk for anxiety disorders during middle adulthood. *Anxiety Disorders, 20,* 408–426.

Johnson, J. G., Cohen, P., Kasen, S., Skodol, A. E., & Oldham, J. M. (2008). Cumulative prevalence of personality disorders between adolescence and adulthood. *Acta Psychiatric Scandanavia, 118,* 410–413.

Johnson, J. G., Cohen, P., Smailes, E., Kasen, S., Oldham, J. M., Skodol, A. E., et al. (2000). Adolescent personality disorders associated with violence and criminal behavior during adolescence and early adulthood. *American Journal of Psychiatry, 157*(9), 1406–1412.

Joiner, T. (2000). Depressions viscious scree: Self-propogating and erosive processes in depression chronicity. *Clinical Psychology: Science and Practice, 7,* 203–218

Joiner, T., E., & Rudd, M. D. (2002). The incremental validity of passive–aggressive personality symptoms rivals or exceeds that of other personality symptoms in suicidal outpatients. *Journal of Personality Assessment, 79*(1), 161–170.

Jones, A., Laurens, K., Herba, C., Barker, G., & Viding, E. (2009). Amygdala hypoactivity to fearful faces in boys with conduct problems and callous–unemotional traits. *American Journal of Psychiatry, 166*(1), 95–102.

Jones, S. H., Burrell-Hodgson, G., & Tate, G. (2007). Relationships between the personality beliefs questionnaire and self-rated personality disorders. *British Journal of Clinical Psychology/British Psychological Society, 46*(2), 247–251.

Joyce, P. R., McKenzie, J. M., Carter, J. D., Rae, A. M., Luty, S. E., Frampton, C. M. A., et al. (2007). Temperament, character and personality disorders as predictors of response to interpersonal psychotherapy and cognitive-behavioural therapy for depression. *British Journal of Psychiatry, 190,* 503–508.

Juni, S., & Semel, S. R. (1982). Person perception as a function of orality and anality. *Journal of Social Psychology, 118,* 99–103.

Kagan, J. (1989). Temperamental contributions to social behavior. *American Psychologist, 44*(4), 668–674.

Kagan, J., Reznick, J. S., & Snidman, N. (1987). The physiology and psychology of behavioral inhibition in children. *Child Development, 58*(6), 1459–1473.

Kampman, M., Keijsers, G. P. J., Hoogduin, C. A. L., & Hendriks, G. J. (2008). Outcome prediction of cognitive behaviour therapy for panic disorder: Initial symptom severity is predictive for treatment outcome, comorbid anxiety or depressive disorder, Cluster

C personality disorders and initial motivation are not. *Behavioural and Cognitive Psychotherapy, 36,* 99–112.

Kantor, M. (2002). *Passive–aggression. A guide for the therapist, the patient, and the victim.* Westport, CT: Greenwood.

Kaplan, M. S., Asnis, G. M., Sanderson, W. C., & Keswani, L. (1994). Suicide assessment: Clinical interview vs. self report. *Journal of Clinical Psychology, 50*(2), 294–298.

Kapur, S., Phillips, A. G., & Insel, T. R. (2012). Why has it taken so long for biological psychiatry to develop clinical tests and what to do about it? *Molecular Psychiatry, 17*(12), 1174–1179.

Kaufman, A. R., & Way, B. (2010). North Carolina resident psychiatrists' knowledge of the commitment statutes: Do they stray from the legal standard in the hypothetical application of involuntary commitment criteria? *Psychiatric Quarterly, 81,* 363–367.

Kazantzis, N., Whittington, C., & Dattilio, F. (2010). Meta-analysis of homework effects in cognitive and behavioral therapy: A replication and extension. *Clinical Psychology: Science and Practice, 17,* 144–156.

Kelly, G. (1955). *The psychology of personal constructs.* New York: Norton.

Kendler, K. S., Myers, J., Torgersen, S., Neale, M. C., & Reichborn-Kjennerud, T. (2007). The heritability of cluster A personality disorders assessed by both personal interview and questionnaire. *Psychological Medicine, 37*(5), 655–666.

Kendler, K. S., Prescott, C. A., Myers, J., & Neale, M. C. (2003). The structure of genetic and environmental risk factors for common psychiatric and substance use disorders in men and women. *Archives of General Psychiatry, 60*(9), 929–937.

Kernis, M. (2005). Measuring self-esteem in context: The importance of stability of self-esteem in psychological functioning. *Journal of Personality, 73,* 1–37.

Kessler, R. C., Chiu, W. T., Demler, O., & Walters, E. E. (2005). Prevalence, severity, and comorbidity of 12-month DSM-IV disorders in the National Comorbidity Survey Replication. *Archives of General Psychiatry, 62*(6), 617–627.

Keulen-de Vos, M. K., Bernstein, D. P., & Arntz, A. (2014). Schema therapy for aggressive offenders with personality disorders. In R. C. Tafrate & D. Mitchell (Eds.), *Forensic CBT: A handbook for clinical practice* (pp. 66–83). Chichester, UK: Wiley.

Khalifa, N., Duggan, C., Stoffers, J., Huband, N., Völlm, B. A., Ferriter, M., et al. (2010). Pharmacological interventions for antisocial personality disorder. *Cochrane Database of Systematic Reviews,* Article No. CD007667. DOI: 10.1002/14651858.CD007667.pub2.

Kiehl, K. A., Smith, A. M., Hare, R. D., Mendrek, A., Forster, B. B., Brink, J., et al. (2001). Limbic abnormalities in affective processing by criminal psychopaths as revealed by functional magnetic resonance imaging. *Biological Psychiatry, 50*(9), 677–684.

Kimmerling, R., Zeiss, A., & Zeiss, R. (2000). Therapist emotional responses to patients: Building a learning-based language. *Cognitive and Behavioral Practice, 7,* 312–321.

Kincade, S. R., & McBride, D. (2009). CBT and autism spectrum disorders: A comprehensive literature review. Retrieved from *http://files.eric.ed.gov/fulltext/ED506298.pdf.*

King-Casas, B., & Chiu, P. H. (2012). Understanding interpersonal function in psychiatric illness through multiplayer economic games. *Biological Psychiatry, 72*(2), 119–125.

King-Casas, B., Sharp, C., Lomax-Bream, L., Lohrenz, T., Fonagy, P., & Montague, P. R. (2008). The rupture and repair of cooperation in borderline personality disorder. *Science, 321*(5890), 806–810.

Kleespies, P. M., Deleppo, J. D., Gallagher, P. L., & Niles, B. L. (1999). Managing suicidal emergencies: Recommendations for the practitioner. *Professional Psychology: Research and Practice, 30*(5), 454–463.

Kleespies, P. M., & Dettmer, E. L. (2000). The stress of patient emergencies for the clinician: Incidence, impact, and means of coping. *Journal of Clinical Psychology, 56*(10), 1353–1369.

Kleespies, P. M., Marshall, S., Pokrajac, T., & Amodio, R. (1994). Case consultation: The transition from inpatient to outpatient care: Comment. *Suicide and Life-Threatening Behavior, 24*, 305–307.

Kleespies, P. M., Penk, W. E., & Forsyth, J. P. (1993). The stress of patient suicidal behavior during clinical training: Incidence, impact, and recovery. *Professional Psychology, Research and Practice, 24*(3), 293–303.

Kleespies, P. M., & Richmond, J. S. (2009). Evaluating behavioral emergencies: The clinical interview. In P. M. Kleespies (Ed.), *Behavioral emergencies: An evidence-based resource for evaluating and managing risk of suicide, violence, and victimization* (pp. 33–55). Washington, DC: American Psychological Association.

Kleespies, P. M., Van Orden, K. A., Bongar, B., Bridegman, D., Bufka. L. F., Galper, D. I., et al. (2011). Psychologist suicide: Incidence, impact, and suggestions for prevention, intervention, and postvention. *Professional Psychology, 42*(3), 244–251.

Klein, D. N. (1999). Commentary on Ryder and Bagby's "Diagnostic viability of depressive personality disorder: Theoretical and conceptual issues." *Journal of Personality Disorders, 118*, 118–127.

Klein, D. N., & Shih, J. H. (1998). Depressive personality: Associations with DSM-III-R mood and personality disorders and negative and positive affectivity, 30-month stability, and prediction of course of Axis I depressive disorders. *Journal of Abnormal Psychology, 107*, 319–327.

Kliem, S., Kröger, C., & Kosfelder, J. (2010). Dialectical behavior therapy for borderline personality disorder: A meta-analysis using mixed-effects modeling. *Journal of Consulting and Clinical Psychology, 78*, 936–951.

Knight, K., Garner, B. R., Simpson, D. D., Morey, J. T., & Flynn, P. M. (2006). An assessment for criminal thinking. *Crime and Delinquency, 52*, 159–177.

Koch, C. (2012). Modular biological complexity. *Science, 337*, 531–532.

Koocher, G., & Keith-Spiegel, P. (1998). *Ethics in psychology: Professional standards and cases* (2nd ed.). New York: Oxford University Press.

Kool, S., Dekker, J., Duijsens, I. J., de Jonghe, F., & Puite, B. (2003). Changes in personality pathology after pharmacotherapy and combined therapy for depressed patients. *Jounal of Personality Disorders, 17*, 60–72.

Kraepelin, E. (1921). *Manic-depressive insanity and paranoia.* Edinburgh, UK: Livingstone.

Kramlinger, K. G., & Post, R. (1996). Ultra-rapid and ultradian cycling in bipolar affective illness. *British Journal of Psychiatry, 168*, 314–323.

Krause-Utz, A., Oei, N., Niedtfeld, I., Bohus, M., Spinhoven, P., Schmahl, C., et al. (2011). Influence of emotional distraction on working memory performance in borderline personality disorder. *Psychological Medicine, 42*(10), 2181–2192.

Kroner, D. G., & Morgan, R. D. (2014). An overview of strategies for the assessment and treatment of criminal thinking. In R. C. Tafrate & D. Mitchell (Eds.), *Forensic CBT: A handbook for clinical practice* (pp. 87–103). Chichester, UK: Wiley.

Kropp, P. R. (2008). Intimate partner violence risk assessment and management. *Violence and Victims, 23*(2), 202–220.

Krueger, R. F. (2005). Continuity of Axes I and II: Toward a unified model of personality, personality disorders, and clinical disorders. *Journal of Personality Disorders, 19*(3), 233–261.

Krueger, R. F., Derringer, J., Markon, K. E., Watson, D., & Skodol, A. E. (2012). Initial construction of a maladaptive personality trait model and inventory for DSM-5. *Psychological Medicine, 42*(9), 1879–1890.

Krueger, R. F., & Tackett, J. L. (2003). Personality and psychopathology: Working toward the bigger picture. *Journal of Personality Disorders, 17*(2), 109–128.

Krysinska, K., Heller, T. S., & De Leo, D. (2006). Suicide and deliberate self-harm in personality disorders. *Current Opinion in Psychiatry, 19*(1), 95–101.

Kuyken, W., Kurzer, N., DeRubeis, R. J., Beck, A. T., & Brown, G. K. (2001). Response to cognitive therapy in depression: The role of maladaptive beliefs and personality disorders. *Journal of Consulting and Clinical Psychology, 69*(3), 560–566.

Kuyken, W., Padesky, C. A., & Dudley, R. (2009). *Collaborative case conceptualization: Working effectively with clients in cognitive-behavioral therapy.* New York: Guilford Press.

Kwon, J. S., Kim, Y.-M., Chang, G.-C., Park, B.-J., Kim, L., Yoon, D. J., et al. (2000). Three-year follow-up of women with the sole diagnosis of depressive personality disorder: Subsequent development of dysthymia and major depression. *American Journal of Psychiatry, 157,* 1966–1972.

Lahey, B. B. (2007). Public health significance of neuroticism. *American Psychologist, 64,* 241–256.

Lahti, J., Raikkonen, K., Sovio, U., Miettunen, J., Hartikainen, A. L., Pouta, A., et al. (2009). Early-life origins of schizotypal traits in adulthood. *British Journal of Psychiatry, 195,* 132–137.

Lam, D. H., Jones, S. H., & Hayward, P. (2010). *Cognitive therapy for bipolar disorder: A therapist's guide to concepts, methods, and practice* (2nd ed.). Oxford, UK: Wiley.

Lambert, M. (2003). Suicide risk assessment and management: Focus on personality disorders. *Current Opinion in Psychiatry, 16*(1), 71–76.

Landenberger, N. A., & Lipsey, M. W. (2005). The positive effects of cognitive behavioral programs for offenders: A meta-analysis of factors associated with effective treatment. *Journal of Experimental Criminology, 1,* 451–476.

Laptook, R. S., Klein, D. N., & Dougherty, L. R. (2006). Ten-year stability of depressive personality disorder in depressed outpatients. *American Journal of Psychiatry, 163,* 865–871.

La Roche, M. J. (2005). The cultural context and the psychotherapeutic process: Toward a culturally sensitive psychotherapy. *Journal of Psychotherapy Integration, 15*(2), 169–185.

Latessa, E., Smith, P., Lemke, R., Makarios, M., & Lowenkamp, C. (2009). *Creation and validation of the Ohio Risk Assessment System Final Report.* Cincinnati, OH: University of Cincinnati. Available at *www.ocjs.ohio.gov/ORAS_FinalReport.pdf.*

Latessa, E. J. (2004). The challenge of change: Correctional programs and evidence-based practices. *Criminology and Public Policy, 3,* 547–559.

Layden, M. A., Newman, C. F., Freeman, A., & Morse, S. B. (1993). *Cognitive therapy of borderline personality disorder.* Boston: Allyn & Bacon.

Lazare, A., Klerman, G. L., & Armor, D. (1966). Oral, obsessive, and hysterical personality patterns. *Archives of General Psychiatry, 14,* 624–630.

Lazarus, R. S. (1991). *Emotion and adaptation.* New York: Oxford University Press.

Leahy, R. L. (2001). *Overcoming resistance in cognitive therapy.* New York: Guilford Press.

Leahy, R. L. (2006). *The worry cure: Seven steps to stop worry from stopping you.* New York: Harmony.

Leahy, R. L. (2010). *Beat the blues before they beat you: How to overcome depression.* Carlsbad, CA: Hay House.

Lee, C. W., Taylor, G., & Dunn, J. (1999). Factor structure of the Schema Questionnaire in a large clinical sample. *Cognitive Therapy and Research, 23,* 441–451.

Leichsenring, F., Leibing, E., Kruse, J., New, A. S., & Leweke, F. (2011). Borderline personality disorder. *Lancet, 377,* 74–84.

Leichsenring, F., & Rabung, S. (2011). Long-term psychodynamic psychotherapy in complex mental disorders: Update of a meta-analysis. *British Journal of Psychiatry, 199*(1), 15–22.

Lenzenweger, M. F., & Korfine, L. (1992). Confirming the latent structure and base rate of schizotypy: A taxometric analysis. *Journal of Abnormal Psychology, 101*(3), 567–571.

Lenzenweger, M. F., Lane, M. C., Loranger, A. W., & Kessler, R. C. (2007). DSM-IV personality disorders in the National Comorbidity Survey Replication. *Biological Psychiatry, 62*(6), 553–564.

Levenson, J. C., Wallace, M. L., Fournier, J. C., Rucci, P., & Frank, E. (2012). The role of personality pathology in depression treatment outcome with psychotherapy and pharmacotherapy. *Journal of Consulting and Clinical Psychology, 80*(5), 719–729.

The Lewin Group. (2013). Becoming a high reliability organization: Operational advice for hospital leaders. Prepared for Agency for Healthcare Research and Quality U.S. Department of Health and Human Services. Retrieved from *www.ahrq.gov/ professionals/quality-patient-safety/quality-resources/tools/hroadvice/hroadvice.pdf.*

Lewinsohn, P. M., Joiner, T. E., & Rohde, P. (2001). Evaluation of cognitive diathesis–stress models in predicting major depression in adolescents. *Journal of Abnormal Psychology, 110*, 203–215.

Lewis, D. A., & Gonzalez-Burgos, G. (2008). Neuroplasticity of neocortical circuits in schizophrenia. *Neuropsychopharmacology, 33*(1), 141–165.

Lewis-Fernández, R., & Kleinman, A. (1994). Culture, personality, and psychopathology. *Journal of Abnormal Psychology, 103*(1), 67–71.

Leyton, M., Boileau, I., Benkelfat, C., Diksic, M., Baker, G., & Dagher, A. (2002). Amphetamine-induced increases in extracellular dopamine, drug wanting, and novelty seeking: A PET/[11C]raclopride study in healthy men. *Neuropsychopharmacology, 27*(6), 1027–1035.

Lieb, K., Völlm, B., Rücker, G., Timmer, A., & Stoffers, J. M. (2010). Pharmacotherapy for borderline personality disorder: Cochrane systematic review of randomised trials. *British Journal of Psychiatry, 196*(1), 4–12.

Lieb, K., Zanarini, M. C., Schmahl, C., Linehan, M. M., & Bohus, M. (2004). Borderline personality disorder. *Lancet, 364*, 453–461.

Linehan, M. M. (1993). *Cognitive-behavioral treatment of borderline personality disorder.* New York: Guilford Press.

Linehan, M. M., Armstrong, H. E., Suarez, A., Allmon, D., & Heard, H. L. (1991). Cognitive-behavioral treatment of chronically parasuicidal borderline patients. *Archives of General Psychiatry, 48*, 1060–1064.

Linehan, M. M., & Heard, H. L. (1999). Borderline personality disorder: Costs, course, and treatment outcomes. In N. E. Miller & K. M. Magruder (Eds.), *Cost-effectiveness of psychotherapy: A guide for practitioners, researchers, and policymakers* (pp. 291–305). New York: Oxford University Press.

Links, P. S. (1996). *Clinical assessment and management of severe personality disorder.* Washington, DC: American Psychiatric Press.

Links, P. S. (2013). Pathological narcissism and the risk of suicide. In J. S. Ogrodniczuk (Ed.), *Understanding and treating pathological narcissism* (pp. 167–181). Washington, DC: American Psychological Association.

Lipsey, M. W., Chapman, G. L., & Landenberger, N. A. (2001). Cognitive-behavioral programs for offenders. *Annals of the American Academy of Political and Social Science, 578*, 144–147.

Livesley, W. J. (1990). *DAPP-BQ Personality Questionnaire Clinical Version.* Vancouver, British Columbia, Canada: University of British Columbia.

Livesley, W. J. (1998). Suggestions for a framework for an empirically based classification of personality disorder. *Canadian Journal of Psychiatry, 43*(2), 137–147.

Livesley, W. J., & Jang, K. L. (2000). Toward an empirically based classification of personality disorder. *Journal of Personality Disorders, 14*(2), 137–151.

Lloyd, B. T. (2002). A conceptual framework for examining adolescent identity, media influence and social development. *Review of General Psychology, 6*(1), 73–91.

Lohr, J. M., Hamberger, L. K., & Bonge, D. (1988). The nature of irrational beliefs in different personality clusters of spouse abusers. *Journal of Rational-Emotive and Cognitive-Behavior Therapy, 6*(4), 273–285.

Loranger, A., Sartorius, N., Andreoli, A., Berger, P., Buchheim, P., Channabasavanna, S., et al. (1994). The International Personality Disorder Examination: The World Health Organization/Alcohol, Drug Abuse, and Mental Health Administration International Pilot Study of Personality Disorders. *Archives of General Psychiatry, 51*(3), 215–224.

Loranger, A. W. (1990). The impact of DSM-III on diagnostic practice in a university hospital: A comparison of DSM-II and DSM-III in 10,914 patients. *Archives of General Psychiatry, 47*, 672–675.

Loranger, A. W., Lenzenweger, M. F., Gartner, A. F., Lehman, S. V., Herzig, J., Zammit, G. K., et al. (1991). Trait–state artifacts and the diagnosis of personality disorders. *Archives of General Psychiatry, 48*, 720–728.

Loranger, P. (1989). *The Personality Disorders Examination (PDE) manual.* Yonkers, NY: DV Communications.

Lugnegård, T., Hallerbäck, M. U., & Gillberg, C. (2011). Personality disorders and autism spectrum disorders: What are the connections? *Comprehensive Psychiatry, 53*, 333–340.

Luxton, D. D., June, J. D., & Comtois, K. A. (2013). Can postdischarge follow-up contacts prevent suicide and suicidal behavior? *Crisis, 34*(1), 32–41.

Lynch, T. R. (2014). *Radically open-dialectical behavior therapy for disorders of overcontrol.* New York: Guilford Press.

Lynch, T. R., Cheavens, J. S., Cukrowicz, K. C., Thorp, S. R., Bronner, L., & Beyer, J. (2007). Treatment of older adults with co-morbid personality disorder and depression: A dialectical behavior therapy approach. *International Journal of Geriatric Psychiatry, 22*(2), 131–143.

Lynch, T. R., Gray, K. L. H., Hempel, R. J., Titley, M., Chen, E. Y., & O'Mahen, H. A. (2013). Radically open-dialectical behavior therapy for adult anorexia nervosa: Feasibility and outcomes from an inpatient program. *BMC Psychiatry, 13*, 293–310.

MacKenzie, K. R. (1997). *Time-managed group psychotherapy: Effective clinical applications.* Washington, DC: American Psychiatric Press.

Maddux, R. E., Riso, L. P., Klein, D. N., Markowitz, J. C., Rothbaum, B. O., Arnow, B. A., et al. (2009). Select comorbid personality disorders and the treatment of chronic depression with nefazodone, targeted psychotherapy, or their combination. *Journal of Affective Disorders, 117*, 174–179.

Maffei, C., Fossati, A., Agnostoni, I., Barraco, A., Bagnato, M., Deborah, D., et al. (1997). Interrater reliability and internal consistency of the Structured Clinical Interview for DSM-IV Axis II Personality Disorders (SCID-II), version 2.0. *Journal of Personality Disorders, 11*(3), 279–284.

Mahoney, M. (1984). Behaviorism, cognitivism, and human change processes. In M. A. Reda & M. Mahoney (Eds.), *Cognitive psychotherapies: Recent developments in theory, research, and practice* (pp. 3–30). Cambridge, MA: Ballinger.

Malinow, K. (1981). Passive–aggressive personality. In J. Lion (Ed.), *Personality disorders diagnosis and management* (2nd ed., pp. 121–132). Baltimore: Williams & Wilkins.

Mandracchia, J. T., Morgan, R. D., Garos, S., & Garland, J. T. (2007). Inmate thinking patterns: An empirical investigation. *Criminal Justice and Behavior, 34*, 1029–1043.

Mankiewicz, P. D. (2013). Cognitive behavioural symptom-oriented understanding of psychosis: Abandoning the disease paradigm of schizophrenia. *Counseling Psychology Review, 28*, 53–63.

Mankiewicz, P. D., Gresswell, D. M., & Turner, C. (2013). Subjective wellbeing in psychosis. Mediating effects of psychological distress on happiness levels amongst individuals diagnosed with paranoid schizophrenia. *International Journal of Wellbeing, 3*(1), 35–59.

Manlick, C., Black, D., Stumpf, A., McCormick, B., & Allen, J. (2012). Symptoms of migraine and its relationship to personality disorder in a non-patient sample. *Journal of Psychosomatic Research, 73*, 479–480.

Markon, K. E., Quilty, L. C., Bagby, R. M., & Krueger, R. F. (2013). The development and psychometric properties of an informant-report form of the Personality Inventory for DSM-5 (PID-5). *Assessment, 20*(3), 370–383.

Markowitz, J. C., Moran, M. E., Kocsis, J. H., & Frances, A. J. (1992). Prevalence and comorbidity of dysthymic disorder among psychiatric outpatients. *Journal of Affective Disorders, 24,* 63–71.

Marsh, A., Finger, E., Mitchell, D., Reid, M., Sims, C., Kosson, D., et al. (2008). Reduced amygdala response to fearful expressions in children and adolescents with callous–unemotional traits and disruptive behavior disorders. *American Journal of Psychiatry, 165*(6), 712–720.

Martell, C. R., Addis, M. E., & Jacobson, N. S. (2001). *Depression in context: Strategies for guided action.* New York: Norton.

Martino, S., Carrroll, K., Kostas, D., Perkins, J., & Rounsaville, B. (2002). Dual diagnosis motivational interviewing: A modification of motivational interviewing for substance-abusing patients with psychotic disorders. *Journal of Substance Abuse Treatment, 23,* 297–308.

Mathew, A. R., Chamberlain, L. D., Szafranski, D. D., Smith, A. H., & Norton, P. J. (2013). Prognostic indicators of treatment response in adults with anxiety. In E. A. Storch & D. McKay (Eds.), *Handbook of treating variants and complications in anxiety disorders* (pp. 23–35). New York: Springer.

Matthews, G., Deary, I. J., & Whiteman, M. C. (2003). *Personality traits.* Cambridge, UK: Cambridge University Press.

Mattia, J. I., & Zimmerman, M. (2001). Epidemiology. In W. J. Livesley (Ed.), *Handbook of personality disorders: Theory, research, and treatment* (pp. 107–123). New York: Guilford Press.

Matusiewicz, A., Hopwood, C., Banducci, A., & Lejuez, C. (2010). The effectiveness of cognitive behavioral therapy for personality disorders. *Psychiatric Clinics of North America, 33*(3), 657–685.

Mayberg, H. S., Lozano, A. M., Voon, V., McNeely, H. E., Seminowicz, D., Hamani, C., et al. (2005). Deep brain stimulation for treatment-resistant depression. *Neuron, 45*(5), 651–660.

Mays, D. T. (1985). Behavior therapy with borderline personality disorders: One clinician's perspective. In D. T. Mays & C. M. Franks (Eds.), *Negative outcome in psychotherapy and what to do about it* (pp. 301–311). New York: Springer.

McCann, J. T. (1988). Passive–aggressive personality disorder: A review. *Journal of Personality Disorders, 2*(2), 170–179.

McCann, J. T. (2009). Obsessive-compulsive and negativistic personality disorders. In P. Blaney & T. Millon (Eds.), *Oxford textbook of psychopathology* (2nd ed., pp. 671–691). New York: Oxford University Press.

McCranie, E., & Bass, J. (1984). Childhood family antecedents of dependency and self-criticism. *Journal of Abnormal Psychology, 93,* 3–8.

McDermut, W., Zimmerman, M., & Chelminski, I. (2003). The construct validity of depressive personality disorder. *Journal of Abnormal Psychology, 112,* 49–60.

McDougall, W. (1921). *An introduction to social psychology* (14th ed.). Boston: Luce.

McGarvey, E. L., Leon-Verdin, M., Wanchek, T. N., & Bonnie, R. J. (2013). Decisions to initiate involuntary commitment: The role of intensive community services and other factors. *Psychiatric Services, 64,* 120–126.

McGilloway, A., Hall, R. E., Lee, T., & Bhui, K. S. (2010). A systematic review of personality disorder, race and ethnicity: Prevalence, aetiology and treatment. *BMC Psychiatry, 10*(1), 33.

McGinn, L. K., & Young, J. E. (1996). Schema-focused therapy. In P. M. Salkovskis (Ed.), *Frontiers of cognitive therapy* (pp. 182–207). New York: Guilford Press.

McGlashan, T. H., Grilo, C. M., Skodol, A. E., Gunderson, J. G., Shea, M. T., Morey, L.

C., et al. (2000). The Collaborative Longitudinal Personality Disorders Study: Baseline Axis I/II and II/II diagnostic co-occurrence. *Acta Psychiatrica Scandinavica, 102,* 256–264.

McKay, D., Neziroglu, F., Todaro, J., & Yaryura-Tobias, J. A. (1996). Changes in personality disorders following behavior therapy for obsessive–compulsive disorder. *Journal of Anxiety Disorders, 10*(1), 47–57.

McMurran, M., & Christopher, G. (2008). Dysfunctional beliefs and antisocial personality disorder. *Journal of Forensic Psychiatry and Psychology, 19*(4), 533–542.

McMurran, M., Huband, N., & Overton, E. (2010). Non-completion of personality disorder treatments: A systematic review of correlates, consequences, and interventions. *Clinical Psychology Review, 30,* 277–287.

McNeil, D. E. (2009). Assessment and management of acute risk of violence in adult patients. In P. M. Kleespies (Ed.), *Behavioral emergencies: An evidence-based resource for evaluating and managing risk of suicide, violence, and victimization* (pp. 125–145). Washington, DC: American Psychological Association.

McNeil, D. E., Binder, R. L., & Greenfield, T. K. (1988). Predictors of violence in civilly committed acute psychiatric patients. *American Journal of Psychiatry, 145,* 965–970.

McNeil, D. E., Weaver, C. M., & Hall, S. E. (2007). Base rates of firearm possession by hospitalized patients. *Psychiatric Services, 58,* 551–553.

Mennin, D. S., & Heimberg, R. G. (2000). The impact of comorbid mood and personality disorders in the cognitive-behavioral treatment of panic disorder. *Clinical Psychology Review, 20,* 339–357.

Miller, J. D., Campbell, W. K., & Widiger, T. A. (2010). Narcissistic personality disorder and the DSM-V. *Journal of Abnormal Psychology, 119*(4), 640–649.

Miller, P. R. (2001). Inpatient diagnostic assessments: 2. Interrater reliability and outcomes of structured vs. unstructured interviews. *Psychiatry Research, 105*(3), 265–271.

Miller, W. R., & Rollnick, S. (2002). *Motivational interviewing: Preparing people for change* (2nd ed.). New York: Guilford Press.

Miller, W. R., & Rollnick, S. (2013). *Motivational interviewing: Helping people change* (3rd ed.). New York: Guilford Press.

Millon, T. (1969). *Modern psychopathology: A biosocial approach to maladaptive learning and functioning.* Philadelphia: Saunders.

Millon, T. (1981). *Disorders of personality: DSM-III, Axis II.* New York: Wiley.

Millon, T. (1993). Negativistic (passive–aggressive) personality disorder. *Journal of Personality Disorders, 7*(1), 78–85.

Millon, T. (1994). *Manual for the MCMI-III.* Minneapolis, MN: National Computer Systems.

Millon, T. (1999). *Personality-guided therapy.* New York: Wiley-Interscience.

Millon, T. (2011). Further thoughts on the relation of personality and psychopathology. *World Psychiatry, 10,* 107–108.

Millon, T., & Davis, R. (1996). *Disorders of personality: DSM-IV and beyond* (2nd ed.). Oxford, UK: Wiley.

Millon, T., & Davis, R. D. (2000). *Personality disorders in modern life.* Hoboken, NJ: Wiley.

Millon, T., & Grossman, S. (2007). *Overcoming resistant personality disorders: A personalized psychotherapy approach.* Hoboken, NJ: Wiley.

Millon, T., Grossman, S., Millon, C., Meagher, S., & Ramnath, R. (2004). *Personality disorders in modern life.* Hoboken, NJ: Wiley.

Millon, T., Millon, C., Davis, R., & Grossman, S. (2009). *MCMI-III manual* (4th ed.). Minneapolis, MN: Pearson Education.

Millon, T., Millon, C. M., Meagher, S., Grossman, S., & Ramnath, R. (2004). *Personality disorders in modern life* (2nd ed.). Hoboken, NJ: Wiley.

Mills, J. F., Kroner, D. G., & Forth, A. E. (2002). Measures of criminal attitudes and associates (MCAA): Development, factor structure, reliability, and validity. *Assessment, 9,* 240–253.

Minichiello, W. E., Baer, L., & Jenike, M. A. (1987). Schizotypal personality disorder: A poor prognostic indicator for behavior therapy in the treatment of obsessive–compulsive disorder. *Journal of Anxiety Disorders, 1*, 273–276.

Mitchell, D., & Tafrate, R. C. (2012). Conceptualization and measurement of criminal thinking: Initial validation of the Criminogenic Thinking Profile. *International Journal of Offender Therapy and Comparative Criminology, 56*, 1080–1102.

Mittal, V. A., Kalus, O., Bernstein, D. P., & Siever, L. J. (2007). Schizoid personality disorder. In W. O'Donohue, K. A. Fowler, & S. O. Lilenfeld (Eds.), *Personality disorders: Toward the DSM-V* (pp. 63–80). Thousand Oaks, CA: Sage.

Monroe, S. M. (2008). Modern approaches to conceptualizing and measuring human life stress. *Annual Review of Clinical Psychology, 4*, 33–52.

Mooney, K. A., & Padesky, C. A. (2000). Applying client creativity to recurrent problems: Constructing possibilities and tolerating doubt. *Journal of Cognitive Psychotherapy: An International Quarterly, 14*(2), 149–161.

Moran, P., Leese, M., Lee, T., Walters, P., Thornicroft, G., & Mann, A. (2003). Standardised Assessment of Personality—Abbreviated Scale (SAPAS): Preliminary validation of a brief screen for personality disorder. *British Journal of Psychiatry: Journal of Mental Science, 183*, 228–232.

Morana, H. C. P., & Camara, F. P. (2006). International guidelines for the management of personality disorders. *Current Opinion in Psychiatry, 19*(5), 539–543.

Morey, L. C., Gunderson, J., Quigley, B. D., & Lyons, M. (2000). Dimensions and categories: The "big five" factors and the DSM personality disorders. *Assessment, 7*(3), 203–216.

Morey, L. C., Hopwood, C. J., & Klein, D. N. (2007). Passive–aggressive, depressive, and sadistic personality disorders. In W. O'Donohue, K. A. Fowler, & S. O. Lilienfeld (Eds.), *Personality disorders: Toward the DSM-V* (pp. 353–374). Thousand Oaks, CA: Sage.

Morey, L. C., Krueger, R. F., & Skodol, A. E. (2013). The hierarchical structure of clinician ratings of proposed DSM-5 pathological personality traits. *Journal of Abnormal Psychology, 122*(3), 836–841.

Morey, L. C., Lowmaster, S. E., & Hopwood, C. J. (2010). A pilot study of manual-assisted cognitive therapy with a therapeutic assessment augmentation for borderline personality disorder. *Psychiatry Research, 178*(3), 531–535.

Morrison, A. P., Renton, J. C., French, P., & Bentall, R. P. (2008). *Think you're crazy?: Think again: A resource book for cognitive therapy for psychosis*. London: Routledge.

Morton, J., Snowdon, S., Gopold, M., & Guymer, E. (2012). Acceptance and commitment therapy group treatment for symptoms of borderline personality disorder: A public sector pilot study. *Cognitive and Behavioral Practice, 19*(4), 527–544.

Moscicki, E. K. (1997). Identification of suicide risk factors using epidemiologic studies. *Psychiatric Clinics of North America, 20*, 171–177.

Motto, J. A., & Bostrom, A. G. (2001). A randomized controlled trial of postcrisis suicide prevention. *Psychiatric Services, 52*(6), 828–833.

Moyers, T. B., Martin, T., Houck, J. M., Christopher, P. J., & Tonigan, J. S. (2009). From in-session behaviors to drinking outcomes: A causal chain for motivational interviewing. *Journal of Consulting and Clinical Psychology, 77*, 1113–1124.

Mueser, K. T., Gottlieb J. D., Cather, C., Glynn S. M., Zarate, R., Smith, L. F., et al. (2012). Antisocial personality disorder in people with co-occurring severe mental illness and substance use disorders: Clinical, functional, and family relationship correlates. *Psychosis, 4*, 52–62.

Mulder, R. T. (2002). Personality pathology and treatment outcome in major depression: A review. *American Journal of Psychiatry, 159*, 359–371.

Mulder, R. T., Joyce, P. R., & Frampton, C. M. A. (2010). Personality disorders improve in patients treated for major depression. *Acta Psychiatrica Scandinavica, 122*(3), 219–225.

Müller, J. L., Sommer, M., Wagner, V., Lange, K., Taschler, H., Röder, C. H., et al. (2003). Abnormalities in emotion processing within cortical and subcortical regions in criminal psychopaths: Evidence from a functional magnetic resonance imaging study using pictures with emotional content. *Biological Psychiatry, 54*(2), 152–162.

Muran, J., Safran, J., Samstag, L., Wallner, L., & Winston, A. (2005). Evaluating an alliance-focused treatment for personality disorders. *Psychotherapy: Theory, Research, Practice, Training, 42*(4), 532–545.

Muroff, J. (2007). Cultural diversity and cognitive behavior therapy. In T. Ronen & A. Freeman (Eds.), *Cognitive behavior therapy in clinical social work practice* (pp. 109–146). New York: Springer.

Murphy, C., Meyer, S., & O'Leary, K. (1994). Dependency characteristics of partner assaultive men. *Journal of Abnormal Psychology, 103*(4), 729–735.

Naeem, F., Waheed, W., Gobbi, M., Ayub, M., & Kingdon, D. (2011). Preliminary evaluation of culturally sensitive CBT for depression in Pakistan: Findings from Developing Culturally-Sensitive CBT Project (DCCP). *Behavioural and Cognitive Psychotherapy, 39*(2), 165–173.

National Alliance on Mental Illness. (2013). Retrieved from *www.nami.org/template. cfm?section=About_NAMI*.

Neff, K. D. (2011). Self-compassion, self-esteem and well-being. *Social and Personality Compass, 5*, 1–12.

Nestadt, G., Di, C., Samuels, J. F., Bienvenu, O. J., Reti, I. M., Costa, P., et al. (2010). The stability of DSM personality disorders over twelve to eighteen years. *Journal of Psychiatric Research, 44*(1), 1–7.

Nett, D. E., & Gross, M. (2011). How can we help masochistic inpatients not to sabotage psychiatric treatment before it even starts? *Journal of Psychiatric Practice, 17*(2), 124–128.

Newman, C. (1997). Maintaining professionalism in the face of emotional abuse from clients. *Cognitive and Behavioral Practice, 4*, 1–29.

Newman, C. F. (2011). When clients' morbid avoidance and chronic anger impeded their response to cognitive-behavioral therapy for depression. *Cognitive and Behavioral Practice, 18*, 350–361.

Newman, C. F., Leahy, R. L., Beck, A. T., Reilly-Harrington, N. A., & Gyulai, L. (2002). Moderating mania and hypomania in bipolar disorder. In C. F. Newman, R. L. Leahy, A. T. Beck, N. A. Harrington, & L. Gyulai (Eds.), *Bipolar disorder: A cognitive therapy approach* (pp. 47–77). Washington, DC: American Psychological Association.

Newton-Howes, G., Weaver, T., & Tyrer, P. (2008). Attitudes of staff towards patients with personality disorder in community mental health teams. *Australian and New Zealand Journal of Psychiatry, 42*, 572–577.

Ng, H., & Bornstein, R. (2005). Comorbidity of dependent personality disorder and anxiety disorders: A meta-analytic review. *Clinical Psychology: Science and Practice, 21*(4), 395–406.

Ng, R. M. (2005). Cognitive therapy for obsessive–compulsive personality disorder—a pilot study in Hong Kong Chinese patients. *Hong Kong Journal of Psychiatry, 15*(2), 50.

NICE. (2009). Borderline personality disorder: Treatment and management. NICE clinical guideline 78. British Psychological Society and Royal College of Psychiatrists. Available at *www.guidance.nice.org.uk/cg78*.

Nicolo, G., Semerari, A., Lysaker, P. H., Dimaggio, G., Conti, L., D'Angerio, S., et al. (2011). Alexithymia in personality disorders: Correlations with symptoms and interpersonal functioning. *Psychiatry Research, 190*, 37–42.

Northpointe Institute for Public Management. (1996). *COMPAS*. Traverse City, MI: Author.

O'Connor, B. P., & Dyce, J. A. (1998). A test of models of personality disorder configuration. *Journal of Abnormal Psychology, 107*(1), 3–16.

Oei, T. P., & Baranoff, J. (2007). Young Schema Questionnaire: Review of psychometric and measurement issues. *Australian Journal of Psychology, 59*(2), 78–86.

Ogloff, J. R. P. (2006). Psychopathy/antisocial personality disorder continuum. *Australian and New Zealand Journal of Psychiatry, 40*, 519–528.

Olin, S. S., Raine, A., Cannon, T. D., & Parnas, J. (1997). Childhood behavior precursors of schizotypal personality disorder. *Schizophrenia Bulletin, 23*, 93–103.

Oltmanns, T. F., & Balsis, S. (2011). Personality disorders in later life: Questions about the measurement, course, and impact of disorders. *Annual Review of Clinical Psychology, 7*, 321–349.

Oltmanns, T. F., & Turkheimer, E. (2009). Person perception and personality pathology. *Current Directions in Psychological Science, 18*(1), 32–36.

Ørstavik, R. E., Kendler, K. S., Czajkowski, N., Tambs, K., & Reichborn-Kjennerud, T. (2007). The relationship between depressive personality disorder and major depressive disorder: A population-based twin study. *American Journal of Psychiatry, 164*, 1866–1872.

Othmer, E., & Othmer, S. (2002). *The Clinical Interview using DSM-IV: Vol. 1. Fundamentals* (2nd ed.) Washington, DC: American Psychiatric Press.

Ottaviani, R. (1990). Passive–aggressive personality disorder. In A. T. Beck, A. Freeman, & Associates (Eds.), *Cognitive therapy of personality disorders* (pp. 333–349). New York: Guilford Press.

Ottenbreit, N. D., & Dobson, K. S. (2008). Avoidance. In K. S. Dobson & D. J. A. Dozois (Eds.), *Risk factors in depression* (pp. 447–470). New York: Guilford Press.

Pabian, Y. L., Welfel, E., & Beebe, R. S. (2009). Psychologists' knowledge of their states' laws pertaining to Tarasoff-type situations. *Professional Psychology: Research and Practice, 40*(1), 8–14.

Padesky, C. A. (1986, September 18–20). *Personality disorders: Cognitive therapy into the 90's.* Paper presented at the Second International Conference on Cognitive Psychotherapy, Umeå, Sweden.

Padesky, C. A. (1993a). Schema as self prejudice. *International Cognitive Therapy Newsletter, 5/6*, 16–17.

Padesky, C. A. (1993b, September 24). *Socratic questioning: Changing minds or guided discovery?* Keynote address delivered at the European Congress of Behavioural and Cognitive Therapies, London, United Kingdom.

Padesky, C. A. (1994). Schema change processes in cognitive therapy. *Clinical Psychology and Psychotherapy, 1*, 267–278.

Padesky, C. A. (1997). A more effective treatment focus for social phobia. *International Cognitive Therapy Newsletter, 11*(1), 1–3.

Padesky, C. A., & Beck, A. T. (2003). Science and philosophy: Comparison of cognitive therapy and rational emotive behavior therapy. *Journal of Cognitive Psychotherapy, 17*, 211–224.

Padesky, C. A. (with Greenberger, D.). (1995). *Clinician's guide to mind over mood.* New York: Guilford Press.

Padesky, C. A., & Mooney, K. A. (2012). Strengths-based cognitive-behavioural therapy: A four-step model to build resilience. *Clinical Psychology and Psychotherapy, 19*(4), 283–290.

Palmer, S., Davidson, K., Tyrer, P., Gumley, A., Tata, P., Norrie, J., et al. (2006). The cost-effectiveness of cognitive behavior therapy for borderline personality disorder: Results from the BOSCOT trial. *Journal of Personality Disorders, 20*, 466–481.

Papas, R. K., Sidle, J. E., Martino, S., Baliddawa, J. B., Songole, R., Omolo, O. E., et al. (2010). Systematic cultural adaptation of cognitive-behavioral therapy to reduce alcohol use among HIV-infected outpatients in western Kenya. *AIDS and Behavior, 14*(3), 669–678.

Parhar, K. K., Wormith, J. S., Derkzen, D. M., & Beauregard, A. M. (2008). Offender coercion in treatment: A meta-analysis of effectiveness. *Criminal Justice and Behavior, 35,* 1109–1135.

Paris, J. (1993). The treatment of borderline personality disorder in light of the research on its long term outcome. *Canadian Journal of Psychiatry, 38*(Suppl. 1), S28–S34.

Paris, J. (1998). Psychotherapy for personality disorders: Working with traits. *Bulletin of the Menninger Clinic, 62*(3), 287–297.

Paris, J. (2005). Borderline personality disorder. *Canadian Medical Association Journal, 172,* 1579–1583.

Paris, J., & Lis, E. (2012). Can sociocultural and historical mechanisms influence the development of borderline personality disorder? *Transcultural Psychiatry, 50*(1), 140–151.

Parker, G., Tupling, H., & Brown, L. (1979). A parental bonding insrument. *British Journal of Medical Psychology, 52,* 1–10.

Pasieczny, N., & Connor, J. (2011). The effectiveness of dialectical behaviour therapy in routine public mental health settings: An Australian controlled trial. *Behaviour Research and Therapy, 49*(1), 4–10.

Paukert, A. L., Phillips, L., Cully, J. A., Loboprabhu, S. M., Lomax, J. W., & Stanley, M. A. (2009). Integration of religion into cognitive-behavioral therapy for geriatric anxiety and depression. *Journal of Psychiatric Practice, 15*(2), 103–112.

Paul, G. L. (1967). Strategy of outcome in research in psychotherapy. *Journal of Consulting Psychology, 31*(2), 109–118.

Pepper, C. M., Klein, D. N., Anderson, R. L., Riso, L. P., Ouimette, P. C., & Lizardi, H. (1995). DSM-III-R Axis II comorbidity in dysthymia and major depression. *American Journal of Psychiatry, 152,* 239–247.

Perez, M., Pettit, J., David, C., Kistner, J., & Joiner, T. (2001). The interpersonal consequences of inflated self-esteem in an inpatient psychiatric youth sample. *Journal of Consulting and Clinical Psychology, 69*(4), 712–716.

Perlis, M. L., Jungquist, C., Smith, M. T., & Posner, D. (2005). *Cognitive behavioral treatment of insomnia: A session-by-session guide.* New York: Springer.

Perry, J., & Corner, A. (2011). Impulsive phenomena, the impulsive character [der triebhafte charakter] and DSM personality disorders. *Journal of Personality Disorders, 25*(5), 586–606.

Perry, J., & Flannery, R. (1982). Passive–aggressive personality disorder treatment implications of a clinical typology. *Journal of Nervous and Mental Disease, 170*(3), 164–173.

Persons, J. B., Burns, B. D., & Perloff, J. M. (1988). Predictors of drop-out and outcome in cognitive therapy for depression in a private practice setting. *Cognitive Therapy and Research, 12,* 557–575.

Perugi, G., Angst, J., Azorin, J. M., Bowden, C., Vieta, E., & Young, A. H. (2012). Is comorbid borderline personality disorder in patients with major depressive episode and bipolarity a developmental subtype? Findings from the international BRIDGE study. *Journal of Affective Disorders, 144,* 72–78.

Pfohl, B. (1999). Axis I and Axis II: Comorbidity or confusion? In C. Robert Cloninger (Ed.), *Personality and psychopathology* (pp. 83–98). Washington, DC: American Psychiatric Press.

Pfohl, B., Barrash, J., True, B., & Alexander, B. (1989). Failure of two Axis II measures to predict medication noncompliance among hypertensive outpatients. *Journal of Personality Disorders, 3,* 45–52.

Pfohl, B., Blum, N., & Zimmerman, M. (1997). *Structured Interview for DSM-IV Personality.* Washington, DC: American Psychiatric Press.

Phelps, E. A., & LeDoux, J. E. (2005). Contributions of the amygdala to emotion processing: From animal models to human behavior. *Neuron, 48*(2), 175–187.

Phillips, K. A., Gunderson, J. G., Triebwasser, J., Kimble, C. R., Faedda, G., Lyoo, I. K., et al. (1998). Reliability and validity of depressive personality disorder. *American Journal of Psychiatry, 155,* 1044–1048.

Piaget, J. (1926). *The language and thought of the child.* New York: Harcourt, Brace.

Piaget, J. (1952). *The origin of intelligence in children.* New York: International Universities Press. (Original work published 1936)

Pietrzak, R., Wagner, J., & Petry, N. (2007). DSM-IV personality disorders and coronary heart disease in older adults: Results from the National Epidemiological Survey on Alcohol and Related Conditions. *Journals on Gerontology, Series B: Psychological Sciences and Social Sciences, 62B,* 295–299.

Pilkonis, P. A., & Frank, E. (1988). Personality pathology in recurrent depression: Nature, prevalence, and relationship to treatment response. *American Journal of Psychiatry, 145,* 435–441.

Pinto, A., Liebowitz, M. R., Foa, E. B., & Simpson, H. B. (2011). Obsessive compulsive personality disorder as a predictor of exposure and ritual prevention outcome for obsessive compulsive disorder. *Behaviour Research and Therapy, 49,* 453–458.

Plante, D. T., & Winkelman, J. W. (2008). Sleep disturbance in bipolar disorder: Therapeutic implications. *American Journal of Psychiatry, 165,* 830–843.

Player, M. J., Taylor, J. L., Weickert, C. S., Alonzo, A., Sachdev, P., Martin, D., et al. (2013). Neuroplasticity in depressed individuals compared with healthy controls. *Neuropsychopharmacology, 38*(11), 2101–2108.

Podolsky, E. (1970). The passive–aggressive alcoholic personality. *Samiksa, 17*(4), 198–206.

Pompili, M., Girardi, P., Ruberto, A., & Tatarelli, R. (2005). Suicide in borderline personality disorder: A meta-analysis. *Nordic Journal of Psychiatry, 59,* 319–324.

Pope, K., & Tabachnick, B. (1993). Therapists' anger, hate, fear, and sexual feelings: National survey of therapist responses, client characteristics, critical events, formal complaints, and training. *Professional Psychology: Research and Practice, 24,* 142–152.

Posner, K., Brown, G., Stanley, B., Brent, D., Yershova, K., Oquendo, M., et al. (2011). The Columbia-Suicide Severity Rating Scale (C-SSRS): Initial validity and internal consistency findings from three multi-site studies with adolescents and adults. *American Journal of Psychiatry, 168,* 1266–1277.

Potter, N. N. (2006). What is manipulative behavior, anyway? *Journal of Personality Disorders, 20*(2), 139–156.

Pretzer, J. (1990). Borderline personality disorder. In A. T. Beck, A. Freeman, & Associates (Eds.), *Cognitive therapy of personality disorders* (pp. 176–207). New York: Guilford Press.

Pretzer, J., Beck, A. T., & Newman, C. F. (1989). Stress and stress management: A cognitive view. *Journal of Cognitive Psychotherapy: An International Quarterly, 3,* 163–179.

Pretzer, J., & Hampl, S. (1994). Cognitive behavioural treatment of obsessive compulsive personality disorder. *Clinical Psychology and Psychotherapy, 1*(5), 298–307.

Prinstein, M. (2014, January 6). Is iPhone raising your child? Blog post to *The Modern Teen.* Retrieved from *www.psychologytoday.com/blog/the-modern-teen/201401/is-iphone-raising-your-child.*

Prout, M., & Platt, J. (1983). The development and maintenance of passive–aggressiveness: The behavioral approach. In R. Parsons & R. Wicks (Eds.), *Passive aggressiveness theory and practice* (pp. 25–43). New York: Brunner/Mazel.

Pujara, M., Motzkin, J. C., Newman, J. P., Kiehl, K. A., & Koenigs, M. (2014). Neural correlates of reward and loss sensitivity in psychopathy. *Social Cognitive and Affective Neuroscience, 9*(6), 794–801.

Pukrop, R., Steinbring, I., Gentil, I., Schulte, C., Larstone, R., & Livesley, J. W. (2009). Clinical validity of the "Dimensional Assessment of Personality Pathology (DAPP)" for psychiatric patients with and without a personality disorder diagnosis. *Journal of Personality Disorders, 23*(6), 572–586.

Purnell, L. D. (2013). Transcultural diversity and health care. In L. D. Purnell (Ed.), *Transcultural health care: A culturally competent approach* (4th ed., pp. 3–14). Philadelphia: Davis.

Qin, P., & Nordentoft, M. (2005). Suicide risk in relation to psychiatric hospitalization. *Archives of General Psychiatry, 62,* 427–432.

Quilty, L. C., Ayearst, L., Chmielewski, M., Pollock, B. G., & Bagby, R. M. (2013). The psychometric properties of the Personality Inventory for DSM-5 in an APA DSM-5 field trial sample. *Assessment, 20*(3), 362–369.

Raskin, R., Novacek, J., & Hogan, R. (1991). Narcissistic self-esteem management. *Journal of Personality and Social Psychology, 60,* 911–918.

Raskin, R. N., & Terry, H. (1988). A principle components analysis of the Narcissistic Personality Inventory and further evidence of its construct validity. *Journal of Personality and Social Psychology, 54,* 890–902.

Rasmussen, P. R. (2005). The negativistic prototype. In T. Millon (Ed.), *Personality-guided therapy to cognitive behavioral therapy* (pp. 275–290). Washington, DC: American Psychological Association.

Rasmussen, S., & Tsuang, M. (1986). Clinical characteristics and family history in DSM-III obsessive–compulsive disorder. *American Journal of Psychiatry, 143,* 317–322.

Rathod, S., Kingdon, D., Phiri, P., & Gobbi, M. (2010). Developing culturally sensitive cognitive behaviour therapy for psychosis for ethnic minority patients by exploration and incorporation of service users' and health professionals' views and opinions. *Behavioural and Cognitive Psychotherapy, 38*(5), 511–533.

Rathod, S., Phiri, P., Harris, S., Underwood, C., Thagadur, M., Padmanabi, U., et al. (2013). Cognitive behaviour therapy for psychosis can be adapted for minority ethnic groups: A randomised controlled trial. *Schizophrenia Research, 143*(2–3), 319–326.

Ready, R. E., Watson, D., & Clark, L. A. (2002). Psychiatric patient- and informant-reported personality: Predicting concurrent and future behavior. *Assessment, 9*(4), 361–372.

Rees, C. S., & Pritchard, R. (in press). Brief cognitive therapy for avoidant personality disorder. *Psychotherapy.*

Reich, J., & Green, A. (1991). Effect of personality disorders on outcome of treatment. *Journal of Nervous and Mental Disease, 179,* 74–82.

Reichborn-Kjennerud, T., Czajkowski, N., Neale, M. C., Ørstavik, R. E., Torgersen, S., Tambs, K., et al. (2007). Genetic and environmental influences on dimensional representations of DSM-IV cluster C personality disorders: A population-based multivariate twin study. *Psychological Medicine, 37*(5), 645–654.

Renneberg, B., Goldstein, A. J., Phillips, D., & Chambless, D. L. (1990). Intensive behavioral group treatment of avoidant personality disorder. *Behavior Therapy, 21*(3), 363–377.

Renner, F., van Goor, M., Huibers, M., Arntz, A., Butz, B., & Bernstein, D. (2013). Short-term group schema cognitive-behavioral therapy for young adults with personality disorders and personality disorder features: Associations with changes in symptomatic distress, schemas, schema modes and coping styles. *Behaviour Research and Therapy, 51*(8), 487–492.

Renton, J. C. (2002). Cognitive therapy for paranoia. In A. P. Morrison (Ed.), *A casebook of cognitive therapy for psychosis* (pp. 19–36). London: Routledge.

Rey, J. M., Morris-Yates, A., Singh, M., Andrews, G., & Stewart, G. W. (1995). Continuities between psychiatric disorders in adolescents and personality disorders in young adults. *American Journal of Psychiatry, 152*(6), 895–900.

Rilling, J. K., Glenn, A. L., Jairam, M. R., Pagnoni, G., Goldsmith, D. R., Elfenbein, H. A., et al. (2007). Neural correlates of social cooperation and non-cooperation as a function of psychopathy. *Biological Psychiatry, 61*(11), 1260–1271.

Roberts, A. (2000). *Crisis intervention handbook* (2nd ed.). New York: Oxford University Press.

Roberts, A. (2005). *Crisis intervention handbook* (3rd ed.). New York: Oxford University Press.

Robertson, J. (1988). *Psychiatric malpractice: Liability of mental health professionals.* New York: Wiley.

Robinson, D. J. (2005). *Disordered personalities.* Port Huron, MI: Rapid Psychler Press.

Rodebaugh, T. L., Chambless, D. L., Renneberg, B., & Fydrich, T. (2005). The factor structure of the DSM-III-R personality disorders: An evaluation of competing models. *International Journal of Methods in Psychiatric Research, 14*(1), 43–55.

Rogers, P., Watt, A., Gray, N., MacCulloch, M., & Gournay, K. (2002). Content of command hallucinations predicts self-harm but not violence in a medium secure unit. *Journal of Forensic Psychiatry, 13*(2), 251–262.

Roggenbaum, S., Christy, A., & LeBlanc, A. (2012). Suicide assessment and prevention during and after emergency commitment. *Community Mental Health Journal, 48,* 741–745.

Rohner, R. P. (1984). Toward a conception of culture for cross-cultural psychology. *Journal of Cross-Cultural Psychology, 15*(2), 111–138.

Rosen, H. (1988). The constructivist–development paradigm. In R. A. Dorfman (Ed.), *Paradigms of clinical social work* (pp. 317–355). New York: Brunner/Mazel.

Rosenbluth, M., MacQueen, G., McIntyre, R. S., Beaulieu, S., & Schaffer, A. (2012). The Canadian Network for Mood and Anxiety Treatments (CANMAT) task force recommendations for the management of patients with mood disorders and comorbid personality disorders. *Annals of Clinical Psychiatry, 24,* 56–68.

Rosengren, D. B. (2009). *Building motivational interviewing skills.* New York: Guilford Press.

Ross, J. M., & Babcock, J. C. (2009). Proactive and reactive violence among intimate partner violent men diagnosed with antisocial and borderline personality disorder. *Journal of Family Violence, 24,* 607–617.

Rotenstein, O. H., McDermut, W., Bergman, A., Young, D., Zimmerman, M., & Chelminski, I. (2007). The validity of DSM-IV passive–aggressive (negativistic) personality disorder. *Journal of Personality Disorders, 21*(1), 28–41.

Rothbaum, F., Morling, B., & Rusk, N. (2009). How goals and beliefs lead people into and out of depression. *Review of General Psychology, 13,* 302–314.

Ruscio, J., & Ruscio, A. M. (2004). Clarifying boundary issues in psychopathology: The role of taxometrics in a comprehensive program of structural research. *Journal of Abnormal Psychology, 113*(1), 24–38.

Ryder, A. G., & Bagby, R. M. (1999). Diagnostic viability of depressive personality disorder: Theoretical and conceptual issues. *Journal of Personality Disorders, 13,* 99–117.

Ryder, A. G., Quilty, L. C., Vachon, D. D., & Bagby, R. M. (2010). Depressive personality and treatment outcome in major depressive disorder. *Journal of Personality Disorders, 24,* 392–404.

Ryder, A. G., Schuller, D. R., & Bagby, R. M. (2006). Depressive personality and dysthymia: Evaluating symptom and syndrome overlap. *Journal of Affective Disorders, 91,* 217–227.

Salkovskis, P. (Ed.). (1996). *Frontiers of cognitive therapy.* New York: Guilford Press.

Samuel, D. B., & Ball, S. A. (2013). The factor structure and concurrent validity of the Early Maladaptive Schema Questionnaire: Research Version. *Cognitive Therapy and Research, 37*(1), 150–159.

Samuel, D. B., Hopwood, C. J., Krueger, R. F., Thomas, K. M., & Ruggero, C. J. (2013). Comparing methods for scoring personality disorder types using maladaptive traits in DSM-5. *Assessment, 20*(3), 353–361.

Samuels, J., Eaton, W. W., Bienvenu, J., Brown, C. H., Costa, P. T., Jr., & Nestadt, G. (2002). Prevalence and correlates of personality disorders in a community sample. *British Journal of Psychiatry, 180,* 536–542.

Sansone, R. A., Farukhi, S., & Wiederman, M. W. (2011). Utilization of primary care physicians in borderline personality. *General Hospital Psychiatry, 33*, 343–346.

Sansone, R. A., & Sansone, L. A. (2013). Disruptive office behaviors in the medical setting. *Innovations in Clinical Neuroscience, 10*, 35–39.

Satel, S., & Lilienfeld, S. O. (2013). *Brainwashed: The seductive appeal of mindless neuroscience.* New York: Basic Books.

Saulsman, L. M., Coall, D. A., & Nathan, P. R. (2006). The association between depressive personality and treatment outcome for depression following a group cognitive-behavioral intervention. *Journal of Clinical Psychology, 62*, 1181–1196.

Saulsman, L. M., & Page, A. C. (2004). The five-factor model and personality disorder empirical literature: A meta-analytic review. *Clinical Psychology Review, 23*(8), 1055–1085.

Sava, F. (2009). Maladaptive schemas, irrational beliefs, and their relationship with the five-factor personality model. *Journal of Cognitive and Behavioral Psychotherapies, 9*(2), 135–147.

Scarr, S. (1987). Personality and experience: Individual encounters with the world. In J. Aronoff, A. I. Robin, & R. A. Zucker (Eds.), *The emergence of personality* (pp. 66–70). New York: Springer.

Schindler, A., Hiller, W., & Witthöft, M. (2013). What predicts outcome, response, and drop-out in CBT of depressive adults?: A naturalistic study. *Behavioural and Cognitive Psychotherapy, 41*(3), 365–370.

Schmidt, N. B., Joiner, T. E., Young, J. E., & Telch, M. J. (1995). The Schema Questionnaire: Investigation of psychometric properties and the hierarchical structure of a measure of maladaptive schemas. *Cognitive Therapy and Research, 19*, 295–321.

Schmitz, W. M., Allen, M. H., Feldman, B. N., Gutin, N. J., Jahn, D. R., Kleespies, P. M., et al. (2012). Preventing suicide through improved training in suicide risk assessment and care: An American Association of Suicidology task force report addressing serious gaps in U.S. mental health training. *Suicide and Life-Threatening Behavior, 42*(3), 292–304.

Schneider, B., Schnabel, A., Wetterling, T., Bartusch, B., Weber, B., & Georgi, K. (2008). How do personality disorders modify suicide risk? *Journal of Personality Disorders, 22*(3), 233–245.

Schneider, B., Wetterling, T., Sargk, D., Schenider, F., Schnabel, A., Maurer, K., et al. (2006). Axis I disorders and personality disorders as risk factors for suicide. *European Archives of Psychiatry and Clinical Neuroscience, 256*, 17–27.

Schneider, K. (1958). *Psychopathic personalities* (M. Hamilton, Trans.). Springfield, IL: Thomas. (Original work published 1923)

Schultz, W. D. P., & Montague, P. R. (1997). A neural substrate of prediction and reward. *Science, 275*(5306), 1593–1599.

Schwartz, C. E., Wright, C. I., Shin, L. M., Kagan, J., & Rauch, S. L. (2003). Inhibited and uninhibited infants "grown up": Adult amygdalar response to novelty. *Science, 300*(5627), 1952–1953.

Seeler, L., Freeman, A., DiGuiseppe, R., & Mitchell, D. (2014). Traditional cognitive-behavioral therapy models for antisocial patterns. In R. C. Tafrate & D. Mitchell (Eds.), *Forensic CBT: A handbook for clinical practice* (pp. 15–42). Chichester, UK: Wiley.

Segal, D. L., Coolidge, F. L., & Rosowsky, E. (2006). *Personality disorders and older adults: Diagnosis, assessment, and treatment.* Hoboken, NJ: Wiley.

Segal, Z. V., Williams, J. M. G., & Teasdale, J. D. (2002). *Mindfulness-based cognitive therapy for depression: A new approach to preventing relapse.* New York: Guilford Press.

Segall, M. H., Dasen, P. R., Berry, J. W., & Poortinga Y. H. (1990). *Human behaviour in global perspective: An introduction to cross-cultural psychology.* New York: Pergamon.

Segar, M. (1997). Coping: A survival guide for people with Asperger syndrome. Available at *www-users.cs.york.ac.uk/~alistair/survival*.

Sehiralti, M., & Er, R. A. (2012). Decisions of psychiatric nurses about duty to warn, compulsory hospitalization, and competence of patients. *Nursing Ethics, 20*(1), 41–50.

Seres, I., Unoka, Z., & Keri, S. (2009). The broken trust and cooperation in borderline personality disorder. *NeuroReport, 20*(4), 388–392.

Shapiro, D. (1965). *Neurotic styles.* New York: Basic Books.

Shea, M. T., Glass, D. R., Pilkonis, P. A., Watkins, J., & Docherty, J. P. (1987). Frequency and implications of personality disorders in a sample of depressed outpatients. *Journal of Personality Disorders, 1*, 27–42.

Shea, M. T., Stout, R. L., Yen, S., Pagano, M. E., Skodol, A. E., Morey, L. C., et al. (2004). Associations in the course of personality disorders and Axis I disorders over time. *Journal of Abnormal Psychology, 113*, 499–508.

Siegle, G. J., Steinhauer, S. R., Thase, M. E., Stenger, V. A., & Carter, C. S. (2002). Can't shake that feeling: Event-related fMRI assessment of sustained amygdala activity in response to emotional information in depressed individuals. *Biological Psychiatry, 51*(9), 693–707.

Simone, S., & Fulero, S. M. (2005). Tarasoff and the duty to protect. *Journal of Aggression, Maltreatment and Trauma, 11*(1/2), 145–168.

Simourd, D. J. (1997). The Criminal Sentiments Scale—Modified and Pride in Delinquency Scale: Psychometric properties and construct validity of two measures of criminal attitudes. *Criminal Justice and Behavior, 24*, 52–70.

Skodol, A. E. (2005). Manifestations, clinical diagnosis, and comorbidity. In J. M. Oldham, A. E. Skodol, & D. S. Bender (Eds.), *Textbook of personality disorders* (pp. 57–87). Washington, DC: American Psychiatric Publishing.

Skodol, A. E. (2008). Longitudinal course and outcome of personality disorders. *Psychiatric Clinics of North America, 31*(3), 495–503.

Skodol, A. E. (2012). Personality disorders in DSM-5. *Annual Review of Clinical Psychology, 8*, 317–344.

Skodol, A. E., Grilo, C. M., Keyes, K. M., Geier, T., Grant, B. F., & Hasin, D. S. (2011). Relationship of personality disorders to the course of major depressive disorder in a nationally representative sample. *American Journal of Psychiatry, 168*, 257–264.

Skodol, A. E., Oldham, J. M., Bender, D. S., Dyck, I. R., Stout, R. L., Morey, L. C., et al. (2005). Dimensional representations of DSM-IV personality disorders: Relationships to functional impairment. *American Journal of Psychiatry, 162*(10), 1919–1925.

Skodol, A. E., Stout, R. L., McGlashan, T. H., Grilo, C. M., Shea, M. T., Morey, L. C., et al. (1999). Co-occurrence of mood and personality disorders: A report from the Collaborative Longitudinal Personality Disorders Study (CLPS). *Depression and Anxiety, 10*, 175–182.

Small, I., Small, J., Alig, V., & Moore, D. (1970). Passive–aggressive personality disorder: A search for a syndrome. *American Journal of Psychiatry, 126*(7), 973–983.

Smit, Y., Huibers, M. J., Ioannidis, J., van Dyck, R., van Tilburg, W., & Arntz, A. (2012). The effectiveness of long-term psychoanalytic psychotherapy: A meta-analysis of randomized controlled trials. *Clinical Psychology Review, 32*(2), 81–92.

Smith, J. M., Grandin, L. D., Alloy, L. B., & Abramson, L. Y. (2006). Cognitive vulnerability to depression and Axis II personality dysfunction. *Cognitive Therapy and Research, 30*, 609–621.

Smokler, I. A., & Shevrin, H. (1979). Cerebral lateralization and personality style. *Archives of General Psychiatry, 36*, 949–954.

Soeteman, D. I., Verheul, R., Meerman, A. M., Ziegler, U., Rossum, B. V., Delimon, J., et al. (2011). Cost-effectiveness of psychotherapy for Cluster C personality disorders: A decision–analytic model in the Netherlands. *Journal of Clinical Psychiatry, 72*(1), 51.

Soloff, P. H. (1994). Is there any drug treatment of choice for the borderline patient? *Acta Psychiatrica Scandinavica, 379,* 50–55.

Soloff, P. H., Lynch, K. G., Kelly, T. M., Malone, K. M., & Mann, J. J. (2000). Characteristics of suicide attempts of patients with major depressive episode and borderline personality disorder: A comparative study. *American Journal of Psychiatry, 157,* 601–608.

Sperry, L. (2006). *Cognitive behavior therapy of DSM-IV-TR personality disorders: Highly effective interventions for the most common personality disorders* (2nd ed., pp. 165–187). New York: Routledge.

Spörrle, M., Strobel, M., & Tumasjan, A. (2010). On the incremental validity of irrational beliefs to predict subjective well-being while controlling for personality factors. *Psicothema, 22*(4), 543–548.

Springer, T., Lohr, N. E., Buchtel, H. A., & Silk, K. R. (1996). A preliminary report of short-term cognitive-behavioral group therapy for inpatients with personality disorders. *Journal of Psychotherapy Practice and Research, 5,* 57–71.

Sprock, J., & Hunsucker, L. (1998). Symptoms of prototypic patients with passive–aggressive personality disorder: DSM-III-R versus DSM-IV negativistic. *Comprehensive Psychiatry, 395,* 287–295.

Standage, K., Bilsbury, C., Jain, S., & Smith, D. (1984). An investigation of role-taking in histrionic personalities. *Canadian Journal of Psychiatry, 29,* 407–411.

Steckler, J. A. (2013). People of German heritage. In L. D. Purnell (Ed.), *Transcultural health care: A culturally competent approach* (4th ed., pp. 250–268). Philadelphia: Davis.

Steiner, J. L., Tebes, J. K., Sledge, W. H., Walker, W. H., & Loukides, M. (1995). A comparison of the Structured Clinical Interview for DSM-III-R and clinical diagnoses. *Journal of Nervous and Mental Disease, 183*(6), 365–369.

Steketee, G., & Shapiro, L. J. (1995). Predicting behavioral treatment outcome for agoraphobia and obsessive–compulsive disorder. *Clinical Psychology Review, 15,* 315–346.

Stepp, S. D., Whalen, D. J., Pilkonis, P. A., Hipwell, A. E., & Levine, M. D. (2011). Children of mothers with borderline personality disorder: Identifying parenting behaviors as potential targets for intervention. *Personality Disorders, 3,* 76–91.

Stinson, F. S., Dawson, D. A., Goldstein, R. B., Chou, S. P., Huang, B., Smith, S. M., et al. (2008). Prevalence, correlates, disability, and comorbidity of DSM-IV narcissistic personality disorder: Results from the Wave 2 National Epidemiologic Survey on Alcohol and Related Conditions. *Journal of Clinical Psychiatry, 69,* 1033–1045.

Stoffers J., Völlm, B. A., Rücker, G., Timmer, A., Huband, N., & Lieb K. (2010). Pharmacological interventions for borderline personality disorder. *Cochrane Database of Systematic Reviews, 6.* Available at *www.thecochranelibrary.com.*

Stoffers, J. M., Völlm, B. A., Rücker, G., Timmer, A., Huband, N., & Lieb, K. (2012). Psychological therapies for people with borderline personality disorder (Review). *Cochrane Database of Systematic Reviews,* Article No. CD005652.

Stone, M. (1993a). *Abnormalities of personality: Within and beyond the realm of treatment.* New York: Norton.

Stone, M. (1993b). Long-term outcome in personality disorders. *British Journal of Psychiatry, 162,* 299–313.

Strauss, J. L., Hayes, A. M., Johnson, S. L., Newman, C. F., Brown, G. K., Barber, J. P., et al. (2006). Early alliance, alliance ruptures, and symptom change in a nonrandomized trial of cognitive therapy for avoidant and obsessive–compulsive personality disorders. *Journal of Consulting and Clinical Psychology, 74*(2), 337–345.

Strosahl, K. D., Hayes, S. C., Wilson, K. G., & Gifford, E. V. (2004). An ACT primer: Core therapy processes, intervention strategies, and therapist competencies. In S. C. Hayes & K. D. Strosahl (Eds.), *A practical guide to acceptance and commitment therapy* (pp. 31–58). New York: Springer.

Sullivan, G. R., & Bongar, B. (2009). Assessing suicide risk in the adult patient. In P. M.

Kleespies (Ed.), *Behavioral emergencies: An evidence-based resource for evaluating and managing risk of suicide, violence, and victimization* (pp. 59–78). Washington, DC: American Psychological Association.

Sun, K. (2014). Treating depression and PTSD behind bars: An interaction schemas approach. In R. C. Tafrate & D. Mitchell (Eds.), *Forensic CBT: A handbook for clinical practice* (pp. 456–470). Chichester, UK: Wiley.

Sungur, M. (2013). The role of cultural factors in the course and treatment of sexual problems. In K. S. Hall & C. A. Graham (Eds.), *The cultural context of sexual pleasure and problems* (pp. 308–332). New York: Routledge.

Swann, W. B., & Read, S. J. (1981). Self-verification processes: How we sustain our self-conceptions. *Journal of Experimental Social Psychology, 17*, 351–372.

Swann, W. B., Wenzlaff, R. M., Krull, D. S., & Pelham, B. W. (1992). Allure of negative feedback: Self-verification strivings among depressed persons. *Journal of Abnormal Psychology, 101*, 293–306.

Szentagotai, A., & Freeman, A. (2007). An analysis of the relationship between irrational beliefs and automatic thoughts in predicting distress. *Journal of Cognitive and Behavioral Psychotherapies, 1*, 1–11.

Szentagotai, A., Schnur, J., DiGiuseppe R., Macavei, B., Kallay, E., & David, D. (2005). The organization and the nature of irrational beliefs: Schemas or appraisal? *Journal of Cognitive and Behavioral Psychotherapies, 2*, 139–158.

Tafrate, R. C., & Luther, J. D. (2014). Integrating motivational interviewing with forensic CBT: Promoting treatment engagement and behavior change with justice-involved clients. In R. C. Tafrate & D. Mitchell (Eds.), *Forensic CBT: A handbook for clinical practice* (pp. 411–435). Chichester, UK: Wiley.

Tafrate, R. C., Mitchell, D., & Novaco, R. W. (2014). Forensic CBT: Five recommendations for clinical practice and five topics in need of more attention. In R. C. Tafrate & D. Mitchell (Eds.), *Forensic CBT: A handbook for clinical practice* (pp. 473–486). Chichester, UK: Wiley.

Tai, S., & Turkington, D. (2009). The evolution of cognitive behaviour therapy for schizophrenia: Current practice and recent developments. *Schizophrenia Bulletin, 35*(5), 865–873.

Tangney, J. P., Steuwig, J., Furukawa, E., Kopelovich, S., Meyer, P. J., & Crosby, B. (2012). Reliability, validity, and predictive utility of the 25-item Criminogenic Cognitions Scale (CCS). *Criminal Justice and Behavior, 39*, 1340–1360.

Tardiff, K., Marzuk, P. M., Leon, A. C., & Portera, L. (1997). A prospective study of violence by psychiatric patients after hospital discharge. *Psychiatric Services, 48*(5), 678–681.

Tartakovsky, M. (2011). What to do when you think someone is suicidal. *Psych Central.* Retrieved from *http://psychcentral.com/lib/what-to-do-when-you-think-someone-is-suicidal/0007461.*

Tebaldi, C. (2012). Understanding involuntary hospitalization and use of seclusion and restraint. *Nurse Practitioner, 37*(6), 13–16.

Thomas, G. (1994). Mixed personality disorder with passive–aggressive and avoidant features. In P. T. Costa & T. A. Widiger (Eds.), *Personality disorders and the five-factor model of personality* (pp. 211–215). Washington, DC: American Psychological Association.

Thompson, R., & Zuroff, D. (1998). Dependent and self-critical mothers' responses to adolescent autonomy and competence. *Personality and Individual Differences, 24*(3), 311–324.

Timmons, K. A., & Joiner, T. E. (2008). Reassurance seeking and negative feedback seeking. In K. S. Dobson & D. J. A. Dozois (Eds.), *Risk factors in depression* (pp. 429–446). New York: Guilford Press.

Tolin, D. F. (2010). Is cognitive-behavioral therapy more effective than other therapies?: A meta-analytic review. *Clinical Psychology Review, 15*, 315–346.

Tomko, R. L., Trull, T. J., Wood, P. K., & Sher, K. J. (2013). Characteristics of borderline personality disorder in a community sample: Comorbidity, treatment utilization, and general functioning. *Journal of Personality Disorders, 27,* 1–17.

Torgerson, S. (1980). The oral, obsessive and hysterical personality syndromes. *Archives of General Psychiatry, 37,* 1272–1277.

Torgersen, S. (2009). The nature (and nurture) of personality disorders. *Scandanavian Journal of Psychology, 50,* 624–632.

Torgersen, S., Kringlen, E., & Cramer, V. (2001). The prevalence of personality disorders in a community sample. *Archives of General Psychiatry, 58*(6), 590–596.

Torgersen, S., Lygren, S., Oien, P., Skre, I., Onstad, S., Edvardsen, J., et al. (2000). A twin study of personality disorders. *Comprehensive Psychiatry, 41,* 416–425.

Torgersen, S., Myers, J., Reichborn-Kjennerud, T., Røysamb, E., Kubarych, T. S., Kendler, K. S. (2012). The heritability of cluster B personality disorders assessed both by personal interview and questionnaire. *Journal of Personality Disorders, 26*(6), 848.

Town, J. M., Abbass, A., & Hardy, G. (2011). Short-term psychodynamic psychotherapy for personality disorders: A critical review of randomized controlled trials. *Journal of Personality Disorders, 25*(6), 723–740.

Treadway, M. T., & Buckholtz, J. W. (2011). On the use and misuse of genomic and neuroimaging science in forensic psychiatry: Current roles and future directions. *Child and Adolescent Psychiatric Clinics of North America, 20*(3), 533–546.

Treadway, M. T., Buckholtz, J. W., Cowan, R. L., Woodward, N. D., Li, R., Ansari, M. S., et al. (2012). Dopaminergic mechanisms of individual differences in human effort-based decision-making. *Journal of Neuroscience, 32*(18), 6170–6176.

Treloar, A. J., & Lewis, A. J. (2008). Targeted clinical education for staff attitudes towards deliberate self-harm in borderline personality disorder: Randomized controlled trial. *Australian and New Zealand Journal of Psychiatry, 42,* 981–988.

Trull, T. J. (2001). Structural relations between borderline personality disorder features and putative etiological correlates. *Journal of Abnormal Psychology, 110,* 471–481.

Trull, T. J., Sher, K. J., Minks-Brown, C., Durbin, J., & Burr, R. (2000). Borderline personality disorder and substance use disorders: A review and integration. *Clinical Psychology Review, 20*(2), 235–253.

Trull, T. J., Widiger, T. A., & Burr, R. (2001). A structured interview for the assessment of the five-factor model of personality: Facet-level relations to the Axis II personality disorders. *Journal of Personality, 69*(2), 175–198.

Turkat, I. D., & Maisto, S. A. (1985). Personality disorders: Application of the experimental method to the formulation and modification of personality disorders. In D. H. Barlow (Ed.), *Clinical handbook of psychological disorders: A step-by-step treatment manual* (pp. 503–570). New York: Guilford Press.

Turner, R. M. (1987). The effects of personality disorder diagnosis on the outcome of social anxiety symptom reduction. *Journal of Personality Disorders, 1,* 136–143.

Twenge, J., Konrath, S., Foster, J. D., Campbell, W. K., & Bushman, B. J. (2008). Egos inflating over time: A cross temporal meta-analysis of the Narcissistic Personality Inventory. *Journal of Personality, 76*(4), 875–902.

Tyrer, P., Coombs, N., Ibrahimi, F., Mathilakath, A., Bajaj, P., Ranger, M., et al. (2007). Critical developments in the assessment of personality disorder. *British Journal of Psychiatry. 49*(Suppl.), 51–59.

Unoka, Z., Seres, I., Aspan, N., Bodi, N., & Keri, S. (2009). Trust game reveals restricted interpersonal transactions in patients with borderline personality disorder. *Journal of Personality Disorders, 23*(4), 399–409.

van Asselt, A. D. I., Dirksen, C. D., Arntz, A., Giesen-Bloo, J. H., van Dyck, R., Spinhoven, P., et al. (2008). Out-patient psychotherapy for borderline personality disorder: Cost-effectiveness of schema-focused therapy v. transference-focused psychotherapy. *British Journal of Psychiatry, 192,* 450–457.

van Asselt, A. D. I., Dirksen, C. D., Arntz, A., & Severens, J. L. (2007). The cost of border-line personality disorder: Societal cost of illness in BPD-patients. *European Psychiatry, 22*, 354–361.

van Velzen, C. J. M., & Emmelkamp, P. M. G. (1996). The assessment of personality disor-ders: Implications for cognitive and behavior therapy. *Behaviour Research and Ther-apy, 34*(8), 655–668.

van't Wout, M., Chang, L. J., & Sanfey, A. G. (2010). The influence of emotion regulation on social interactive decision-making. *Emotion, 10*(6), 815.

Vereycken, J., Vertommen, H., & Corveleyn, J. (2002). Authority conflicts and personality disorders. *Journal of Personality Disorders, 16*(1), 41–51.

Verheul, R., Bartak, A., & Widiger, T. (2007). Prevalence and construct validity of personal-ity disorder not otherwise specified (PDNOS). *Journal of Personality Disorders, 21*(4), 359–370.

Vickerman, K. A., & Margolin, G. (2008). Trajectories of physical and emotional marital aggression in midlife couples. *Violence and Victims, 23*, 18–34.

Walters, G. D. (1995). The Psychological Inventory of Criminal Thinking Styles: I. Reliabil-ity and preliminary validity. *Criminal Justice and Behavior, 22*, 307–325.

Ward, R. (2004). Assessment and management of personality disorders. *American Family Physician, 70*(8), 1505–1512.

Ward, T., & Brown, M. (2004). The good lives model and conceptual issues in offender rehabilitation. *Psychology, Crime and Law, 10*(3), 243–257.

Watkins, E. R., Scott, J., Wingrove, J., Rimes, K. A., Bathurst, N., Steiner, H., et al. (2007). Rumination focused cognitive behaviour therapy for residual depression: A case series. *Behaviour Research and Therapy, 45*, 2144–2154.

Watson, D., & Clark, L. A. (2006). Clinical diagnosis at the crossroads. *Clinical Psychology: Science and Practice, 13*(3), 210–215.

Weaver, T., & Clum, G. (1993). Early family environments and traumatic experiences associ-ated with borderline personality disorder. *Journal of Consulting and Clinical Psychol-ogy, 61*, 1068–1075.

Wegener, I., Alfter, S., Geiser, F., Liedtke, R., & Conrad, R. (2013). Schema change without schema therapy: The role of early maladaptive schemata for a successful treatment of major depression. *Psychiatry: Interpersonal and Biological Processes, 76*(1), 1–17.

Weiner, A. S., & Bardenstein, K. K. (2000). *Personality disorders in children and adoles-cents*. New York: Basic Books.

Weinberg, I., Gunderson, J. G., Hennen, J., & Cutter, C. J., Jr. (2006). Manual assisted cog-nitive treatment for deliberate self-harm in borderline personality disorder. *Journal of Personality Disorders, 20*, 482–492.

Weiner, B. (1985). An attribution theory of achievement motivation and emotion. *Psycho-logical Review, 92*, 548–573.

Weiss, M., Zelkowitz, P., Feldman, R. B., Vogel, J., Heyman, M., & Paris, J. (1996). Psycho-pathology in offspring of mothers with borderline personality disorder: A pilot study. *Canadian Journal of Psychiatry, 41*, 285–290.

Weissman, A. (1979). *Dysfunctional Attitude Scale: A validation study*. Unpublished doc-toral dissertation, University of Pennsylvania, Philadelphia.

Wellburn, K., Coristine, M., Dagg, P., Pontefract, A., & Jordan, S. (2002). The Schema Questionnaire—Short Form: Factor analysis and relationship between schemas and symptoms. *Cognitive Therapy and Research, 26*(4), 519–530.

Wessler, R. L. (1982). Varieties of cognitions in the cognitively-oriented psychotherapies. *Rational Living, 17*, 3–10.

West, M., Rose, S., & Sheldon-Keller, A. (1994). Assessment of patterns of insecure attach-ment in adults and application to dependent and schizoid personality disorders. *Jour-nal of Personality Disorders, 8*, 249–256.

Westen, D. (1997). Divergences between clinical and research methods for assessing personality disorders: Implications for research and the evolution of Axis II. *American Journal of Psychiatry, 154*, 895–903.

Westen, D., & Shedler, J. (1999a). Revising and assessing Axis-II: Part I. Developing a clinically and empirically valid assessment method. *American Journal of Psychiatry, 156*, 258–272.

Westen, D., & Shedler, J. (1999b). Revising and assessing Axis-II: Part II. Toward a clinically based and empirically useful classification of personality disorders. *American Journal of Psychiatry, 156*, 273–285.

Westen, D., Shedler, J., Bradley, B., & DeFife, J. A. (2012). An empirically derived taxonomy for personality diagnosis: Bridging science and practice in conceptualizing personality. *American Journal of Psychiatry, 169*, 273–284.

Wetzler, S., & Jose, A. (2012). Passive–aggressive personality disorder: The demise of a syndrome. In T. Widiger (Ed.), *The Oxford handbook of personality disorders* (pp. 674–693). New York: Oxford University Press.

Wetzler, S., & Morey, L. C. (1999). Passive–aggressive personality disorder: The demise of a syndrome. *Psychiatry: Interpersonal and Biological Processes, 62*(1), 49–59.

Whisman, M. A., & Schonbrun, Y. C. (2009). Social consequences of borderline personality disorder symptoms in a population-based survey: Marital distress, marital violence, and marital disruption. *Journal of Personality Disorders, 23*, 410–415.

White, A. (2010). Managing behavioral emergencies: Striving toward evidence-based practice. *Journal of Emergency Nursing, 36*(5), 455–459.

Whitman, R., Trosman, H., & Koenig, R. (1954). Clinical assessment of passive–aggressive personality. *Archives of Neurology and Psychiatry, 72*, 540–549.

Widiger, T., Frances A. J., Harris, M., Jacobsberg, L., Fyer, M., & Manning, D. (1991). Comorbidity among Axis II disorders. In J. M. Oldham (Ed.), *Personality disorders: New perspectives on diagnostic validity* (pp. 165–185). Washington, DC: American Psychiatric Association.

Widiger, T. A. (2003). Personality disorder and Axis I psychopathology: The problematic boundary of Axis I and Axis II. *Journal of Personality Disorders, 17*(2), 90–108.

Widiger, T. A., & Clark, L. A. (2000). Toward DSM-V and the classification of psychopathology [Special issue]. *Psychological Bulletin: Psychology in the 21st Century, 126*(6), 946–963.

Widiger, T. A., & Costa, P. T. (1994). Personality and personality disorders [Special issue]. *Journal of Abnormal Psychology: Personality and Psychopathology, 103*(1), 78–91.

Widiger, T. A., Costa, P. T., Jr., & McCrae, R. R. (2002). A proposal for Axis II: Diagnosing personality disorders using the five-factor model. In P. T. Costa, Jr. & T. A. Widiger (Eds.), *Personality disorders and the five-factor model of personality* (2nd ed., pp. 431–456). Washington, DC: American Psychological Association.

Widiger, T. A., & Samuel, D. B. (2005a). Diagnostic categories or dimensions?: A question for the diagnostic and statistical manual of mental disorders—fifth edition [Special issue]. *Journal of Abnormal Psychology: Toward a Dimensionally Based Taxonomy of Psychopathology, 114*(4), 494–504.

Widiger, T. A., & Samuel, D. B. (2005b). Evidence-based assessment of personality disorders. *Psychological Assessment, 17*(3), 278–287.

Widiger, T. A., & Samuel, D. B. (2009). Evidence-based assessment of personality disorders. *Personality Disorders: Theory, Research, and Treatment, 5*(1), 3–17.

Widiger, T. A., & Simonsen, E. (2005). Alternative dimensional models of personality disorder: Finding a common ground. *Journal of Personality Disorders, 19*(2), 110–130.

Widiger, T. A., Simonsen, E., Krueger, R., Livesley, W. J., & Verheul, R. (2005). Personality disorder research agenda for the DSM-V. *Journal of Personality Disorders, 19*(3), 315–338.

Widiger, T. A., & Smith, G. T. (2008). Personality and psychopathology. In O. P. John, R.

W. Robins, & L. A. Pervin (Eds.), *Handbook of personality: Theory and research* (3rd ed., pp. 743–769). New York: Guilford Press.

Wiggins, J. (1982). Circumplex models of interpersonal behavior in clinical psychology. In P. C. Kendall & J. N. Butler (Eds.), *Handbook of research methods in clinical psychology* (pp. 183–221). New York: Wiley.

Wink, P. (1991). Two faces of narcissism. *Journal of Personality and Social Psychology, 61,* 590–597.

Wirz-Justice, A., & Van den Hoofdakker, R. H. (1999). Sleep deprivation in depression: What do we know, where do we go? *Biological Psychiatry, 46,* 445–453.

Woodin, E. M., & O'Leary, K. D. (2010). A brief motivational intervention for physically aggressive dating couples. *Prevention Science, 11*(4), 371–383.

Woodward, N. D., Cowan, R. L., Park, S., Ansari, M. S., Baldwin, R. M., Li, R., et al. (2011). Correlation of individual differences in schizotypal personality traits with amphetamine-induced dopamine release in striatal and extrastriatal brain regions. *American Journal of Psychiatry, 168*(4), 418–426.

Woody, G. E., McLellan, A. T., Luborsky, L., & O'Brien, C. P. (1985). Sociopathy and psychotherapy outcome. *Archives of General Psychiatry, 42,* 1081–1086.

World Health Organization. (1992). *The ICD-10 classification of mental and behavioural disorders: Clinical descriptions and diagnostic guidelines.* Geneva, Switzerland: Author.

World Health Organization. (2010). International classification of diseases—version 2010. Retrieved from *http://apps.who.int/classifiations/icd10/brwose/2010/en#/F60.8.*

World Health Organization. (2013). *International classification of diseases and related health problems* (10th rev.). Geneva, Switzerland: Author.

Wright, A. G. C., Thomas, K. M., Hopwood, C. J., Markon, K. E., Pincus, A. L., & Krueger, R. F. (2012). The hierarchical structure of DSM-5 pathological personality traits. *Journal of Abnormal Psychology, 121*(4), 951–957.

Wright, J. H., Basco, M. R., & Thase, M. E. (2006). *Learning cognitive-behavior therapy: An illustrated guide.* Washington, DC: American Psychiatric Association.

Wu, T., Luo, Y., Broster, L. S., Gu, R., & Luo, Y.-J. (2013). The impact of anxiety on social decision-making: Behavioral and electrodermal findings. *Social Neuroscience, 8*(1), 11–21.

Yalom, I. (1985). *The theory and practice of group psychotherapy* (3rd ed.). New York: Basic Books.

Yalom, I. (1995). *The theory and practice of group psychotherapy* (4th ed.). New York: Basic Books.

Yanes, P. K., Tiffany, S. T., & Roberts, J. E. (2010). Cognitive therapy for co-occurring depression and behaviors associated with passive–aggressive personality disorder. *Clinical Case Studies, 9*(5), 369–382.

Yang, M. Y., Wong, S. C. P., & Coid, J. (2010). The efficacy of violence prediction: A meta-analytic comparison of nine risk assessment tools. *Psychological Bulletin, 136*(5), 740–767.

Yen, S., Shea, M. T., Pagano, M., Sanislow, C. A., Grilo, C. M., McGlashan, T. H., et al. (2003). Axis I and Axis II disorders as predictors of prospective suicide attempts: Findings from the Collaborative Longitudinal Personality Disorders Study. *Journal of Abnormal Psychology, 112,* 375–381.

Yen, S., Shea, M. T., Sanislow, C. A., Skodol, A. E., Grilo, C. M., Edelen, M. O., et al. (2009). Personality traits as prospective predictors of suicide attempts. *Acta Psychiatrica Scandinavica, 120,* 222–229.

Young, J. E. (1990). *Cognitive therapy for personality disorders: A schema-focused approach.* Sarasota, FL: Professional Resource Exchange.

Young, J. E. (1998). *Young Schema Questionnaire Short Form.* New York: Cognitive Therapy Center.

Young, J. E. (1999). *Cognitive therapy for personality disorders: A schema-focused approach* (3rd ed.). Sarasota, FL: Professional Resource Press/Professional Resource Exchange.

Young, J. E. (2006). *Young Schema Questionnaire–3*. New York: Cognitive Therapy Center.

Young, J. E., & Brown, G. (1994). Young Schema Questionnaire (2nd ed.). In J. E. Young (Ed.), *Cognitive therapy for personality disorders: A schema-focused approach* (rev. ed.). Sarasota, FL: Professional Resource Exchange.

Young, J. E., Klosko, J., & Weishaar, M. E. (2003). *Schema therapy: A practitioner's guide*. New York: Guilford Press.

Zald, D. H., Cowan, R. L., Riccardi, P., Baldwin, R. M., Ansari, M. S., Li, R., et al. (2008). Midbrain dopamine receptor availability is inversely associated with novelty-seeking traits in humans. *Journal of Neuroscience, 28*(53), 14372–14378.

Zanarini, M. C., Jacoby, R. J., Frankenburg, F. R., Reich, D. B., & Fitzmaurice, G. (2009). The 10-year course of social security disability income reported by patients with borderline personality disorder and Axis II comparison subjects. *Journal of Personality Disorders, 23*, 346–356.

Zimmerman, M. (1994). Diagnosing personality disorders: A review. *Archives of General Psychiatry, 51*, 225–245.

Zimmerman, M., & Coryell, W. (1989). The reliability of personality disorder diagnoses in a nonpatient sample. *Journal of Personality Disorders, 3*, 53–57.

Zimmerman, M., Pfohl, B., Coryell, W., Stangl, D., & Corenthal, C. (1988). Diagnosing personality disorder in depressed patients. *Archives of General Psychiatry, 45*, 733–737.

Zimmerman, M., Rothschild, L., & Chelminski, I. (2005). The prevalence of DSM-IV personality disorders in psychiatric outpatients. *American Journal of Psychiatry, 162*, 1911–1918.

Index

Page numbers in *italic* indicate a figure or table

importance of creating high standards
for practice, 415
importance of maintaining awareness of
the patient's environment, 434–435
importance of realistic self-evaluation,
437
self-care. *See* Clinician self-care
suicide assessment and, 419–420
therapist-related variables affecting
therapeutic outcomes, 413–414
See also Treatment teams
Therapy assignments, importance of
anticipating problems with the
completion of, 434. *See also*
Homework
Therapy-interfering beliefs/behaviors
addressing, 133–135
avoidant patients and, 182–183
Thinking Helpsheet, 360–362
Thinking styles, 59–60
Third-wave CBT, 7
Thought records
with avoidant patients, 200
with schizotypal patients, 262
using in therapy, 110
Threats
avoidant personality disorder, 49
dependent personality disorder, 50
obsessive–compulsive personality
disorder, 52
paranoid personality disorder, 53
passive–aggressive personality disorder,
51
Time and routine management, 118
Traits. *See* Personality traits
Transdiagnostic approach, 18
Transference
discussion of, 127–128
erotic transference, 335
with histrionic patients, 335, 344
occurrence in treatment, 431–432
using in therapy, 108, 432
Treatment effectiveness, culture and,
143–144. *See also* Therapeutic
outcomes
Treatment goals
antisocial personality disorder, 351–355
avoidant personality disorder, 184–185
borderline personality disorder, 374–375
dependent personality disorder, 160–161
depressive personality disorder,
233–234, 241
histrionic personality disorder, 333–334

importance of maintaining a realistic
perspective on, 437
importance of therapist and patient
agreement on, 430–431
narcissistic personality disorder, 313
obsessive–compulsive personality
disorder, 211–213
paranoid and schizotypal personality
disorders, 245
passive–aggressive personality disorder,
286–288, 298
schizoid personality disorder, 245,
269–270
Treatment teams
clinical management case example,
409–411, 427
importance of assessing negative staff
perception toward those with
personality disorders, 415
importance of training and support for,
414–415
See also Clinical management
Trophy mode, 310–311
Two-player economic "games," 92

U

Unconditional beliefs, 34
Unconscious information processing, 9
Unrelenting standards schema, 305
"Unspecified personality disorder," 64–65
Unstructured clinical interviews, 71–72,
80

V

Validation, in therapy with histrionic
patients, 336–337
Values
discussing with antisocial patients, 358
distinguished from goals, 358
Values clarification, 122–123
Vector approach, to personality disorders,
42
Verbal reattribution, 273
"Very important person" mode, 310
View of others
in an evolutionary model of personality
disorders, 60–62
antisocial personality disorder, 46, 54
avoidant personality disorder, 44, 48